Computational Intelligence for Medical Internet of Things (MIoT) Applications

Advances in ubiquitous sensing applications for healthcare

Computational Intelligence for Medical Internet of Things (MIoT) Applications

Volume 14

Machine Intelligence Applications for IoT in Healthcare

Edited by

Yassine Maleh

Ahmed A. Abd El-Latif

Kevin Curran

Patrick Siarry

Series Editor

Nilanjan Dey

Amira Ashour

Simon James Fong

ELSEVIER

ACADEMIC PRESS

An imprint of Elsevier

Academic Press is an imprint of Elsevier
125 London Wall, London EC2Y 5AS, United Kingdom
525 B Street, Suite 1650, San Diego, CA 92101, United States
50 Hampshire Street, 5th Floor, Cambridge, MA 02139, United States
The Boulevard, Langford Lane, Kidlington, Oxford OX5 1GB, United Kingdom

ISBN: 978-0-323-99421-7

For information on all Academic Press publications visit our website at https://www.elsevier.com/books-and-journals

Publisher: Mara E. Conner
Acquisitions Editor: Carrie L. Bolger
Editorial Project Manager: Michael Nicholls
Production Project Manager: Fizza Fathima
Cover Designer: Matthew Limbert

Typeset by TNQ Technologies

Contents

List of contributors

Arshad Ali
Department of Computer Science, FAST University, Lahore, Pakistan

Paola Ariza-Colpas
Universidad De la Costa, CUC Barranquilla, Colombia

Marina Bagić Babac
University of Zagreb, Faculty of Electrical Engineering and Computing, Zagreb, Croatia

Mohamed Bahaj
Faculty of Sciences and Techniques, Hassan 1st University, Settat, Morocco

Abderrahim Bajit
Laboratory of Advanced Systems Engineering (ISA), National School of Applied Sciences, Ibn Tofail University, Kenitra, Morocco

Zohra Bakoury
École Mohammadia d'Ingénieurs, Mohammed V University in Rabat, Rabat, Morocco

Anass Barodi
Laboratory of Advanced Systems Engineering (ISA), National School of Applied Sciences, Ibn Tofail University, Kenitra, Morocco

Siham Beloualid
Laboratory of Advanced Systems Engineering (ISA), National School of Applied Sciences, Ibn Tofail University, Kenitra, Morocco

Dominik Bezić
University of Zagreb, Faculty of Electrical Engineering and Computing, Zagreb, Croatia

Anirban Bhowmik
Department of Computer Science, M.U.C. Women's College, Purba Bardhaman, West Bengal, India

Shariq Aziz Butt
Department of Computer Science, The University of Lahore, Lahore, Pakistan

Alae Elalami
Faculty of Sciences and Techniques, Hassan 1st University, Settat, Morocco

Abdelhadi El Allali
Laboratory of Advanced Systems Engineering (ISA), National School of Applied Sciences, Ibn Tofail University, Kenitra, Morocco

Fatima Ez Zahra El Arbaoui
SI2M Laboratory, National Institute of Statistics and Applied Economics (INSEA), Rabat, Morocco

Said El Kafhali
Hassan 1st University of Settat, Faculty of Sciences and Techniques, Computer, Networks, Modeling, and Mobility Laboratory (IR2M), Settat, Morocco

Iman El Mir
Hassan 1st University of Settat, Institute of Sport Sciences, Computer, Networks, Mobility and Modeling Laboratory (IR2M), Settat, Morocco

Omar Er-Remyly
Faculty of Sciences and Techniques, Hassan 1st University, Settat, Morocco

Xiaohua Feng
School of Computer Science and Technology, University of Bedfordshire, Bedfordshire, Luton, United Kingdom

Javid Ghahremani-Nahr
Faculty Member of Academic Center for Education, Culture and Research (ACECR), Tabriz, Iran

Raman Goel
Media.Net Software Services (India) Private Limited, Mumbai, Maharashtra, India

Kaoutar El Hari
SI2M Laboratory, National Institute of Statistics and Applied Economics (INSEA), Rabat, Morocco

Sunil Karforma
Department of Computer Science, The University of Burdwan, Purba Bardhaman, West Bengal, India

Abbas Khalid
Department of Computer Science, The University of Lahore, Lahore, Pakistan

Youness Khourdifi
Polydisciplinary Faculty of Khouribga, Sultan Moulay Slimane University, Beni Mellal, Morocco

Tejpal Kumar
Central University of Rajasthan, Ajmer, Rajasthan, India

Ilham Morino
Laboratory of Advanced Systems Engineering (ISA), National School of Applied Sciences, Ibn Tofail University, Kenitra, Morocco

Dimitrios V. Moysidis
Hippokration University Hospital, Aristotle University of Thessaloniki, Thessaloniki, Greece

Anurag Mudgil
Media.Net Software Services (India) Private Limited, Mumbai, Maharashtra, India

Fadi Muheidat
Computer Science and Engineering, California State University, San Bernardino, San Bernardino, CA, United States

Esmaeil Najafi
Department of Industrial Engineering, Science and Research Branch, Islamic Azad University, Tehran, Iran

Anvit Negi
Gas Authority of India Limited (GAIL), India

Hamed Nozari
School of Industrial Engineering, College of Engineering, University of Tehran, Tehran, Iran

Salma Ait Oussous
Laboratory of Advanced Systems Engineering (ISA), National School of Applied Sciences, Ibn Tofail University, Kenitra, Morocco

Andreas S. Papazoglou
Athens Naval Hospital, Athens, Greece

Kritesh Rauniyar
Department of Computer Science and Engineering, Delhi Technological University, New Delhi, India

Rehab A. Rayan
Department of Epidemiology, High Institute of Public Health, Alexandria University, Alexandria, Egypt

Rajaa Saidi
SI2M Laboratory, National Institute of Statistics and Applied Economics (INSEA), Rabat, Morocco

Sajidha S. A.
School of Computer Science and Engineering, Vellore Institute of Technology, Chennai, Tamilnadu, India

Qaisar Shaheen
Department of Computer Science, University of South Asia, Lahore, Pakistan

Muhammad Shiraz
Department of Computer Science, Federal Urdu University of Arts, Sciences and Technology, Islamabad, Pakistan

Krishan Pal Singh
Jaipur National University, School of Computer and System Sciences, Jaipur, Rajasthan, India

Sanskar Srivastava
School of Computer Science and Engineering, Vellore Institute of Technology, Chennai, Tamilnadu, India

Reza Tavakkoli-Moghaddam
School of Industrial Engineering, College of Engineering, University of Tehran, Tehran, Iran

Loai A. Tawalbeh
Department of Computer Engineering, Jordan University of Science and Technology, Irbid, Jordan

Surendrabikram Thapa
Department of Computer Science and Engineering, Delhi Technological University, New Delhi, India; Department of Computer Science, Virginia Tech, Blacksburg, VA, United States

Shubham Tomar
Central University of Rajasthan, Ajmer, Rajasthan, India

Christos Tsagkaris
Faculty of Medicine, University of Crete, Rethymno, Greece

Amit Kumar Tyagi
School of Computer Science and Engineering, Vellore Institute of Technology, Chennai, Tamilnadu, India; Centre for Advanced Data Science, Vellore Institute of Technology, Chennai, Tamilnadu, India

Imran Zafar
Department of Bioinformatics and Computational Biology, Virtual University of Pakistan, Lahore, Punjab, Pakistan

Hayat Zaydi
École Mohammadia d'Ingénieurs, Mohammed V University in Rabat, Rabat, Morocco

Mounia Zaydi
Faculty of Sciences and Techniques, Hassan 1st University, Settat, Morocco

About the editors

Prof. Yassine Maleh is a cybersecurity professor and practitioner with industry and academic experience. He holds a PhD in Computer Science. Since 2019, he has worked as Professor of Cybersecurity at Sultan Moulay Slimane University, Morocco. He worked for the National Port agency (ANP) in Morocco as Senior Security Analyst from 2012 to 2019. He is a senior member of IEEE, and a member of the International Association of Engineers and the Machine Intelligence Research Labs. Dr. Maleh has made contributions in information security and privacy, Internet of Things (IoT) security, and wireless and constrained network security. His research interests include information security and privacy, IoT, networks security, information systems, and IT governance. He has published over 100 papers (book chapters, international journals, and conferences/workshops), 20 edited books, and 3 authored books. He is Editor-in-Chief of the International Journal of Information Security and Privacy (IJISP). He serves as Associate Editor for IEEE Access (2019 Impact Factor 4.098), the International Journal of Digital Crime and Forensics, and the International Journal of Information Security and Privacy. He was also a guest editor of a special issue on "Recent Advances on Cyber Security and Privacy for Cloud-of-Things" of the International Journal of Digital Crime and Forensics, Volume 10, Issue 3, July—September 2019. He has served and continues to serve on executive and technical program committees and as a reviewer of numerous international conferences and journals such as Elsevier Ad Hoc Networks, IEEE Network Magazine, IEEE Sensor Journal, ICT Express, and Springer Cluster Computing. He was the publicity chair of BCCA 2019 and the general chair of the MLBDACP 19/20/21 symposiums and ICI2C′21 conference.

Prof. Ahmed Abd El-Latif holds a BSc with honor rank in Mathematics and Computer Science (2005), MSc in Computer Science (2010), and PhD in Computer Science and Technology at Harbin Institute of Technology, Harbin, China (2013). He is Associate Professor of Computer Science at Menoufia University, Egypt, and School of Information Technology and Computer Science, Nile University, Egypt. He is author and coauthor of more than 140 indexed papers. He is a referee of many referred journals and conferences of international repute. He has received many awards, such as the State Encouragement Award in Engineering Sciences (2016), Arab Republic of Egypt; the best PhD student award from Harbin Institute of Technology, China (2013); and the Young Scientific Award, Menoufia University, Egypt (2014). He is a fellow at Academy of Scientific Research and Technology, Egypt. Dr. Abd El-Latif is also an associate editor in several Scopus Journals and leading many special issues in SCI journals.

Prof. Kevin Curran is Professor of Cyber Security, Executive Codirector of the Legal Innovation Centre, and Group Leader of the Ambient Intelligence and Web Technologies Research Group at Ulster University. He is also a Senior Member of the IEEE. Prof. Curran is globally recognized as a security Top Influencer "IFSEC Global influencers in security and fire 2020" in the category Security Thought Leadership. He was ranked second. Prof Curran is perhaps most well-known for his work on internet security and location positioning evidenced by over 800 published works. His expertise has been acknowledged by invitations to present his work at international conferences, overseas universities, and research laboratories. He is a regular contributor on television, radio, and in trade and consumer IT magazines with 1000+ interviews in recent years. He is currently the recipient of an Royal Academy of Engineering Senior Research Fellowship and is an IEEE Technical Expert for Internet Security. Professor Curran has performed external panel duties for various Higher Education Institutions and public bodies such as OFCOM and the National Institute for Health Research (NIHR).

Prof. Patrick Siarry was born in France in 1952. He received his PhD in Computer Science and Optimization from University Paris VI, Paris, France, in 1986, and his Doctorate of Sciences (Habilitation) in Computer Science and Optimization from University Paris XI, Orsay, France, in 1994. He was first involved in the development of analog and digital models of nuclear power plants with Electricité de France, Paris. Since 1995, he has been a Professor of Automatics and Informatics with Université Paris-Est Créteil, Créteil, France. His main research interests include computer-aided design of electronic circuits, cognitive intelligence, and applications of new stochastic global optimization heuristics to various engineering fields, also including the fitting of process models to experimental data, the learning of fuzzy rule bases, and of neural networks.

Preface

Computational intelligence is a powerful methodology for addressing complex real-world problems to which mathematical or traditional modeling can be useless. Computational intelligence paradigms comprising numerous branches, including neural networks, swarm intelligence, expert systems, evolutionary computation, fuzzy systems, and learning systems, can play a vital role in handling the different aspects of healthcare.

With the advances in Medical Internet of Things (MIoT), it becomes feasible to design numerous automated diagnostic models for early stage diagnostic of different diseases. Machine learning models have been broadly employed to evaluate biomedical data collected from MIoT. But these models need effective feature extraction and selection approaches as a preprocessing tool to evaluate the collected biomedical data. Therefore, the feature extraction and selection approaches may hinder the performance of machine learning-based biomedical data analysis.

Therefore, deep learning models have been implemented to evaluate the biomedical data collected from MIoT. These models apply numerous filters at each layer to automatically extract and select the potential features of biomedical data. These models have achieved considerably better results than machine learning models, but the model-building process is extremely expensive, both in terms of resources and time. Additionally, deep learning models perform efficiently when a huge amount of data is available.

Computational Intelligence for Medical Internet of Things (MIoT) Applications explores the machine intelligence techniques necessary for effective MIoT research and practice, taking a practical approach for practitioners and students entering the field. This book lays a good foundation for MIoT and applications' core concepts and applications, walking the reader through the fundamental ideas with expert ease. The book progresses on the topics in a step-by-step manner. It reinforces theory with a full-fledged pedagogy designed to enhance the researchers' understanding and offer them a practical insight into its applications.

This book comprises a number of state-of-the-art contributions from both scientists and practitioners working in computational intelligence for MIoT. It aspires to provide a relevant reference for students, researchers, engineers, and professionals working in this particular area or those interested in grasping its diverse facets and exploring the latest advances computational intelligence for MIoT applications. More specifically, the book consists of 15 contributions classified into three pivotal sections. Section 1, "Computational Intelligence for Medical Internet of Things (MIoT): Current States and Challenges," introduces the state-of-the-art computational intelligence for MIoT architectures, futures trends, and exploring the effectiveness of the cloud, Internet of Things (IoT), and fog computing for healthcare monitoring systems. Section 2, "Computational Intelligence for Medical Internet of Things (MIoT): Applications," offers the latest architectures, applications, and uses cases of computational intelligence for MIoT. Section 3, "Computational Intelligence for Medical Internet of Things (MIoT): Security and Privacy," explores security and privacy in MIoT applications.

We want to take this opportunity and express our thanks to the contributors of this volume and the editorial board for their great efforts in reviewing and providing interesting feedback. The editors would like to thank Ms. Mariana Kühl Leme (Senior Editorial Project Manager) and Ms. Carrie Bolger (Acquisitions Editor) for the editorial assistance and support to produce this important scientific work. Without this collective effort, this book would not have been possible.

Prof. Yassine Maleh
Prof. Ahmed A. Abd El-Latif
Prof. Kevin Curran
Prof. Patrick Siarry

SECTION

1

Computational Intelligence for Medical Internet of Things (MIoT): Current States and Challenges

CHAPTER

AI and IoT working for healthcare: general aspects and application examples

1

Hayat Zaydi[1], Mounia Zaydi[2], Zohra Bakoury[1]

[1]*École Mohammadia d'Ingénieurs, Mohammed V University in Rabat, Rabat, Morocco;* [2]*Faculty of Sciences and Techniques, Hassan 1st University, Settat, Morocco*

1.1 Introduction

The computing power and memory needed to collect large amounts of data and implement machine learning algorithms usually exceed the capabilities of a typical IT infrastructure of nonspecialized enterprises. The alternative for them is cloud computing. It is a service consisting of the provision of IT resources, including servers, databases, networks, and software that can be accessed via the internet.

Edge computing is about processing data at the edge of the network, i.e., as close to its source as possible. This is especially true for those where the speed of the analysis is of key importance—the proximity of the source allows for their processing in real-time. The remaining data, for example, subject to historical analysis, is sent to the cloud. Fog computing, in turn, is a solution that introduces an intermediary layer between Internet of Things (IoT) devices and the cloud. Thanks to this, a dispersed IT infrastructure is created, allowing you to use the computing power of the cloud closer to the data source (Dimitrov, 2016).

The combination of technology, data, artificial intelligence, and machine learning in healthcare is helping to improve the way patient care is delivered. By responding to patient needs that are both more focused and in real-time, the IoT can help healthcare professionals improve the patient experience. Most engineers admit that they are comfortable working in a team, although they would appreciate having more contact with peers outside their own company. That impulse may have once been satisfied by attending fairs and conferences, but the COVID-19 pandemic has shut it down completely. It also made contact with peers in companies difficult.

The paradigms enunciated by Hippocrates and reinforced by Galen regarding the clinical method (near the bed) conditioned the practice of medicine until the seventeenth century, which was based on the interpretation of information exclusively collected through simple observation, interrogation, and the direct examination of the sick person to arrive at the diagnosis and treatment of diseases (Elhoseny, 2021).

Computational Intelligence for Medical Internet of Things (MIoT) Applications
https://doi.org/10.1016/B978-0-323-99421-7.00018-0

The incorporation of technology into medical practice began with the discovery by the Dutchman Janssen, through the microscope, of the existence of tiny "bugs" that Pasteur would later identify as responsible for certain infectious diseases. The medical *armamentarium* uses radiant energy (called X-rays) for the exploration of the interior of the organism.

This is how the development of technology has provided valuable support for the accurate diagnosis and timely treatment of conditions. Currently, Information and Communication Technologies (ICTs) have not been alienating to this task, providing new and different applications to the practice of medicine:

- Dissemination and universal availability of up-to-date knowledge
- Communication and consultation online, remotely and in real time between doctors
- Unlimited handling of clinical files
- Direct referral of laboratory test results to the physician
- Remote surgery with robots
- Surgery using a microscope or endoscopy
- Microprocessor devices for modifying bodily functions
- Automatic dispensers for medications or intravenous fluids, among many others (Tsai, 2014)

1.2 Methodology

This work aims to show and bring together the different facets of the implication of artificial intelligence (AI) technologies, IoT, and sciences that revolve in the same orbit in the field of healthcare through examples, use cases, and other methods. The study focused on a number of articles and book chapters on these areas, but also others dealing with the ethical aspect and good practices in this regard, over seven years.

These documents deal with AI and IoT, IoT and health, AI and IoT and health, plus others on ethics and deontology in this field, given the sensitivity of the health field, which involves individuals and their private lives. The following Fig. 1.1 highlights this approach:

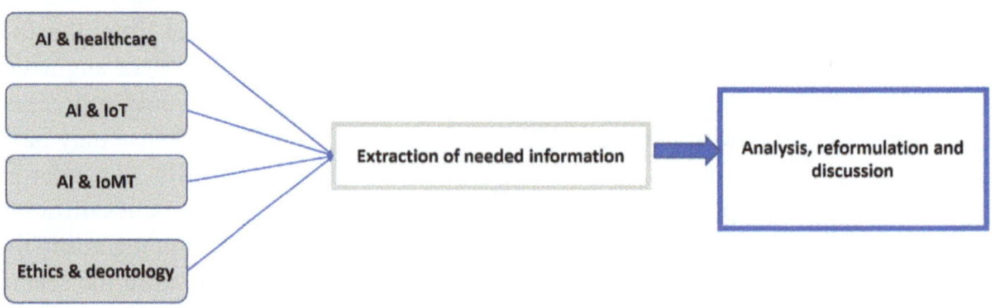

FIGURE 1.1

Followed methodology.

Gaurav described the World Economic Fund meeting held at the beginning of 2016 as focused on this issue, since, as highlighted by its president, Klaus Schwab, "now, with the dramatic increase in global mobile connectivity and the incorporation of sensors, robots and data analysis, we are facing the emergence of technologies that can create a new cycle of innovation and global economic activity. The convergence of the digital, human and physical domains will result in software eating the world." (Gaurav, 2022).

The concept of the IoT was first proposed in 1999 by a pioneer in sensor technology, the British Kevin Ashton, as "a system of objects in the physical world that are connected to the Internet through sensors." Today, the most widely accepted definition in the medium is the one proposed by Vermesan and Friess: "Communication infrastructure in a global and dynamic network with self-configuration capabilities, based on standard and interoperable communication protocols, where physical and virtual things have an identity, physical attributes and a virtual personality. These same things use smart interfaces and are tightly integrated into an information network system."

Edge devices include all entities that are not in the cloud, from simple devices connected to nodes that group them according to a certain hierarchy, which goes from the least performing to the most efficient as the operator gets closer to the cloud. We must consider the profile and characteristics of each of the nodes, namely their storage and computing capacity, as well as the capacity of the network (wired, Wi-Fi, or cellular) to deploy the various applications and processing tasks to the optimal place. One of the main difficulties is the great diversity of objects that can be connected to the same network. The digital turn of companies will further accentuate the trend of connected objects, among other things by the addition of sensors taking frequent measurements at regular intervals and whose measurements will be used to control actuators which may in some cases require rapid decision-making. Local preprocessing of this data before final storage in the cloud would save on cloud costs in addition to significantly reducing latency (Akhtar, 2021).

1.2.1 IoT in practice

IoT is a general, collective term for various hardware and software solutions and technologies. Complementing each other, they support the most important aspects of IoT, forming a layered structure together. Thanks to it, connecting things into a network with access to the internet makes sense, as it allows you to obtain useful information from the data generated on IoT and to take specific actions based on it.

The individual IoT layers are therefore responsible for: recording, transmitting, preprocessing (filtering) and analyzing data and reacting to it. The lowest of these are IoT devices. They are at the same time the starting point, providing the measurement results from the sensors and the target point thanks to the actuators. As for the latter, depending on the application, they perform different functions, most often turning off or on a device.

Many of the connected object applications of tomorrow require a response speed that edge computing can improve (Ugandran, 2021).

Initially, solutions in this area were primarily aimed at helping manufacturing companies gather sensor information, perform real-time predictive analytics, and then communicate the results to the decision-maker or directly to the control system. Today we know the field of applications of IoT is huge and that it can be used in fields such as medicine, agriculture, smart cities, or transport. The IoT market is expected to grow intensely by 2025, reaching 25.2 billion connections by 2025 and $1100 billion in investment. Some researchers used a special approach to IoT. The internet stuff is extremely important; we face this area of technology-specific expectations and we attach our hopes for the future to it. There is now a greater emphasis on certain strategies to help customers design their production resources and optimize the entire production value chain. Delivered, there are also tools to help you design products and automation (Singh, 2020, pp. 102364–102370).

1.2.2 IoT in healthcare

Several factors contribute to the popularization of the IoT in healthcare. First of all, it is one of the conditions for the digital transformation of this sector. Moreover, the awareness of the need to take care of health is growing widely, which is accompanied by a greater interest in the possibility of controlling its condition remotely and on one's own. Moreover, it is important to strive to reduce expenditure on healthcare, while improving its quality.

It is predicted that IoT in the healthcare sector will develop mainly in several directions. One of them is remote health monitoring—currently, it is the largest segment of Internet of Healthcare Things (IoHT) in terms of expenditure. The tendency to relieve healthcare facilities (hospitals, ambulance services) by performing medical procedures at home, which are possible in this way, is becoming more and more evident. This is for a number of reasons.

IoHT is a concept that concerns devices used in the medical field that are connected to the internet and can communicate with each other. These solutions allow, for example, to locate and obtain information on your assets in real-time, and manage them remotely or automatically. This not only results in high-quality care and significant time savings, but also in increased patient safety. Thanks to the IoHT, the management of healthcare facilities becomes more efficient: you are always connected to your devices, to the necessary data and patient information. The most important features of most IoHT solutions are flexibility and customization: the systems can adapt to any structure, regardless of specialization or size. It is also possible to integrate them with existing, connected, and modified technologies and software.

- Quick and easy notification to the staff of any problems, received from patients or a device
- Continuous monitoring of patients' conditions and saving of their parameters
- Increased safety thanks to remote medical assistance to detect anomalous events
- Faster and more effective access to medical care and therefore to diagnosis and treatment

- Comprehensive assistance outside of medical facilities
- Automatic transfer and analysis of data collected by devices
- Remote medical consultations
- Automatic reminders

By 2022, the global Internet of Medical Things (IoMT) market is expected to reach $158 billion, up from $41 billion in 2017, and to far exceed those sums of money by 2025.

IoT offers performance optimization software. Data collected thanks to IoT can be reused in design software, enabling future improvement products. This creates a feedback loop. You can combine production data, product data, and product life cycle management data. In turn, the operating system intended for IoT supports data analysis harvested from machinery and physical infrastructure, helping to create new services and business models, save costs and use existing resources more efficiently. Ultimately, Industrial Internet of Things (IIoT) will enable the creation of smart factories with advanced production models. In the factories these machines will be largely automatically "programmed" based on incoming orders (Yang, 2019). They will be backed up by chains logistics, arranged in logical sequences, using ready-made rules, supplying raw materials and assembly materials to production lines and sending finished goods. The implementation of IoT technology is part of modern companies "journey" toward the next stage of modernization of production and logistics. Is a part of philosophy known as Industry 4.0, the fourth industrial revolution, characterized by cyber-physical systems and using digital twin technology? But for many, if not most modern factories, the "journey" toward modernization is more evolution rather than revolution. Cloud-based platforms, can accelerate your progress while reducing at the same time costs of technological changes. With the advances in the IoMT, it has become practical to plan various robotized demonstrative models for beginning phase finding of various sicknesses. AI models have been extensively utilized to assess biomedical information gathered from IoMT. Be that as it may, these models need viable component extraction and choice methodologies as a prehandling apparatus to assess the gathered biomedical information. Thus, the element extraction and determination approaches might upset the presentation of AI-based biomedical information examination. In this way, profound learning models have been executed to assess the biomedical information gathered from IoMT. These models apply various channels at each layer to naturally remove and select the expected highlights of biomedical information. These models have accomplished impressively preferred outcomes over AI models, yet the model structure process is incredibly costly, both as far as assets and time. Moreover, profound learning models perform proficiently when a gigantic measure of information is accessible.

IoT will soon be in our immediate vicinity for good. Most of the devices equipped with IoT are in use and will be away from home, although this technology also includes ordinary phones cell phones, tablets, portable devices, refrigerators, and coffee machines for coffee. This technology will have an equally significant impact on individuals' areas of the economy—from agriculture to healthcare. Many IoT devices will be sensors placed in other devices, and even in the body of patients. Multiple uses of the IoT may surprise: from facial recognition in security systems to intelligent traffic lights, optimized energy networks, intelligent water consumption management, parking meters, and thousands of other, yet undiscovered opportunities. IoT has been entering our lives for several years. Contemporary cars rolling off the assembly lines, before they even pass the first kilometer, connect to the internet. Connected to the internet, planes are manufactured by the Airbus aviation plant and Boeing. Also, the oil and gas industry, shipping and smart cities are equipped with IoT. We can also find IoT devices in industry, where it has its name IIoT. There are many applications of IoT in the healthcare industry where physicians can monitor patients remotely through a network of interconnected devices and machines without needing to be in direct contact with them. This is very useful if the patients do not have serious problems or have infectious diseases such as COVID-19. One of the most common uses of IoT in healthcare is the use of robots. These include surgical robots that can help physicians perform surgeries more efficiently with greater precision and control. There are also disinfectant robots that can clean surfaces quickly and thoroughly using high-intensity ultraviolet light (Gyu, 2019).

At the heart of technological developments, AI is a leading edge and is also the principle of human evolution with and through the machine. It is difficult to measure this, as recent AI implementations borrow more from fantasies that have become very real than from the augmented reality of a few software innovations. To date, we can confidently assert that AI will impact our health system in all its dimensions, transform practices, redefine the roles of each actor in the healthcare system and see new ones emerge. Indeed, it concentrates the hopes of precision medicine, individualized, safer as much as it is, for certain ideologues of Silicon Valley, the teleological horizon and the active substance of an imminent evolution of humanity.

The IoMT is the particular application of the IoT in medicine. In the beginning, about 20 years ago, the use of the IoT in the healthcare sector was mainly focused on remotely controlling the correct functioning of large medical machines in hospitals. Over time, thanks to technological innovation and the development of digital health, we have seen how healthcare has managed to leave the hospital context to move to the patient's home, allowing healthcare personnel to monitor vital parameters remotely (e.g., body temperature, blood pressure, heart rate, blood glucose values) and daiquiri health data continuously.

It happens that objects equipped with sensors (such as common wearables) are connected to an internet platform which, in turn, integrates the data from these "objects", analyzes them and shares the information obtained from them with applications created for needs-specific clinics.

To give a few examples: IoT in the healthcare sector is particularly suitable for managing sleep apnea, a potentially dangerous disorder in which breathing stops while someone is sleeping. A remote device can monitor their sleep and alert a doctor if they stop breathing.

But also, in the field of heart disease, where the person with a pacemaker, for example, can monitor their heart behavior and the status of the batteries via wireless connectivity that sends data to the doctor or hospital.

In summary, we can say that IoT in medicine has the advantage of:

- offer more predictive healthcare thanks to instant access to aggregated data that allows you to monitor, inform and notify any critical issues in real time, as well as prevent medical errors;
- facilitate communication between patients and doctors and simplify the entire care experience by making the procedures for managing drugs and therapeutic pathways even simpler;
- collect clinical data through sensors to control the patient remotely by setting up treatment programs and monitoring parameters connected directly to home;
- decrease waiting times in hospitals as well as healthcare costs.

1.2.3 Some tips about artificial intelligence

The origins of AI are often located around the 1950s. Macy's conferences lay the founding stones of cybernetics; Douglas Engelbart's "Mother of All Demos" fascinates; Boltzmann's first machines are invented a few years later with the first coded perceptron, this being the ancestor of neural networks to which we owe recent particularly spectacular results in the field of health. Let us point out, for the record, that Leibniz, abundant in his intelligence in fields such as mathematics, physics, and philosophy, in 1666 in *Dissertatio De Arte Combinatoire* theorized the foundations of a method for the computationally generating new ideas. One could also evoke Leonardo and machine controllers, or the Arab Zairja that the XIVth century thought could break systematic issues to generate automated responses congruent (Sukumaran, 2018).

However, it will be necessary to wait until the beginning of this century to begin to see the potential of AI techniques realized. This is based on the extraordinary production of massive data for which the internet has been the vehicle and the potentializer. Thus, so-called Machine Learning computer techniques have been able to develop by causing machines to ingest gargantuan quantities of data which in return have enabled algorithms to sharpen their profile and increase their predictive power. Our purpose is not to discuss the terms of a canonical definition of AI but rather to outline its scope and put into perspective its potential for application in the health field.

We will say that AI is a set of algorithmic methods aimed at ensuring the automated execution of complex tasks performed by humans in the exercise of their cognitive functions. We will find there a mimetic desire (Girardien) in the achievement of performances usually attached to the human but also their improvement, even their surpassing (Sun, 2018).

Because it is important to realize that, for a very long time, machines are no longer an arrangement of cables and silica at the orders of their programmer, since precisely AI is largely based on Machine Learning, consisting of learning centered on data sets. In short, machines learn from the data they compile. This learning is effective in proportion to the masses of data that they ingest.

If we are to appreciate the comparative capacities of human and machine, we can say that both can integrate a knowledge base, which comes under classical computational capacities, and both can use this knowledge base, to collect usage data—this is the notion of feedback—and thus acquire what is commonly called experience. To put it more succinctly, the algorithm is the gene, and the training data set is the epigen, or the epigenetic environment. Thus, the sum of the computational power and the ability to gain experience brings the horizon closer to the faculties endowing machines with those of humans.

It is here that we can sense the anthropological accents of which AI can be the vector. Because we will see, in this learning phenomenon, the organized transfer of skills and experience from human to machine. Basically, all this is part of the continuity of the anthropological need that humans feel to externalize his faculties, extending his motor skills by those of machines, before perhaps tomorrow to transfer thought to them (Jangid, 2020).

1.2.4 Artificial intelligence for new SoC chips

The world has changed from control-centered to data-centered, forcing the evolution of processor architecture. Today, most processors have the von Neumann architecture (or a modification of it—Harvard) with a single set: control unit, memory, compute unit (and I/O). The advent of AI/machine learning (ML) forces changes in the memory architecture (Iqbal, 2020).

At the heart of the AI application is the multiplication and accumulation (MAC) function or the dot product operation. Two numbers are multiplied and the result is added to the accumulator. Numbers are taken and stored in memory. These operations are repeated many times and constitute the vast majority of time and energy used both for the learning process and for inference. The use of in-memory computation, where coefficients can be stored in memory "next to" the processing element, dramatically reduces data transmission distance. Such a change in memory architecture has great consequences. Some programming models, such as persistent memory (PMEM), require the user to understand where the data is, think about how to transfer it, and ensure that the data is in the right place (Alsheikh, 2016).

AI memory requirements are different from those for GPUs or general-purpose CPUs. There will always be a control element in every system we create. As a result, the architecture of von Neumann does not go away. It is a computer with the most universal application and therefore indispensable. At the same time, many computational workloads are shifting to non−von Neumann architectures. Accelerators and custom cores can do a much better job with much less power consumption. To use this avalanche of information properly. Technology providers have to find a way to get the collection, storage and processing. This solution is AI. Expect the coming years of IoT development to pass on inventing more and more perfected tools for data analysis based on AI and machine learning algorithms. This is a necessity; because of the vast amount of information available now, even when supplying IoT devices, people can't analyze the data, especially in real-time. The development of AI will also allow for better human communication with connected devices in IoT, in particular communication with voice. Solutions like Apple's Siri, Google assistant, Amazon Alexa, and Microsoft Cortana already allow some activities to be performed by voice-over devices. The simplicity of communication with IoT solutions, the possibility of natural voice communication, and giving commands to refrigerators, cars, TV or robot cleaners, will disseminate these solutions and lower the cognitive barrier, and as a result the IoT market will grow more dynamically (Amin, 2018). We have already gotten used to e-commerce, that information flows faster on the internet, that a wider range of products and services is available. It took nearly 10 years for the companies to adjust its operation to the changes brought about by the internet. Time to prepare for what it brings IoT. Companies need to develop strategies and plan to leverage IoT and transform all aspects of their business in such a way in order not to miss the technological revolution. They are waiting because we have fundamental changes in the products we use, and in the operation of companies in a transformative market.

1.2.5 The future of the Internet of things

The future of IoT looks promising and the facts speak for themselves:

- Gartner20 believes the number of devices installed worldwide IoT will reach 20 billion by 2020.
- A study by Accenture21 estimates that IoT does 2030 will bring an increase in global GDP by $ 14 billion (Bhattacharya, 2016).
- Business Insider predicts that there will be over 55 by 2025 billion IoT devices, compared to about 9 billion in 2017. Higher functionality of devices communicating on IoT are causing the growing number of sensors built into the newly digital products manufactured. More and more enterprises will see IoT as a way to attract customers and improve the comfort of use. Spyware allows you to get hold of information about users on the internet, and personal data are often sold not only for marketing purposes. There are similar dangers with the use of IoT. Intelligent infrastructure, devices and autonomous vehicles are becoming targets of attacks by data thieves or saboteurs. The blockchain technology that is already successfully allowing to secure financial transactions can be one with possible solutions to related problems with IoT protection. Although we usually associate blockchain with cryptocurrencies, analysts see it as one major trend to play an important role in the future of IoT (Chang, 2018).

Multiple objects in the real world connected with the help of IoT could be effectively managed, tracked, and coordinated just through blockchain. Connected IoT devices can use this technology to organize, store, and share data streams. Even records in a diverse network and device environment blockchain allow any user with the appropriate permissions to connect and take necessary actions. These cryptographic algorithms are a secure shield to protect consumer data and one of the strongest encryption standards available today (Costa, 2017).

Precisely in order to provide an adequate path of action for professional decisions, techniques such as the "Logic Learning Machine" and the "Decision Tree" have been developed which, to the knowledge extracted from the data, add a representation of the deductive path from which it arose. This form of "transparent" representation, step by step, of the learning of the machine will allow the doctor to understand every aspect of the work of the AI and then provide the patient with the necessary explanations on the reasons that led him to a diagnostic or therapeutic decision. Thus, the automatic learning of the intelligent system is created, which, in this form, becomes a precious tool, increasingly necessary for a modern healthcare system. Human intelligence working with AI—that is, a well-informed clinician, empathetic toward the patient, equipped with rigorous predictive tools and guides in making choices, and relieved of repetitive work—can bring us closer to achieving the authentic goal of medicine: care for the patient. Its potential is to benefit both "ordinary" people as consumers and users of, among other things, portable devices and wearable electronics, which include: medical devices, gadgets such as smart glasses and smart watches, sports pedometers, and even jewelry and clothes with built-in sensors, home automation and smart household appliances, business, and industry; IoT is one of the basic technologies of the fourth industrial revolution (Industry 4.0). IoT is also expected to positively influence society as a whole, thanks to the development of intelligent transport and smart cities. Next, we present IoT perspectives in selected applications.

1.2.6 Requirements for smart sensors

Smart IoT sensors must meet certain criteria. First of all, they should be very cheap so that it is profitable to use them in large numbers. Another condition is small size so that it can be discreetly built into anything. The best form of communication in their case is wireless connectivity. Because it is troublesome to lead a large number of cables, especially in places that are difficult to access (Zafar, 2019).

Wired communication prevents mobility. The next requirement is as little energy consumption as possible, thanks to which the built-in battery should be sufficient for the expected working time of the sensor and/or the possibility of using alternative energy sources, for example by obtaining it from the environment (energy harvesting).

Smart sensors should be maintenance-free not only because they do not require battery replacement, but also in terms of maintenance and calibration. Therefore, their important features are: self-diagnosis, self-repairing ability, and auto-calibration. It is good when the sensor preprocesses the measurement results, because it relieves the higher layers of the IoT system, saving their computing resources.

In addition, it is advantageous to arrange a plurality of measuring elements of different sizes in one housing. This saves space and, because the remaining function blocks do not overlap, reduces the total cost of metering the IoT system (Sun, 2017).

1.2.7 Smart sensor function blocks

Intelligent sensors send the measurement results digitally. For this purpose, they are equipped with the following functional blocks: measuring element (usually in the form of a MEMS sensor integrated with one structure with electronic circuits made in CMOS technology), measurement signals preprocessing system (amplifiers), analog-to-digital converter, processor and memory, transceiver, and local user interface.

The processor is programmed to implement application algorithms that include various application-specific measurement result processing functions, such as filtering and measurement error compensation. In addition, it is responsible for the automatic calibration of the sensor based on the data stored in the memory in the event of a change in measurement conditions (auto-calibration).

1.2.8 Remote diagnostics

Costs, of course, play an important role: the public health service can achieve significant savings by remotely monitoring the health of patients. In addition, it will greatly relieve the medical staff. This is of great importance as the health service in many countries is facing an increasingly serious problem of staff shortages. Both benefits will gain importance with the aging of the population, which is accompanied by a high incidence of chronic disease. The therapeutic aspect is also important, as in home conditions patients are exposed to less stress. Remote health monitoring is also a great help for both the health service and patients who live in hard-to-reach areas. Additionally, data obtained from biosensors and wearable electronics, which can be used to remotely control the health of patients, collected and analyzed centrally can be helpful in research (Tariq, 2019).

1.2.9 Conditions to be met

It is worth mentioning here a few very important issues related to the implementation of IoT. The first is the need to protect your data. Information about the state of health is a tasty morsel for hackers, because there would certainly be enough people willing to obtain it for illegal use, for example for blackmailing or making purchases of medical equipment or drugs on the account of victims, which will later be resold on the black market.

Data accuracy and consistency must also be ensured. The consequences of not meeting this condition may be serious if, for example, due to incorrect results, the doctor prescribes too much or too little dose of the drug, or an ambulance is not called to the person in need of help. Training medical staff can be a challenge. This is important as employee errors also threaten the confidentiality, accuracy, and integrity of data on IoHT networks (Xu, 2016).

1.2.10 Smart stethoscopes and smart tablets

Thanks to IoT, it will also be possible to use smart medical devices, for example, digital stethoscopes, allowing the transmission of murmurs, for example in the heart or lungs, which will allow for their processing (amplification, reduction of environmental noise). Better sound quality will provide more accurate diagnosis. In addition, IoT will facilitate the inventory of hospital equipment - smart equipment will be easier to locate in the hospital.

Examples of IoT applications in healthcare can be multiplied, from "ordinary", similar to those already presented, to more unusual, such as smart tablets. A solution of this type was approved by the American Food and Drug Administration some time ago. When swallowed, these pills send confirmation of this fact by communicating with a special mobile application. When taken with food, the tablets are digested and the sensors are expelled. The system was developed for mentally ill patients, but in the future, it will also certainly be used by people with other ailments.

High hopes are placed in the IoHT segment of the IoT. This is reflected in the forecasts that the value of its global market may exceed $169 billion in 2020 (according to Technavio) (Yu, 2018).

1.2.11 Artificial intelligence and machine learning in e-health

One of the solutions that streamline the processes taking place within the medical sector is the Medical Analysis Platform (CMAP). CMAP is a central platform that is based on advanced learning algorithms. Its use in medicine provides multifaceted solutions, both in diagnostics and in managing a medical facility. The algorithms on which CMAP is based are able to process large amounts of data and then select them in such a way that the doctor can only obtain information that interests him. The possibility of intelligent selection of medical records is a functionality that works well in the case of Electronic Medical Records (EDM). Self-learning algorithms help to find dependencies in documents containing medical records, and are also useful in long-term monitoring of the patient's condition, such as reading an EKG. The entire observation process can be performed remotely. Thanks to machine learning, the system extracts only those parts of the reading that indicate cardiac dysfunction, sending the information to the attending physician, which significantly reduces the time to review the historical record in its entirety and improves the treatment process (Ding, 2016, pp. 107–121).

Healthcare facilities seem geared toward using IoMT technology in three areas (inventory management, workflow optimization, and device integration), building on what has already happened in retail. The simple adoption of IoMT devices such as wrist bands and identification badges in wireless technology would allow the management of patient information in real time, from the medical record to the drug administration plan, with obvious benefits in terms of personnel management and resource optimization. Returning to the clinical setting, a trend reported in the United States is the integration of consumer devices to transfer patient data directly into the care management cycle. An example is the neonatal ward of the Boston hospital, where each element of the health cycle is constantly monitored. The hospital also uses IoT sensors for security purposes. Babies receive bracelets which make them locatable at any time. If a baby is brought too close to an exit door without authorization, the doors are blocked. In the intensive care unit, nurses receive notifications on their smartphones about patient parameters, such as heart rate and oxygen changes detected by sensors, allowing them to optimize travel and reach beds more quickly in an emergency. In Boston, the benefits of IoMT technology are not limited to clinical applications. For example, the hospital uses a "biodigester," which breaks down food leftovers from the kitchen and which is monitored through IoT technology for constant control of the operation. The hospital has also installed wireless sensors in refrigerators, freezers, and laboratories to ensure that samples of blood, drugs, and other materials are kept at adequate temperatures. The use of IoMT devices in the healthcare sector also allows you to update electronic health records more quickly; it is possible to insert an ECG request, the results of which are automatically transmitted to the archiving system. There, staff members can remotely view the traces and compare them to previous ECGs. The hospital also has more than 600 infusion pumps that allow staff to automatically deliver and change medications in real time over the wireless network. While this hospital's example represents a pinnacle of excellence, glucose meters, blood pressure cuffs and other devices capable of capturing and transmitting patient vital signs data and statistics are now within reach. The basic idea is to collect data in an automated way by applying some decision support rules to intervene in patients at the beginning of the process. Blood pressure cuffs and other devices capable of detecting and transmitting patient vital signs data and statistics are now within reach. Blood pressure cuffs and other devices capable of detecting and transmitting patient vital signs data and statistics are now within reach.

With AI, healthcare facilities have access to a new technology that helps to find unknown correlations between events, diagnostic, demographic, geographic and epidemiological data, as well as useful for optimizing operational workflow. All healthcare - hospitals, doctors, dental clinics and testing labs - can use patient data and medical records intelligently to save more lives and improve their operational processes. The primary goal of healthcare companies is to constantly improve patient outcomes, both diagnostic and therapeutic, and provide better care, but without increasing costs, but on the contrary by simplifying clinical pathways and related workflows. With the new Machine Learning technologies and AI now available, companies in the health sector can provide data-driven solutions that include improved patient outcomes, complaints management, fraud detection and prediction of hospital-acquired infections.

1.3 Activity monitoring during cancer treatment

Memorial Sloan Kettering Cancer Center (MSK) and cloud research company Medidata are testing the use of activity trackers to collect lifestyle data from patients being treated for multiple myeloma. Patients will wear an activity tracker for up to a week before treatment and then continuously for several months during multiple treatments specified by Job Medical.

1.4 Connected inhalers

The most immediate use of IoT technology in healthcare is not to aid diagnosis, but to ensure adherence. Adding sensors to drugs or delivery mechanisms allows physicians to accurately know whether patients are on track with their treatment plan. Fig. 1.2 illustrates an Example of smart, connected inhaler use for children.

1.5 Ingestible sensors

Proteus Digital Health and its ingestible sensors are another example of digital medicine analysis Job Medical. Again, the primary goal of this technology, tested with an antipsychotic and antihypertensive pill, is to monitor adherence. However, in this case, the pill dissolves in the stomach and produces a small signal which is picked up by a sensor worn on the body, which again relays the data to a smartphone application.

1.6 IoMT data security

In addition to the bureaucratic burdens, doctors already have great difficulty managing the data generated by standard devices. This difficulty increases with the spread of new technologies capable of generating masses of information that are often not contextualized and therefore completely meaningless. This huge amount of data can have repercussions in the clinical, forensic, administrative, contractual, logistic, environmental fields and so on. The solution to the problem lies in training. What is

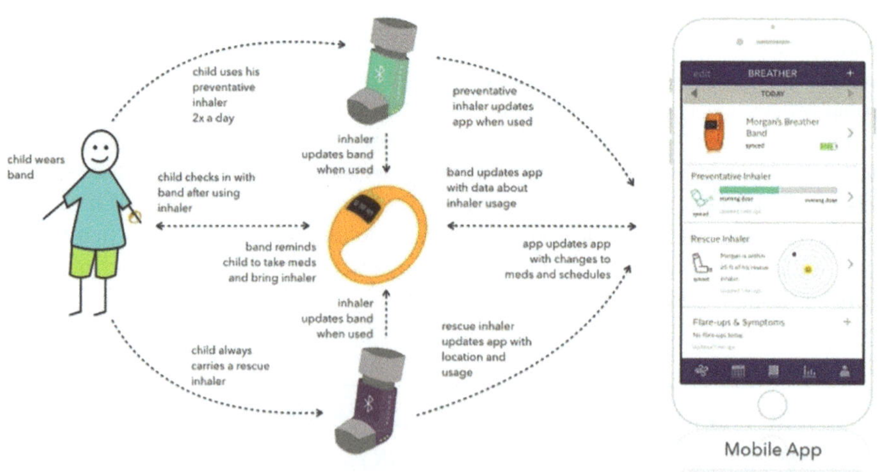

FIGURE 1.2

Example of smart, connected inhaler use for children.

needed are specific professional skills, which allow you to evaluate the data more effectively. For example, the data scientist "Is a figure that already exists in the most advanced health systems". This figure must protect not only the security, but also the interoperability of the data and their usability. According to some analysts, the huge wave of data generated by IoT devices could be overwhelming and only if the industry can find new ways to integrate and deepen the analysis will it be possible to capitalize on the inherent value of IoMT technology. The increased flow of information also carries great vulnerability risks, and healthcare IT professionals are well aware of this problem. In a typical IoMT implementation, it is common to use products and services from multiple vendors. This means a lot of effort from the IT department, forced to manage platforms often unable to communicate with each other and exposed to the risk of attacks. However, the market is reacting quickly. Vendors like Google, Microsoft, Amazon, or VMware are looking to help hospital IT teams through integrated and interoperable solutions. Without certified solutions, IT managers are often hesitant. However, it should not be forgotten that the same situation of vulnerability has been experienced for years in the PC sector, but this has not slowed down the pace of technology adoption. IoT vendors today are investing to keep their firmware up-to-date and, with many of the modern IoT management platforms, to monitor the access and use of information to prevent it from falling into the wrong hands. These risks include breaches that can compromise data security but also patient health. Unauthorized access to a storage or even a device can have effects ranging from tampering with data to tampering with the functionality of, for example, an infusion pump or smart bed. The healthcare community considers this risk increasingly concrete and is starting to address the problem of security and privacy not only from the point of view of the IoT. When it comes to health IoT security issues, the list can seem endless. One of the challenges is related to the multiplicity of channels used by devices to access hospital systems. An example is the so-called "Bring your own device" approach, an expression used to refer to company policies that allow employees to bring their devices to the workplace using them to access confidential information and applications. When this happens, it can be difficult to understand how information is managed, its actual location and the level of confidentiality with which it is treated. Furthermore, since the various devices operate based on different processes, they do not necessarily exploit a common control configuration. This means that you can never be sure that your access has been protected by specific passwords, encryption or hardware/software protection. Another problem, is linked to the fact that autonomous devices exploit networks and connectivity systems in which data transfer can involve real migrations that do not allow to keep track of the paths followed. Such scenarios are worrying and introduce a variety of diversified risks and vulnerabilities. Despite the risks, the health community has understood that IoT is an unavoidable reality. To protect safety as much as possible, there are steps that suppliers and manufacturers must follow. A fundamental prerequisite is device authentication. This process allows limiting access if a certain uniformity to the system platform and standardizing communications. The second aspect is encryption. The data must always be encoded and made illegible in clear text. The third aspect is to follow safe boot processes that automatically set up devices when they are turned on, limiting the user's ability to customize settings. A fourth aspect is to have a clear map of the data, applications and devices that pertain to the system, in order to always know how and where information moves3.

As shown in Fig. 1.3, the IoMT structure is made up of three layers: the perception layer, the network layer, and the application layer.

The perception layer's main purpose is to collect healthcare data from a range of devices.

The network layer, which is made up of wired and wireless systems as well as middleware, processes and transmits the information gathered by the perception layer with the help of technical platforms.

Well-designed transport protocols not only improve transmission efficiency and save energy consumption, but also provide security and privacy.

The application layer integrates medical information resources to provide individualized medical services and meet the demands of end-users, based on the target population's current status and service need.

1.7 Artificial intelligence in healthcare: ethical and legal issues

The application of AI in clinical practice has enormous promise to improve healthcare, but it also poses ethical issues that we must now address.

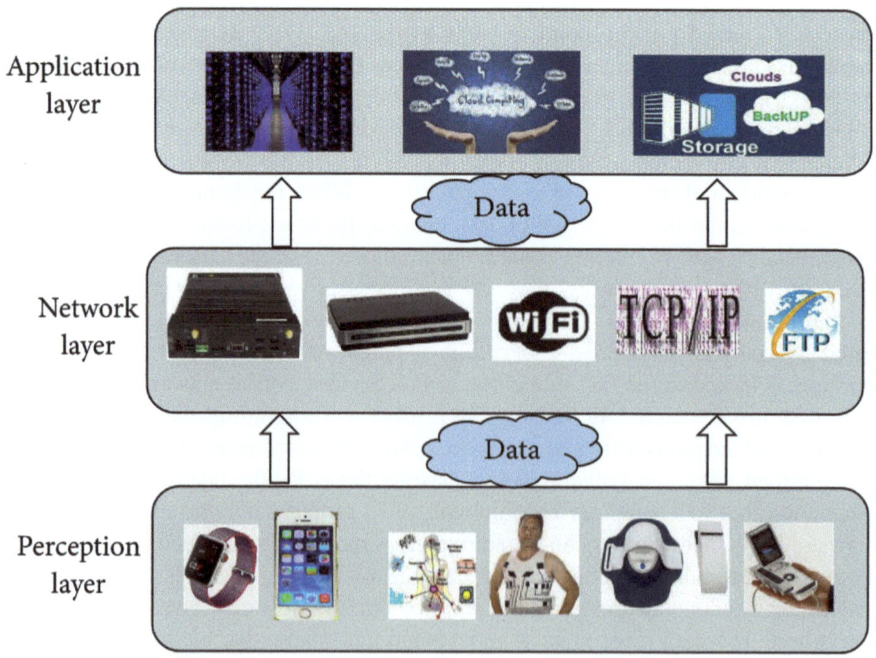

FIGURE 1.3

Medical internet of things structure.

The ethical point of the involvement of AI and all that revolves around it must be treated by laws that govern and regulate the market concerned.

This point diverges from one country to another, from one community to another, depending on the legislation and the level of awareness of the population.

We will attempt to give an overview with some examples, in particular, the United States and the European Union.

1.7.1 United States

The US Government's AI reports during Barack Obama's presidency emphasized, among other things, AI applications for the public good as well as aspects of fairness, safety, and governance.

Fairness, openness, and accountability-by-design, as well as the development of ethical AI, were all underlined in one of the papers.

The US AI strategy has moved to a more free market-oriented approach since Donald Trump's election.

In May 2018, for example, the White House held the AI for American Industry Summit.

The Trump administration wants to reduce regulatory impediments to AI advancements, according to one of the primary findings from the summit breakout conversations.

The White House said in July 2018 that American leadership in AI is one of the Administration's top R&D funding priority topics for 2020.

Trump signed the "Executive Order on Maintaining American Leadership in Artificial Intelligence" in February 2019 in response to accusations that the US has taken a hands-off approach to AI in comparison to other countries like China.

With this executive order, Trump launched the American AI Initiative, a coordinated Federal Government strategy guided by five key areas of focus: (1) investing in AI research and development, (2) unleashing AI resources, (3) setting AI governance standards, (4) building the AI workforce, and (5) international engagement and protecting the US AI advantage.

The White House released proposed recommendations for the regulation of AI applications in January 2020.

It outlines 10 guidelines that organizations should keep in mind while developing AI strategies:

(1) public trust in AI, (2) public participation, (3) scientific integrity and information quality, (4) risk assessment and management, (5) benefits and costs, (6) flexibility, (7) fairness and nondiscrimination, (8) disclosure and transparency, (9) safety and security, and (10) interagency coordination are all important factors to consider.

The White House also released an annual report on the American AI Initiative in February 2020, outlining progress since Trump signed the executive order.

The United States, for example, led historic efforts to develop the Organization for Economic Cooperation and Development (OECD) AI Principles, which were signed by over 40 countries in May 2019 to support innovative and trustworthy AI while respecting democratic ideals and human rights.

The G20 announced AI Principles in June 2019, based on the OECD AI Principles.

1.7.2 Europe

In April 2018, the European Commission adopted its AI strategy for Europe.

The Commission announced a European initiative on AI in this Communication, to ensure a suitable ethical and legal framework, among other things, by forming a European AI Alliance and developing AI ethics standards.

The Ethics Guidelines were issued in April 2019 by the European Commission's High-Level Expert Group on AI (AI HLEG), which was appointed by the European Commission in June 2018 and is also the steering group for the European AI Alliance.

The Guidelines promote the slogan "Trustworthy AI" and include seven key requirements for AI systems to be trustworthy: (1) human agency and oversight, (2) technical robustness and safety, (3) privacy and data governance, (4) transparency, (5) diversity, nondiscrimination, and fairness, (6) environmental and societal well-being, and (7) accountability."

The AI HLEG also issued a document on the definition of AI as part of its deliverables.

In addition, the AI HLEG released another deliverable in June 2019 titled "Policy and Investment Recommendations for Trustworthy AI."

The European Commission urges all EU Member States to adopt a national AI strategy, and several countries, like the United Kingdom (UK) and Germany, have already done so.

In December 2018, the European Commission and the EU Member States, Norway, and Switzerland agreed on a coordinated AI plan to encourage AI development and application in Europe.

The overarching goal of the collaboration is to make Europe the world leader in the development and deployment of "cutting-edge, ethical, and secure AI."

The European Commission produced a White Paper on AI in February 2020, which outlines a European strategy for excellence and trust.

A Communication on a European data strategy and a Report on the liability implications and safety of AI, the IoT, and robotics were also released at the same time by the Commission.

"Europe can combine its technological and industrial strengths with a high-quality digital infrastructure and a regulatory framework based on its basic values to become a global leader in innovation in the data economy and its applications," according to the Commission's White Paper.

In Europe, AI health applications are already available, with more on the way.

Ada, for example, is an AI health app that analyses a person's symptoms and provides advice.

On 14,884 scans, a 94% success rate was achieved.

In the meantime, DeepMind's health team has moved to Google Health, and Moorfield's Eye Hospital is "eager to work with Google Health on the next step to further improve this AI system so it can be utilized by patients all around the world," according to the hospital.

Ultromics is another example.

The University of Oxford team is "committed to reducing misdiagnosis and enabling earlier cardiovascular disease prevention."

Ultromics' EchoGo Pro, for example, is an outcome-based AI system that predicts coronary artery disease at an early stage and has received CE certification in Europe.

Corti is a Danish company's software that uses machine learning to assist emergency dispatchers in making judgments.

By listening in on conversations and evaluating symptoms, voice tone, breathing patterns, and other metadata in real-time, Corti can detect out-of-hospital cardiac arrests (i.e., those that occur in the public or at home) during emergency calls faster and more accurately than humans.

1.8 The main points to remember

IoT is now a mainstream technology that people are familiar with. It is one of those technologies that has changed the way we live our lives. It has also transformed the healthcare industry by introducing smart healthcare apps. Healthcare IoT devices and apps have helped the healthcare industry overcome all limitations and obstacles during the pandemic. IoT application development companies have helped patients, practitioners and service providers reach new levels of quality in healthcare.

The introduction of IoT in healthcare has resulted in reduced death rates and easier access to medical facilities through remote communication. The IoT has proven to be a miracle in health fields with solutions such as telehealth, e-health, telemedicine, etc. Let's dive into some of the healthcare use cases. The rate of adoption of IoT apps and devices has triggered a rising demand curve (Kundhavai, 2016).

Does this article explain how the IoT ushered in a wave of success in healthcare?

Below are some of the use cases of how IoT improves the quality of healthcare.

1.8.1 Remote observation and diagnosis of the patient

One of the most important features of an IoT-enabled telemedicine app is to record vital health parameters to facilitate remote monitoring and diagnostics of patients.

Telemedicine solutions enable doctor–patient consultation via live video and audio call, another form of advanced communication channel, removing the need for the patient to go to the hospital. Other external devices powered by IoT, such as digital oximeters and stethoscopes, are used by patients today during online telemedicine consultations.

Several IoT health monitoring devices are available for use. Devices such as heart rate monitoring cuffs, pulse counters, blood glucose monitors, etc. are used by patients who help physicians observe the health of elderly patients and those with chronic illnesses from a distance. The data accumulated by these devices helps physicians to analyze the correct course of treatment.

1.8.2 Mobile health and wellness

The IoT has taken the quality of healthcare by leaps and bounds. An example would be the use of wearable technologies such as Fitbit trackers, Apple watches which efficiently transmit essential health statistics of a patient through Wi-Fi, Bluetooth, and GPRS networks and display these statistics on smartphones. This is of vital importance for tracking the well-being and vital signs of the body such as body temperature, sleep patterns, blood sugar, heart rate, activity tracking, etc. providing accurate real-time data to physicians, caregivers and patients.

1.8.3 Ingestible IoT-enabled devices

Seeming as if straight out of a sci-fi movie are ingestible sensors in pill form. These are easily usable and when swallowed, they stay inside the human body in a particular place. It sends valuable information to the mobile app that comes with the device. The sensors inside these pills can detect doses of medication taken or forgotten by the patient. These ingestible digestible devices can prevent life-threatening conditions (Neranjan, 2020).

1.8.4 Emergency management

The IoT is well known for its ability to transmit accurate data in real-time, which can be vital for emergency response (ER) medical personnel. In an emergency, it allows the emergency department to stay prepared while the patient is on the way to the hospital, saving valuable time that can be life-saving.

1.8.5 Help surgeries

IoT-powered devices, tools and solutions can prove to be essential and help during surgeries and in the management of postoperative care. IoT sensors efficiently collect data, transmit it in real-time, and analyze the data, which can detect even the smallest health problems and thus avoid surgical complications.

While managing the security of the IoT is complex in other sectors, in healthcare the stakes are much higher. Security vulnerabilities can affect people's safety, or even put their lives at risk altogether.

This hyperconnectivity of ultrasecure "objects" has led to the digital transformation of healthcare establishments. They must now take concrete steps to protect patients, data and the healthcare system against attempted cyberattacks and data hacking (Liu, 2018).

1.8.6 Efficient inventory, staff, and patient tracking

IoT devices contribute in the following ways.

- Wireless ID cards for patients and staff can improve security, manage admissions to secure areas, and effectively manage staff.
- RFID cards are used to track Alzheimer's patients, babies, and are effective for tracking staff in an emergency.
- The IoT integrates the Real-Time Tracking System (RTLS) to manage inventory in healthcare facilities. It uses Bluetooth Low Energy (BLE) and iBeacon to track inventory and supplies in operating rooms.

Managing drugs in the hospital and running the storage facility with the same safety standards is a daunting task and can lead to theft and other such issues. The IoT helps pharmacies manage medications efficiently by ensuring faster medication delivery and retention of medications during transfer.

1.8.7 Critique and analysis

The IoT in healthcare has changed the healthcare service by introducing a wide range of options that are vital for patients, practitioners and healthcare providers. It is high time that more and more healthcare organizations take the initiative and integrate IoT into their healthcare programs, seeing the benefits it can bring to patients.

1.8.8 A glimpse of AI in action

We cannot here exhaust the extent of the potential of AIs and the realized or expected applications. Today, AIs playing video games from which they ignore the rules but which they deduce are being designed, AIs winning over humans for games such as go, reputed to mobilize superior cognitive faculties. The spectacular improvement of the translation engine "Google Translate" is the instance of an AI of which it appears, without even having been programmed for this purpose, that it has developed a kind of own metalanguage. Allowing him to ensure and develop his interpreting skills. Some teams are working on the design of AI capable of transforming any sketch of an invented the machine into a 3D printable machine blueprint.

In the field that interests us, health, AI implementations are numerous and seem to be more and more efficient. Google has developed an AI allowing automated reading of the eye fundus of diabetic subjects. The performances are clear: a sensitivity of around 90% and almost 100% specificity. The same Google is invited into the field of anatomy pathology: the anatomo-pathologist is the ultimate judge to make a diagnosis, and this by means of images of organ removals. His responsibility is major and the reading, sometimes nonconsensual, of the images he processes is complex: the rate of agreement for the same diagnosis made by different doctors is low, barely 50%. However, as part of a work on breast cancer, Google's algorithms were able to correctly locate tumors in 89% of cases, versus 73% for anatomy-pathologists. As a collateral benefit, the diagnosis of the machine, compared to the processing time of an expert, is almost instantaneous.

We could multiply the examples, ranging from the detection of melanomas from images of moles taken by a smartphone to the automated analysis of the scientific literature in order to suggest therapeutic choices, through epidemiological monitoring devices predictive. But let's try to figure out further how AIs will ultimately configure or even conform to the functioning of our health system.

1.8.9 A doctor diminished by an augmented medicine?

The medical examination is a special moment when the patient talks about himself and the doctor investigate in a famous colloquium that is said to be unique, and that it will be even more so because of the increasing digitization of the context in which the patient occurs: doctor-patient interview, online consultation of the Vidal, consultation of consensus conferences, and online entry of the patient file, etc. The patient himself often presents himself to the doctor armed with a mass of medical information consulted on the internet. Internet, or rather the information which is collected there, thus remediates the relations between doctors and patients, in a new balance worked by technology. AI is amplifying this movement and it's a safe bet that, in the near future, the patient will present himself to his doctor with his data set, the result of the collection of data from various connected objects, medical or not. These connected objects, foremost among them the smartphone, produce a considerable amount of data, and this in strongly typed contexts (via metadata): sport, reading, sleep, physical or environmental stressful situation, social dynamics, etc. Symptom monitoring can be done in real-time and in a contextual manner, allowing a more detailed assessment of the impact of behaviors and the environment on their development. Further, whether it is about the effect of the monitored music on the platforms of a situation of physical or environmental stress, social dynamics, etc. Symptoms can be monitored in real-time and in a contextual manner, allowing a more detailed assessment of the impact of behaviors and the environment on their development. Noise stress or pollution via onboard sensors, social interactions via the social graph, medicine, therefore, has new sets of parameters to improve the collection, monitoring and evaluation of physical or physiological manifestations which are no longer the exclusive time of the clinical examination, and to deepen what are the determinants of health.

This permanent monitoring reflects a kind of ambulatory and multisource access to medicine, in front of which are communities of patients, issuing data of all kinds, gathering around forums, data sharing platforms, or ' self-quantify tools.

1.8.10 Automation, conversational robots, and therapeutic innovation with constant pharmacopoeia

Between patients and doctors, technologies are therefore breaking in with all the more impact as they are endowed with AI and, among the promises announced, some should materialize without difficulty within the decade: automated diagnosis in imaging, histology, monitoring of weak signals in epidemiology, cross-referencing of clinical data and therapeutics for personalized medicine with constant pharmacopoeia. This last point is important in that it announces that the masses of data domesticated by AIs make it possible to concentrate part of the research efforts on a better knowledge of human physiology, the evolution of diseases, their environmental determinants, their physio-pathological manifestations, promising a personalized care by using already known therapies.

We should also point out that a trend is rapidly developing in web services: "bots," that is to say, algorithmic entities that take on the role of personal assistants and with which the interaction is done according to a free language, auguring the increase of personalized medicine by a personalized doctor. Finding information, making appointments, virtual secretaries, sorting and referral patients as a first resort are all possibilities. Here, the specter of the redefinition of the role of doctors and of the delegation of competing rather than concurrent tasks between doctors and machines gives rise to concern. Nevertheless, let us see in the new technological situation an opportunity to supplement the quality of medical care.

1.8.11 The Deep Patient

We can expect AIs, in the part they will play in assisting diagnosis or therapeutic choices, that they will improve patient care by anticipating the development of their disease. In this sense, the application of techniques known as "deep neural networks," or Deep Learning, make it possible to design from data from patient files a model known as Deep Patient, capable of accurately predicting the course of the disease and therefore of adapting treatment, thus ushering in the era of personalized and predictive medicine. Of course, the very nature of a medicine that wants to be predictive raises questions in that it would protect us as soon as possible from diseases as much as it would be a way of "pathologizing" the normal. Indeed, the evolutions of AI raise fears of a kind of permanent medicine, where the logic of well-being would be the opportunity to medicalize everyone's daily life, normality becoming a presymptom of the disease, where we would push back the border of death by advancing the definition of disease. And all this is congruent with the economic motivation of private actors, having an interest in pushing the consumption of welfare or health goods.

The medical, societal, and ethical consequences are profound and deserve to be analyzed with care. Today, moreover, it is a question of raising these questions into a major public debate, democratizing access to them, demystifying their often technical terms, so that users of the health system, associations of patients, and the public authorities can discuss their evolutions, measure their contributions and anticipate their drifts.

More generally, ethical and legal questions, in particular that relating to predictive or augmented medicine, robotization, and correlatively to the responsibility of algorithms, seem to us to have to penetrate the minds of decision-makers and in practice integrate the course, if not of training, at least sensitization of health professionals.

1.8.12 The reorganization of the health fabric

The reduction of costs by machines which massively parallel their tasks, which do not get tired and whose processing capacities, were it not for breakdowns, know only little variability, is an element which will not fail to awaken the attention of health authorities. In addition, AI can be expected to result in a substantial reduction in medical errors, and therefore the human and financial costs that they entail. Because, in addition to the intrinsic performance of algorithms, the reproducibility of their execution does not depend on such contingent factors as operator fatigue or training.

Of course, whether it is a question of automation and the savings that can be expected from it, of medical or organizational decision-making assistance, the prospect of better efficiency of the health system seems reasonably achievable. However, in this technological transition, the impacts of which must now be smoothed out, particularly in terms of employment, it is necessary to relate the evidence of the expected savings to the investments required, on the one hand to migrate all of the workers. The current architecture toward a highly digitized and monitored ecosystem on which depends in return on the training and therefore the quality of AIs, and on the other hand to ensure the training and upscaling of skills, with numbers that we hope will also be constant as possible.

From an organizational standpoint, it is no longer improbable that, apart from emergency cases, a large part of medical procedures ultimately fall under last resort medicine, after connected devices operated by AIs have filtered the chaff, physiological normalcy of symptoms. The fundamental movement of the miniaturization of diagnostic tools, to the point of seeing all connected objects, foremost among which is the smartphone, as a sort of laboratory for distributed medical analyzes (a recent publication by *Nature* reports the spectacular diagnostic performance of a mobile application in the detection of melanoma), heralding a radical break in the organization of care itself. The hospital and the doctor's office will no longer be the privileged places of tomorrow's medicine and must reinvent themselves.

By pushing logic further, the hospital could eventually become a third place, integrated into a deeply decentralized whole, powerfully monitored by AIs, whose primary functions would be interventional and whose support function, including the operation. diagnostic, would switch to the cloud. Indeed, the explosion of connected objects combined with the evolution of AI makes it possible to consider that the hospital offers part of its clinical services online: the data collected by the connected objects being analyzed via Application Programming Interfaces (APIs) and referring to a course of action to be taken for the healthcare professional or directly for the patient. In addition, we will see in such a model the opportunity to monetize services: remote diagnosis or concerning private actors, training of AI on data from the healthcare system.

Correspondingly, ethical support for these evolutions is essential because the natural current, in particular evangelized by the ideologies of Silicon Valley, would push the human body to become the object to be connected to machines: we would go, basically, from an examined body to a connected body.

1.8.13 Data-drive medicine

In the future of medicine, data is produced throughout the system, by healthcare structures, healthcare professionals and patients; it is collected by sensors as close as possible to their emitter, as close as possible to the patients, and tomorrow introduced into the patient's own body, and in return these data educate, improve the AI algorithms and will enable robots, located on their own, in the future. Also, as close as possible to the data sources, to ensure a perfectly individualized service, even announcing the detection of presymptoms, the patients being notified at the same time of the action to be taken. Thus, AI makes it possible on the one hand to automate a complex assembly of elementary tasks and, on the other hand, to develop the bases of personalized and predictive medicine. It seems critical to us to note that, in this scheme where data is metabolized to the point of producing feedback mediated by a robot and where the medicine of tomorrow is played out, institutional players are as absent as strategically positioned Google, Apple, Facebook and Amazon (GAFA). Indeed, the technological giants have a marked interest in health, notably vectorized by connected objects. For the moment, they nest their models around well-being, the distinction of which from health will no longer make any sense given the predictive power that AIs will be endowed with. The investment of GAFA in connected objects, their activity of buying home automation start-ups will ultimately represent a way of taking medicine out of the hospital, bypassing it and individualizing it from service applications in a context which moreover will not necessarily be "health-oriented."

It is not too quick to suggest that, until the second half of the 20th century, the hardware has structured qualitative differentiation of industrial supplies, after which the software has emerged. In the economy to come, the element which will confer a competitive advantage will be the training data set, which will in turn define the quality of the software. Like individuals, it is education through data sets that will confer the software quality of the machine.

It is in this sense that the battle for mastery of data is so strategic and that it is up to our institutions to grasp its scope. On a more regal level, our sovereignty depends on it and, in the context of health, the democratic control of the choices that will structure our health system is played out somewhere around AI.

1.8.14 AI and machine training

Mastery of the data, therefore, supposes that we ensure the qualification of software by training them via big data. For that, it is a question of putting as much care into the training of the men as in those of the machines. If medical training relies heavily on mentoring, machines should be integrated into this knowledge transfer scheme. Indeed, the performance of the AIs that equip the machines improves as they are fed with data, which corresponds to the intangible conversion of the experience of the doctor, the patient or any institutional actor in the health system. Carrying out this function of transferring experience from human to the machine will be an essential driving force in raising the predictive performance of AIs and, in return, achieving the medical performance that is expected of them. More globally, it is here that we will situate the stake of a massive "monitoring" of the whole of the health system, that is to say as many sensors equipping medical devices, collecting the physiological parameters of patients equipped with connected objects, metabolizing in an immaterial way the experience of health professionals to return data essential to the management of the entire health system. This learning activity should be one of the major activities of public actors.

1.8.15 Health professionals digested by AI?

Is the Polish plumber of the future the machine? In any case, more than the machine is the future of the Polish plumber. Because if there is one area in which the anxieties of great replacement can find a rationality, it is precisely in the absorption-execution by machines of any work that can be broken down into repetitive tasks. The substitution of human labor for tasks carried out or even controlled by machines gives rise to legitimate fears that human skills will be sidelined.

In the world of health, this will not be reduced to the space of logistic or support functions, and a good attitude of mind consists in considering that all professions will be, as intensive as they are in terms of mobilization of faculty. we would think cognitive therefore superior, partly within reach of machines. AI would thus reduce the threat of diseases to advance it on the employment front, which some fear will cause extinction.

Whether it is health professionals, technicians, logistics or administrative professions, all should be deeply impacted by AI technologies. But if medical care cannot be reduced to decision trees. However, complex they may be, the pace of technological developments is such that it is difficult to predict the professions imminently threatened by machines and it is unfortunately no AI yet to facilitate this exercise which is still divination today.

It is critical for our health system to adapt and balance the potential benefits of the application of these technologies against the risks of job substitution which they will only exaggerate to the extent of our unpreparedness.

In reality, the reinvention of the trades should be an opportunity to hybridize the capacities of human and machine, advantageously complementing the faculty of synthesis of the first by the computational and predictive capacity of the second. This assembly gives birth to the notion of Centaur. Indeed, after Gary Kasparov, the bubbling world chess champion of the 1990s, was defeated by Deep Blue, IBM's AI, teams made up of human—machine pairs were formed and it is then significant that the human—machine pair beats the machine alone.

It appears that the possibility for the expert to detect false positives is low. However, that this probability is more important for the machine and, conversely, the machine seems to be able to avoid false negatives better. We can then bet that human—machine complementarity can lead to the emergence of an effective couple. Further on, some see in this collaboration the starting point of an inevitable hybridization of human and machine, pushing back the boundaries of a human's physiological capacities to the point of singularity, namely "the death of death"—this is the credo of the transhumanist.

As we all know by now, in recent years the technological development in the field of consumer electronics and industrial applications has proved decisive for improving the well-being of people and for greater sustainability of technology in a broad sense. Based on this development, increasingly miniaturized devices (connected both to the internet and to each other) and able to collect and process data everywhere (everywhere computing) are making "the lion's share" in the daily life of many people.

Examples of technologically advanced developments can be represented by fitness trackers, and wearable devices able to accurately measure the movements of the wearer during physical activity (and not only) thanks to the use of integrated sensors. However, it is also necessary to consider other fundamental aspects of the question, such as: the considerable amount of data that these wearable devices can produce and the security aspects that this technological evolution poses. As an example, in 2018 the use of some fitness trackers revealed on the internet the hitherto secret location of some military bases around the world due to the advertising of soldiers' jogging activities.

Other examples can be related to attacks targeting millions of webcams, printers, children's toys and even vacuum cleaners, as well as Distributed Denial-of-Service (DDoS) attacks, to inhibit the availability of certain services. As a consequence of this type of criticality, users' confidence in the technology could be reduced. Therefore, the availability of data collected or produced by such devices must be managed with care, but at the same time it is reasonably impossible for a human person to be able to process such a large amount of information.

For this reason, another line of research that has enabling and positive implications in a large number of scenarios concerns the development of AI and ML algorithms that allow better processing and management of these data.

By way of example, the use of AI and ML mechanisms can allow automatic recognition of faces in particular situations (of danger or safety), remote control (via voice recognition) of connected devices within a home or in a vehicle while driving, or predicting environmental phenomena with some degree of accuracy.

1.9 Discussion

Nowadays, it is almost indisputable the extent that AI and all related sciences take in our lives, all aspects combined; The same is true in the field of health and healthcare; We have, thus, seen through this chapter a panoply of use cases of AI and related sciences in this field. However, the debate is at its peak regarding ethics and deontology in this field.

In this perspective, the questions that arise, among others, are we aware of this magnitude? Will consumers consciously accept AI, or is it quietly infiltrating all aspects of our lives? Do patients readily accept, without resistance or difficulty in understanding, human–AI interactions and consequently the replacement of human doctors by medical AI, or does it remain an unrealistic proposition. The ethical challenges facing AI in the healthcare profession are extensive and complicated. While AI has the potential to improve health and healthcare systems, we must proceed with caution.

The paucity of literature on AI's ethical implications in healthcare and public health also highlights the urgent need for more research into AI's ethical implications in global and public health to ensure that its development and implementation are ethical for everyone, everywhere.

1.10 Conclusion

Internet-connected smart medical devices offer new methods of care. The sensors and devices present in the various equipment allow the collection of numerous information and data on patients. Such data can, for example, help staff prepare for treatments or plan visits, as well as streamline work and improve the quality of care.

The introduction of this technology will make it possible to compensate for the shortage of staff, while the constant cut in local healthcare costs will have little or no impact on the care of patients and the elderly. In the future, it will be more and more widespread, guaranteeing more efficient assistance, without reducing the quality level. Basically, it will be possible to discover causes, connections, and relationships, which will allow us to act quickly thanks to these intelligent systems. Unlike other industrial or service sectors which are exposed to a technological surge of unequaled magnitude - which has imposed in a few years young start-ups in sectors maintained by historic rents - institutional players in health are sheltered by a regulatory microclimate that gives them a certain resilience in the face of water hammer from young shoots, which will bring major innovations, and gives them additional time to adapt. But this time is precious and it must be used with discernment.

Currently, in most large healthcare facilities where AI is being experimented, basic and high-level predictive use cases are being pursued, certainly without replacing human-controlled diagnostic and therapeutic practices or protocols in the clinical setting. sanitary. Over the next few years, more organizations will tackle more advanced use cases that will include the generation of new clinical procedures as capabilities to develop advanced machine learning solutions increase and the industry begins to leverage more sophisticated AI techniques (for example also integrating computer vision, language analysis, etc.). Obviously, these procedures will then be experimented with and subjected to appropriate clinical tests.

Already today, healthcare facilities can use intelligent predictive tools to plan the most appropriate clinical path, recommend personalized therapies and identify patients most at risk. Furthermore, the ability of ML solutions to make qualitative forecasts makes them perfect for supporting medical diagnosis by providing a *second opinion* which, in some clinical and insurance areas, is also mandatory if not strongly recommended.

References

Akhtar, N. (2021). *A holistic analysis of medical internet of things (MIoT). Free and accessible knowledge*.

Alsheikh. (2016). *Mobile big data analytics using deep learning and Apache Spark.*

Amin. (2018). A light weight authentication protocol for IoT-enabled devices in distributed cloud computing environment. *Future Generation Computer Systems*.

Bhattacharya. (2016). Evolutionary optimization: A big data perspective. *J. Journal of Network and Computer Applications*, 416–426.

Chang. (2018). Research investigations on the use or non-use of hearing aids in the smart cities. *Technological Forecasting and Social Change*.

Costa. (2017). A fuzzy-based approach for sensing, coding and transmission configuration of visual sensors in smart city applications. *Sensors*.

Dimitrov. (2016). *Medical internet of things and big data in healthcare*. Healthcare Informatics Research.

Ding. (2016). *Cellular-base-station-assisted device-to-device communications in TV white space*. IEEE.

Elhoseny, M. (2021). Security and privacy issues in medical internet of things: Overview, countermeasures, challenges and future directions. *Sustainability, 13*(21).

Gaurav, A. (2022). Security of cloud-based medical internet of things (MIoTs): A survey. *International Journal of Software Science and Computational Intelligence, 14*(1).

Gyu. (2019). User authentication system based on baseline-corrected ECG for biometrics. *Intelligent Automation and Soft Computing, 25*(1).

Iqbal, R. (2020). Big data analytics: Computational intelligence techniques and application areas. *Technological Forecasting and Social Change, 153*.

Jangid. (2020). Security issues and challenges in healthcare automated devices. In *International Conference on Communication Systems & Networks*.

Kundhavai. (2016). IoT and big data-the current and future technologies: A review. *International Journal of Computer Science and Mobile Computing, 5*(1), 10–14.

Liu. (2018). *A clustering k-anonymity privacy-preserving method for wearable IoT devices. Security and Communication Networks*.

Neranjan, T. (2020). The role of the internet of things in health care: A systematic and comprehensive study. *International Journal of Engineering and Management Research*.

Singh. (2020). Convergence of blockchain and artificial intelligence in IoT network for the sustainable smart city. *Sustainable Cities and Society*.

Sukumaran. (2018). DNA cryptography for secure data storage in cloud. *International Journal of Network Security*.

Sun, W. (2017). *Security and privacy in the medical internet of things: A review*. Security and Communication Network.

Sun. (2018). *Security and privacy in the medical internet of things: A review*. Hindawi Security Communication Networks.

Tariq. (2019). The security of big data in fog-enabled IoT applications including blockchain: A survey. *Sensors*.

Tsai. (2014). *Future internet of things: Open issues and challenges*. Wireless Networks.

Ugandran, I. (2021). A novel cryptosystem using DNA sequencing and contextual array splicing system for Medical Internet of Things. *Computers & Electrical Engineering, 96*.

Xu. (2016). Scalable cloud–sensor architecture for the Internet of Things. *IEEE Internet Things*.

Yang. (2019). Building an open cloud virtual dataspace model for materials scientific data. *Intelligent Automation and Soft Computing*, 615–624.

Yu. (2018). *A survey on the edge computing for the Internet of Things*. IEEE.

Zafar. (2019). Interplay between big spectrum data and mobile internet of things: Current solutions and future challenges. *Computer Networks*.

Further reading

Bennis. (2018). *Ultrareliable and low-latency wireless communication: Tail, risk, and scale*. IEEE.

Doctor. (2016). Type-2 fuzzy sets applied to multivariable self-organizing fuzzy logic controllers for regulating anesthesia. *Applied Soft Computing, 38*, 872–889.

Hitaswi. (2016). *A bio-inspired model to provide data security in cloud storage*. IEEE.

CHAPTER

AIoMT artificial intelligence (AI) and Internet of Medical Things (IoMT): applications, challenges, and future trends

2

Fadi Muheidat[1], **Loai A. Tawalbeh**[2]

[1]*Computer Science and Engineering, California State University, San Bernardino, San Bernardino, CA, United States;* [2]*Department of Computer Engineering, Jordan University of Science and Technology, Irbid, Jordan*

2.1 Introduction

The evolution of technology over the past 20 years has affected how we carry out our daily activities. It is an initiative that has led to positive change in terms of development (Cho & Lee, 2019). One of the things that stood out during the period is the Internet of Things (IoT). IoT entails the physical devices that have an internet connection. This is a key attribute that could be attributed to the change of technology and the spread of the use of the internet. Today, 30% of things that surround us seem to have the internet making it a key point of concern that needs to be positively addressed based on the implication of the practice in our basic well-being (Curran, 2016). IoT seems to run how we reflect on basic concepts and understand how society normally runs. The IoT devices consist of the hardware component that makes it possible for the entity to be a part of an interconnected network. Different devices can be used, some of them include home appliances, healthcare devices, and factory devices. The main aim is to provide sensors that provide physical environmental information such as temperature, humidity, and pollution. The other devices include the actuators such as light switches and displays (Wang et al., 2018). The devices can also be motor-assisted shutters or any device that can be embedded in the computers. The main aim of using IoT devices in a given environment is to ensure that they communicate using different means, such as using the internet. IoT devices have different characteristics. First of all, these devices should actuate and sense the capability of the limiting power and connection to the physical environment (Ahemd et al., 2017). The devices must be fast, provide credible services, and provide a given security level in the network. However, these devices must be protected from the vulnerabilities of external and internal attacks.

Computational Intelligence for Medical Internet of Things (MIoT) Applications
https://doi.org/10.1016/B978-0-323-99421-7.00013-1

IoT, such as IoT medical devices and wearables, is essentially smart devices that can connect to the internet to gather, share, and process data. These devices enable nurses to collect real-time patient data, receive alert notifications, and help with patient monitoring. Instead of running around the hospital checking on patients one by one, they can receive the information they need directly to their phone, a computer, or a wearable device like a smart wristband or smartwatch.

In this paper, we used the traditional (narrative) literature review of the recent advances in the Internet of Medical Things (IoMT) and the use of artificial intelligence in the IoMT applications. It discusses the structure of IoMT systems, applications, security, challenges, and the role of AI methodologies in the advances of IoMT.

2.1.1 Internet of Medical Things

The Medical Internet of Things (MIoT) also known as Internet of Medical Things (IoMT), we will use the two terms interchageably, shares many of the same requirements as the conventional Internet of Things (IoT), especially in terms of managing a large number of devices, dependable communication, and system heterogeneity and interoperability (Islam et al., 2015; Waterman et al., 2020). The Medical Internet of Things (MIoT) is a healthcare system comprised of smart medical devices and software applications. The Internet of Things is helping the flow of information from one device to another, from humans to devices, and from things to things. With the increasing power of connectivity, the IoT is changing the healthcare system, by collecting and sharing data, predicting health issues and diagnosis, telemedicine, patient monitoring, etc. Hence, the birth of the Internet of Medical Things or Medical Internet of Things (MIoT). We will use these terms interchangeably in this chapter.

When health data is collected, communicated, and stored by IoT sensors, data analysis, and intelligent healthcare can be carried out, which can improve risk factor identification, disease diagnosis, treatment, remote monitoring and allow people to self-manage at home, and lower costs. An Integrated Home Assistance (Nugroho et al., 2020) system based on IoMT allows all healthcare systems to move from a traditional model of service delivery, which is often reactive, intermittent, and uncoordinated, toward a more proactive, continuous, and coordinated approach. Such an approach is (Mora et al., 2017) beneficial because it offers the opportunity to provide high-quality care that is both less invasive and attractive to patients and healthcare professionals. Fig. 2.1 is a generalized MIoT environment (Mora et al., 2017).

The generic architecture of IoMT systems consists of four (Dwivedi et al., 2022) or five main layers that integrate different sensors, devices, and technologies interconnected via wired and wireless connection. Fig. 2.2 shows a detailed structure of the MIoT layers (Sun et al., 2020).

1. *Perception Layer(sensor)*: It includes data sources such as smart objects, health monitoring devices, mobile apps, and sensors such as infrared sensors, medical

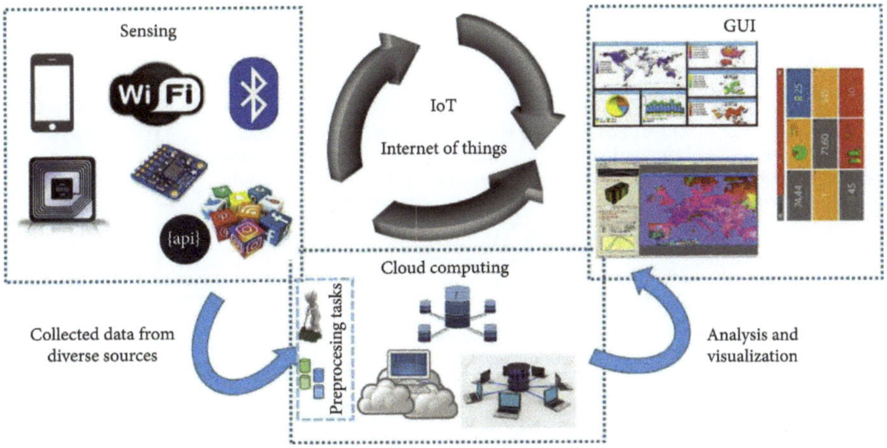

FIGURE 2.1

A generalized MIoT environment.

sensors, smart device sensors, radio frequency identification (RFID) cameras, and global positioning systems (GPS). Sensing systems detect changes in their surroundings and recognize objects, locations, demographics, magnitude, and so on, converting the information into digital signals with the help of a robust, wired, or wireless network transmission infrastructure that serves as a high-performance transport medium. These can also memorize and save data for future use.

2. *Network Layer*: The sensors must be connected to the gateway, which is built by networks that communicate and store information either locally or centrally. The communication can take place over a variety of frequencies and can be either short-range, such as RFID, wireless sensor networks, Bluetooth, ZigBee, low-power Wi-Fi, and mobile communications, or long-range, such as cloud computing, blockchain, and mobile communications. Personal area network (PAN) connections such as ZigBee, Bluetooth, and ultrawideband (UWB), or local area network (LAN) connections such as Ethernet and Wi-Fi are examples of networks. High-frequency fourth-generation (4G) and growing fifth-generation (5G) cellular networks are also gaining popularity due to their ability to link a large number of devices at the same time. The enormous communication potential can enhance the expansion of IoMT applications for health care and emerge as its primary driver.
3. *Business and Data Storage Layer*: The processing of massive raw data to extract relevant information necessitates the use of tools that form the management service or application support layer and can work at a rapid pace using analytics, security controls, process modeling, and device management. This management/application layer manages users, manages data, and analyzes data. Memory analytics assists in the caching of huge amounts of data in random

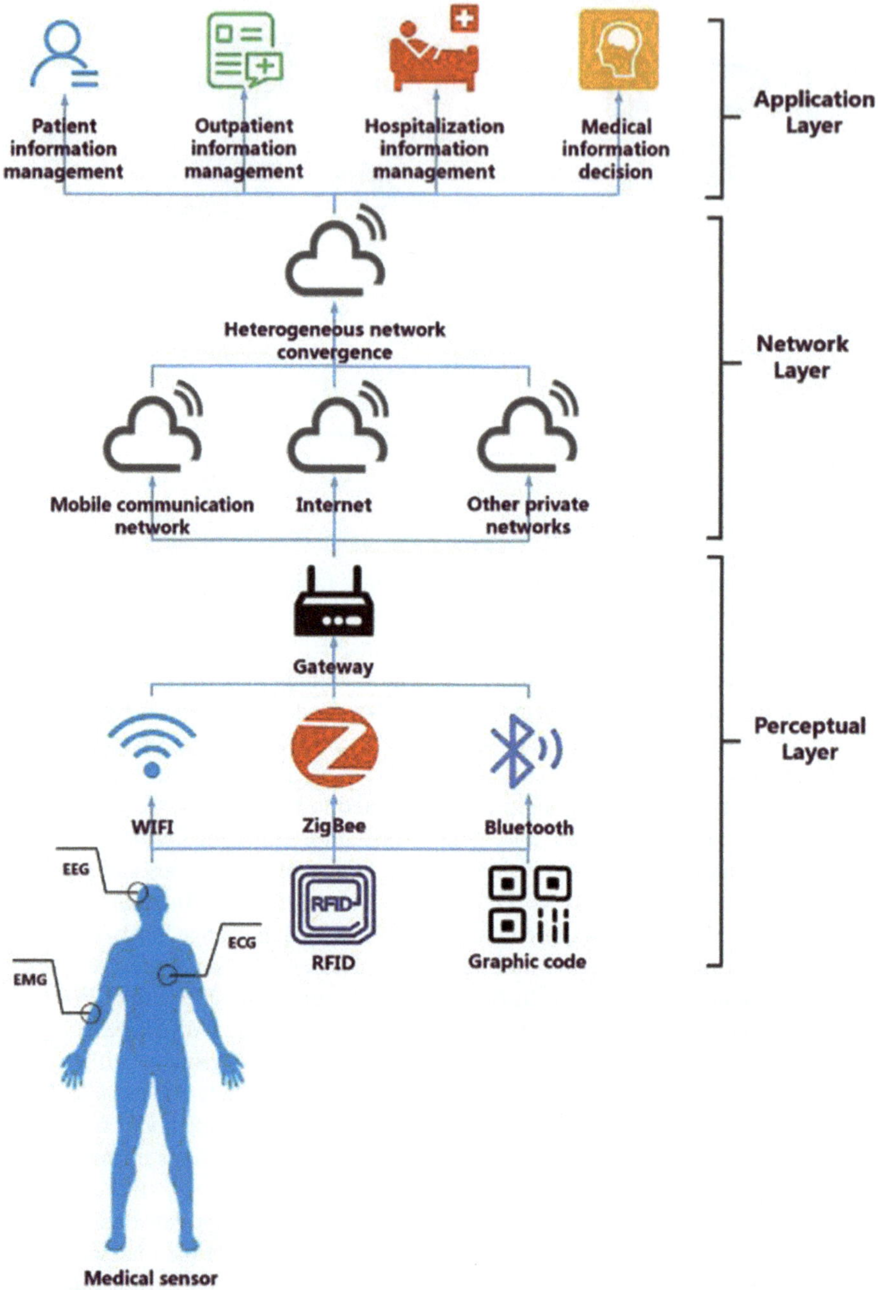

FIGURE 2.2

The architecture of IoMT.

access memory (RAM) format to minimize data query time and accelerate decision-making. Streaming analytics is the examination of data in real-time or data-in-motion to make quick judgments. Scalability and flexibility are provided by web servers and associated gateways such as Apache 2, Flask (Python Web Server Gateway Interface), and others. Databases such as MongoDB (a NoSQL database) allow for greater diversity and sorts of data to be stored. A secure sockets layer application programming interface (SSL API) is used for secure communication. The data that is communicated can be stored locally/decentralized (fog or edge) or centrally in a cloud server. This enables data analysis and processing by IoMT sensors and network gateways (i.e., at the edge). As a result, the scalability of the IoMT device is improved, and the data burden for centralized location is reduced. Another decentralized solution is "blockchain storage," which produces separate collections of information known as blocks, each with a dependent connection. This results in a network governed by patients rather than a third party. The use of the Edge cloud and blockchain in the health care industry is still in its infancy, but it is expected to become an increasing topic of study in the future.

4. *Application and Service Layer*: The application layer's primary job is to understand data and provide application-specific services. The application layer uses Artificial Intelligence (AI) and Deep Machine Learning to grasp EMR data and monitor patterns and changes in the obtained data (data contextualization) via various daily/weekly plots to create decisions regarding diagnosis and/or treatment options. Aside from image analysis, text recognition, and language processing, other scientific applications include health care applications such as drug activity design, risk and gene mutation expression prediction, medical outcomes, diabetes, and mental health management, and prediction of the progression of congestive heart failure, cardiac arrhythmia, bone disease, Alzheimer disease, and benign and malignant tumors.

2.1.2 Artificial intelligence (AI) in IoMT

In large fields of areas such as science, farming, manufacturing, and other discoveries Artificial Intelligence (AI) has started showing good promises. Making every other day reliable and easier for human beings, AI is taking futuristic technologies toward a new era. AI helps in real-life simulation and the expansion of the theories, methodologies, new technologies along with the application system of how the human brain works or thinks and their behavior. With the advancement of the technologies with the help of AI and the applications that uses AI some of the key technologies can be considered as machine learning (ML), natural language processing (NLP), robots, computer version, and an expert system. Among all the technologies ML can be considered as the core technology in AI. It discovers potential clues and codes through learning from a very huge range of information and database to guide human decision-making. As the representative branch of ML, deep learning (DL) supports neural networks. With a strong feature of extraction ability, its structure consists of mostly multilayer perception composed of multiple hidden layers and straightforward to find deep and hidden rules within the knowledge. As one of the most functional and important parts of AI, ML also assists in the health sector by assisting, predicting, and diagnosing diseases, also called artificial diagnosis (Richens et al., 2020).

Some of the most promising medical applications provided by the IoT are through AI (Combi et al., 2015). Scientific applications of artificial intelligence have multiplied, including image analysis, text recognition with NLP, drug activity design, and gene mutation expression prediction (Panch et al., 2019). The AI can read available electronic medical records data, including medical history, physics, laboratory analyses, imaging, and prescription drugs, and contextualize this data to generate decisions and/or options for treatment and/or diagnosis (Topol, 2019).

Medical IoT also uses AI and ML (Perwej, 2015) to support life-changing changes to conventional medical equipment, such as the smart inhaler for asthma sufferers. In reality, in the sense of body area networks, medical sensors and actuators are used as wearable devices. Rather than holding patients in hospitals, these systems can continuously track their health in real-time while still providing them with greater physical versatility and mobility. Medical robots, on the other hand, can be used as surgical robots as well as hospital robots (Beasley, 2012).

During COVID-19 also, considering the need for rapid identification/early screening, several studies have been conducted using AI methods (Yang et al., 2020). AI can facilitate detection, large-scale screening, monitoring, resource allocation, and prediction of possible interactions with the new proposed therapies (Chatterjee et al., 2020).

The AI keyword appeared in much IoMT related research under different names: artificial intelligence, ML, DL, big data, data mining, decision support system, data analytics, classifications, COVID-19, predictive analysis, telemedicine, descriptive analysis, and medical informatics (Secinaro et al., 2021). Fig. 2.3 shows IoMT, big data, and artificial intelligence for COVID-19 mitigation (Aman et al., 2020).

What are the research applications of artificial intelligence for healthcare? In the field of healthcare, AI has shown to be a game-changing technology. AI has aided doctors and medical professionals in the fields of health information systems, geocoding health data, epidemic and syndromic monitoring, predictive modeling and decision assistance, and medical imaging, thanks to its complex algorithms and a variety of applications. There are different opinions on the most beneficial applications of AI for healthcare purposes, ranging from administrative workflows, image analysis, virtual assistance, clinical decision support systems, connected machines, robotic surgery, connected and cognitive devices, personalized medicine, and more (Bohr & Memarzadeh, 2020, pp. 25–60). Here we list the most agreed-upon themes.

1. *Health services management*: AI systems can help healthcare providers access intelligent data and leverage the diverse electronics healthcare records systems, through aggregating heterogeneous data, checking for outliers, and improving patient healthcare by analyzing and predicting diagnostics tests,

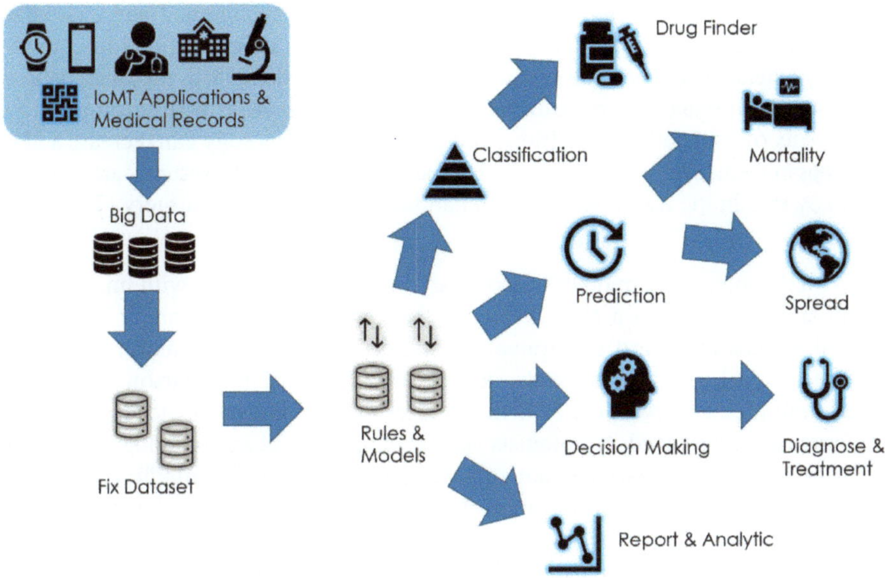

FIGURE 2.3

IoMT, big data, and artificial intelligence for COVID-19 mitigation.

Reproduced from Aman et al. (2020).

risks, and improving outcomes (Shickel et al., 2018). AI systems can provide almost real-time medical information from various sources, including journals, textbooks, and clinical practices (Tran et al., 2019), and through information exchange especially at the times of the pandemics to help mitigate the impacts of COVID-19, for example (Hussain et al., 2020). Healthcare professionals benefit from having more time and concise data to make better patient decisions.

2. *Predictive medicine*: AI systems can design and develop new drugs, monitor patients, and enhance patient treatment plans personalized medicine (PM) by tailoring therapy with the highest safety margin ensuring better patient outcomes (Ahuja, 2019). Central to making precision medicine possible are AI and ML which can make sense of massive amounts of clinical, genomic, and imaging data, thus helping to improve physician efficiency, increase diagnostic accuracy, and personalize treatment. AI systems with their automatic learning power could disrupt medicine, allowing prediction models to be created for drugs and exams that monitor patients over their whole lives (Collins & Moons, 2019).
3. *Clinical decision-making*: AI Systems can help doctors make better clinical decisions in healthcare-specific areas (Jiang et al., 2017). AI algorithms can benefit clinical decisions by accelerating the process and the amount of care provided, positively impacting the cost of health services.

4. *Patient data and diagnostics*: AI systems can help manage and aggregate data generated from clinical activities, such as screening, diagnosis, and treatment assignment, hence helping medical researchers and doctors in the diagnostic process; for example, to realize a high-speed body scan, it will be simpler to have an overall patient condition image. Then, AI technology can recreate a 3D-mapping solution of a patient's body (Jiang et al., 2017). AI systems are playing a key role in the use of robots for rehabilitation therapy and surgery (Tarassoli, 2019).

With the increasing number of radiology images, AI can help with image recognition and analytics, even more, effective than physicians, who cannot handle this load of images in a short timeframe. An important question to answer is, will AI replace medical care professionals, doctors, and radiologists? Pearson (2017) provided multiple narratives: (1) AI will interpret clinical images as accurately as today's most experienced radiologists and eventually replace radiologists; (2) AI will augment radiologists but not replace them; and (3) the middle of the road view that at some point in the future AI will indeed replace radiologists, but it is not worth worrying about as that will happen in the distant future. The most possible narrative is that AI will make the radiologists and physicians work more efficiently, accurately, and valuable despite all its limitations such as engaging in full conversation and engagement with patients, showing empathy and reassurance, not to mention the patient trust to deal with AI avatar for example. AI cannot handle reading and interpreting complex images and cases that require an actual physician with the expertise to figure it out (Krittanawong, 2018).

This will yield to what are the potential risks of Artificial Intelligence in healthcare, as reported in BrookingsInst (2019):

1. *Errors and injuries*: AI systems are prone to errors and sometimes will be wrong, which eventually leads to patient injury or other significant problems. For instance, a patient may take a drug wrongly recommended by the AI system. Likewise, the AI-driven radiological scan may miss a tumor. The wrong allocation of a hospital bed based on AI predictions can lead to injuries and relapse. If AI systems become widespread, an underlying problem in one AI system might result in injuries to thousands of patients rather than the limited number of patients injured by any single provider's error. No family or friend will take it lightly, hearing that their loved one suffered a setback because of a computer error.
2. *Data availability*: Large volumes of data are required to train AI systems from sources such as electronic health records, pharmaceutical records, insurance claims records, or consumer-generated information such as activity trackers or purchase histories. However, health data is frequently problematic. Data is often dispersed across several platforms. Aside from the aforementioned variations, patients frequently see different doctors and transfer insurance carriers, resulting in data fragmentation across many systems and formats. This fragmentation raises the danger of inaccuracy, reduces the comprehensiveness of

data sets, and raises the cost of data collection, limiting the sorts of entities that can create successful healthcare AI.

3. *Privacy concerns*: When it comes to patient data collecting, privacy is a major problem. While researchers have safeguards in place to secure patient data, dangerous hackers are out there attempting to gain access at any cost. If a behemoth like Google can have privacy and patient data issues, it follows that no one in AI should ignore privacy concerns. Another way AI threatens privacy is the system's capacity to forecast information about patients even when the algorithm has not been provided such data.
4. *Bias and inequalities*: Bias is not immune to AI. Even the tiniest trace of prejudice is always reflected in the outcomes. When data from academic medical facilities are incorporated into AI systems, for example, the system may struggle to treat or benefit populations from places other than academic medical centers. Similarly, utilizing speech-recognition AI systems in note transcription may impair the AI's efficiency if the source is of gender or race that is underrepresented in the training data.
5. *Professional reshuffling/realignment*: If AI technology is fully applied, we may see changes in the medical field. Some academics believe that the broad usage of AI will reduce human knowledge and capabilities over time. According to them, it may eventually reach the point where physicians can practically limit AI faults or increase medical expertise.

However, healthcare systems must be aware of the inequalities that may arise as a result of the widespread implementation of MIoT for integrated home care, including people who may not be able to afford or access reliable technological hardware or web services due to geographic location or financial disadvantage. Similarly, if patients and healthcare professionals do not consider the technology to be "simple to use," have bad connections, or do not believe that the effort was planned with their input, this may lead to dissatisfaction and unwillingness to utilize such services (US FDA, 2019).

2.2 IoMT applications

Over time, the Internet of Medical Things (IoMT) has found a variety of real-world applications. During the current COVID-19 epidemic, it has shown to be quite useful as it has expanded the use of several current IoMT-based devices. Today's health monitoring systems have progressed from much basic data gathering systems to complex ones that use AI to make smart decisions. The introduction of newer devices based on IoMT-based technologies has contributed to the transformation of the traditional healthcare system into a smart and personalized one. Some of the IoMT applications:

1. *Remote health monitoring*: many systems have been proposed that collect vital signs; pulse rate, temperature, ECG, GPS, measure heart rate, blood pressure,

through fixed and wearables sensors. The data collected from the sensors is sent to different applications: direct notification to the medical or family personnel, online database, or through smartphone dashboard.

2. *Human behavior prediction*: Xu and Pombo (2019) presents a study of a framework for behavior monitoring that uses noninvasive and privacy-preserving sensors. The data gathered by the sensors is transferred and evaluated with minimal richness in the suggested framework. Various sensors are put in the sensing space for human activity detection, and they are all connected to a Wi-Fi-equipped gateway that allows them to transport data to cloud storage. The architecture may store the acquired data in either the cloud or a local database. Once enough data has been collected, the analysis step begins, which employs classification ML algorithms for trend and anomaly analysis in human behavior. The present human behavior may be anticipated, and the privacy retained data labeled by evaluating the video, which the system first takes using a camera, combined with the data gathered through body area sensors. Fig. 2.4 shows the system architecture (Nazir et al., 2019).
1. *Testing and tracing for disease spread-Covid-19*: Testing and tracing have been the primary concerns for disease spread management over the world, particularly to slow the transmission. Several IoMT-based devices have been used for testing and tracing sick patients, as well as identifying the patient's position to track the probability of disease transmission. such as influenza A (H1N1),

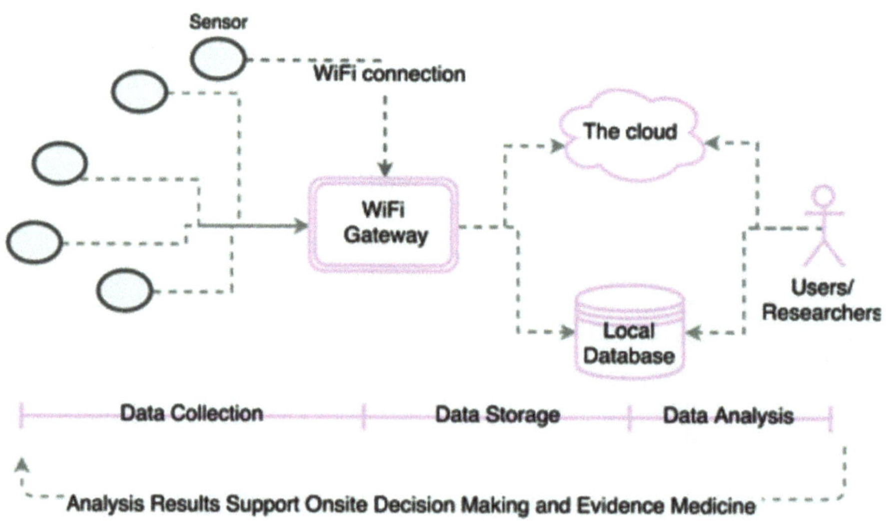

FIGURE 2.4

Human Behavior Prediction System. Five sensors motes installed in an office environment. The different sensors used were: PIR motion sensor, light sensor, infrared obstacle/collision sensor, ultrasonic ranging sensor, and microphone sound detector, all of which are connected to Arduino Industrial 101 board.

human papillomavirus (HPV), Ebola virus disease (EVD), Zika virus (ZIKV), and coronavirus (COVID-19) more efficiently. Using chest X-ray, CT, and ultrasound imaging data, ML and DL approaches such as convolutional neural networks (CNN) were employed to identify early COVID-19 infection with 94.03% accuracy (Yang et al., 2020).

2. *Stress monitoring*: Stress and anxiety problems are becoming more widespread in today's society. As a result, poor stress management can result in stress disorders, psychological anguish, and physical diseases. According to preliminary studies, persons who recovered from COVID-19 saw an increase in anxiety disorders and other mental illnesses. Rabha et al. present a low-cost IoT-based anxiety disorder monitor that extracts emotion characteristics from physiological measurements in a semiimmersive setting. This system's validation findings demonstrated an overall accuracy of 90% in recognizing anxiety disorders. The researchers (Laavanya & Vijayaraghavan, 2020) presented *iMirror*, an ML-based smart gadget that monitors stress levels in users to help the IoMT framework of smart cities and offices. This gadget is intended to lower stress levels, resulting in fewer chronic illnesses induced by numerous stresses. The suggested system makes use of a camera linked to a mirror to recognize a person's face, take photos for stress analysis, and then update the stress level on a mobile application. An automatic data processing unit pulls information from taken photographs of a person (based on a unique ID) to apply an ML model that will identify the user's stress level. The photograph was used to extract four features: eye redness, eye bags, pupil dilation, a scowl on the forehead, and face perspiration. These characteristics are sent into a stress analysis unit, which uses an ML model to describe the stress level and updates the status on the mobile app. The model has an accuracy of around 97% and a precision score of 81.2%, according to experimental data.
3. *Digital biomarkers*: Self-powered IoMT-connected diagnostic devices are being developed to offer real-time monitoring of biomarkers in and on human (or animal) bodily fluids such as sweat, urine, blood, and so on. This can help distinguish between viral and bacterial infections, and customized prediction algorithms can be used to detect infection, sterile inflammation, or the likelihood of recurrence up to hours before observable physical indications appear. The patient's reaction to treatment might be closely monitored, showing whether or not the patient is responding to therapy and perhaps suggesting the presence of resistance, allowing physicians to consider changing their "first line" therapeutic therapy in a timely way (Dwivedi et al., 2022).
4. *Voice assistant*: Sezgin et al. (Sezgin et al., 2020) created voice assistants as an alternate medium for supporting health care during a health crisis/pandemic. The chatbot developed by the Centers for Disease Control and Prevention (CDC) and Microsoft is based on evidence-based information and serves as a COVID-19 text-based platform. The World Health Organization (WHO) recently launched a WhatsApp text-based chatbot to reply to public inquiries regarding COVID-19. Apple's VA app distributes COVID-19 information and

updates via Siri, utilizing CDC resources. Amazon's Alexa VA assists customers in setting up routines during homestays and provides information and assistance on COVID-19.

5. *Fall detection*: Falls and fall-related injuries are common events, particularly among the elderly, putting them at risk of serious injury, functional loss, and healthcare consumption. Many researchers are conducting unique research to avoid this harm in the elderly by employing real-time sensing or monitoring technology to identify or forecast this occurrence. Muheidat et al. (2018) used floor-based sensor system interconnected with remote Jetson Tk1 to host the data and run computational intelligence algorithms to detect falls. In Fadi Muheidat and H. W. Tyrer (2017), the authors used connected component labeling. detect and count the number of people walking on the smart floor. The authors in provide clever real-time camera-based fall detection. This is accomplished by training a support vector machine (SVM) classification algorithm on falling video segments collected from security videotapes to create a data set.
6. *Adverse drug reaction detection*: Aside consequence of taking medicine is referred to as an adverse drug reaction (ADR). The reaction might occur after a single dosage or after a lengthy period of therapy. This is also conceivable as a result of an unfavorable response when two distinct drugs are taken at the same time (Jara et al., 2010). ADR is not affected by the kind of treatment or sickness, and it differs from person to person. A unique identifier/barcode present on each drug to be taken by the patient is the foundation of an IoMT-based ADR system. The information regarding the medicine's compatibility with the patient's body may be validated using a Pharmaceutical Intelligent Information (PII) system, which stores the patient's allergy profile utilizing e-health data. A thorough investigation of the patient's allergy profile and other crucial health facts directs the medication's acceptability (Nakhla et al., 2019).
7. *I-robotics*: A smart environment that includes various interconnected sophisticated integrated systems such as people, robots, and an IoMT system is referred to as an IoMT-aided robotic system. The system primarily employs a cloud-robotic system that can access a vast quantity of data and process it utilizing sensing, processing, and memory to accomplish specified tasks. The system utilizes machine-learning algorithms to create and train robots/machines to operate either based on patient health information data obtained through the network among health professionals or by performing in the medical environment utilizing intelligent computation (Dwivedi et al., 2022), created a healthcare robot (Lio) that avoids collisions on its own using a mix of optical, auditory, ultrasonic, laser, and mechanical sensors. This allows personnel and patients at a hospital to navigate safely. Another IoMT-aided robotic device (ROBIN) allows therapists to capture precise motions that may then be replicated in patients with faulty limb movements. It offers trunk stability during postural alterations and facilitates simple arm and hand movements for reaching and gripping objects (Pavón-Pulido et al., 2020). During COVID-19, Mobile

robots might check for social distance and mask wear in public places, while aerial robotics could supervise quarantine zones (Chamola et al., 2020).

2.3 IoMT security

The development of IoT has seen an increase in the threats and issues related to cyber security. As data is becoming an essential component of the organization, cybercriminals are constantly for new methods of accessing confidential and private information. According to Rahman et al., cyber security is the protection of a society's critical infrastructure, ensuring the governments can pursue policies and bring into account the cyber attackers existing in the global landscape. Therefore, cybersecurity is an essential component in IoT because there are both known and unknown elements threatening organizations' security. The malicious actors pursue different methods of breaching the networks to compromise or steal data. The rapid development and evolution of cybersecurity issues mean that the governments and private sectors must work together. They should ensure that some controls and policies enhance the management of security threats. Manufacturers of different devices are working to ensure that they are designed safely and efficiently. This ensures no significant risks, making it safer and more convenient for the users (Khan & Salah, 2018). However, IoT devices have been ignoring this aspect for a long time and exposing them to severe threats. The occurrence the cyberattacks is a common practice that affects most individuals. Ideally, each person that has a device that is connected to the internet is prone to attacks. It is a progressive appeal that is focused on the presentation of ideas that needs to focus on the outcomes that are essential to reflect upon (Liu et al., 2017). The focus is the creation of a realistic outcome that is focused on the presentation of ideas that are important to reflect upon. One of the common factors that can be identified with the practice is the ransomware that presented a threat to most of the activities within the societal setting. The hack led to a recovery cost of $17 million. This is just an explanation of the common risk that people encounter regularly.

IoT has provided an opportunity for industries to develop practical industrial systems. Different sectors have resulted in adopting intelligent IoT (Al-Turjman et al., 2019). The transport industry is a significant user of this technology. The main application is the monitoring of the vehicles and the movement across different locations. Logistics management has thus found significant development with the application of IoT. It is possible to predict future locations and hence do prior planning (Khan & Salah, 2018). The main reason for applying this technology is to allow the transport industry to collect information that is meaningful automatically. However, compared to the traditional systems, these are more vulnerable and expose information to high risks.

IoT devices have found significant application in the healthcare sector. This is most especially in the devices that are used in monitoring and assessment of the patients. Monitoring the patient condition requires that the patients receive devices planted in their body or are used externally. Personal medical devices are becoming widespread, primarily due to the growth of Telehealth. Due to the COVID-19 pandemic, the global Medical Device Technologies market size is estimated to be worth USD 336,760 million in 2022 and is forecast to a readjusted size of USD 438,560 million by 2028 with a CAGR of 4.5% during the review period, according to report by MarketWatch (2022). These are wireless devices that communicate with the base station used to read the device status and the medical reports and update the status. Therefore, the patient and the doctor can monitor aspects such as blood pressure and sugar levels. This approach has made the management of these chronic conditions easier. The wireless interface is, however, a concern, primarily because of security issues. According to HIPAA, all electronic systems and database information must be protected to ensure privacy is maintained (Wang et al., 2018). Therefore, healthcare's primary goal is to enhance the security of the network to prevent malicious attacks. The attack on these devices has a malicious goal. The aim is to utilize the resources or to shut down the monitoring services. The primary forms of attack in medical devices include eavesdropping to alter the availability and the gritty of information. The most significant security of personal medical devices is that there is no authentication mechanism. This means that unauthorized people can easily access the information (Petrakis et al., 2018). This also means that there can be a hostile denial of service attack. The patient data being sent can be intercepted and altered by attackers.

The IoT devices are connected, and hence they provide the services at the same time in any place. The device is connected to the internet and lacks proper security measures in place. This means that the aspects such as data integrity, confidentiality, and authenticity may not work in this environment (Mukherjee et al., 2017). The IoT requires that some security requirements are fulfilled to ensure that malicious attacks are prevented. Different characteristics must be fulfilled.

1. *Resilience:* Resilience is the capability of a system to recover from the crashes that occur during data transmission. This means that the system should be strong enough to protect itself from intruders' actions (Al Hayajneh et al., 2020). Such an approach would ensure that the system protects itself against eavesdropping without intimation and without users knowing about the down status.
2. *Data authentication:* All information in a system should be authenticated. This is the process that helps to ensure that the data that is transmitted is from authentic sources. Authentication processes ensure that the attackers do not send malicious codes in the form of messages.
3. *Access control:* In an organization, only authorized persons should have access to the information in a system. The same case should occur with IoT devices. Although there is more data due to these devices' networking, it is essential to maintain physical control. The primary threat of IoT and access control is cyber terrorism. Terrorists can use IoT devices to attack critical infrastructure and cause a stoppage of services.

4. *Client privacy:* The IoT systems should ensure that the data is always in safe hands. The authorized individuals should only access personal data. Through authentication, there is no irrelevant user who can access the system.

The security and privacy of data acquired by MIoT devices, either during transmission to or storage in a cloud, remain important unresolved problems, and more work is needed.

2.4 Current challenges

Several issues and consequences exist now that must be solved before the widespread use of IoMT, such as data privacy and security, data management, scalability and upgradability, legislation, interoperability, and cost-effectiveness. The usage of IoMT devices in integrated home help will increasingly rely on a clear and rigorous code of behavior for data management, privacy, confidentiality, and IT security (Cyber Security Report, 2021). Clinical standards on digital health prescriptions, as well as a rigorous compensation strategy, are required from the standpoint of the healthcare system for integrated home help services supplied through the IoMT (Adler-Waxman, 2017).

To integrate data from IoMT devices into electronic health records, interested parties must actively negotiate current barriers. By seeing IoMT devices as active components of a linked digital integrated healthcare and home aid infrastructure, diverse commercial, personal, professional, and healthcare system interests may be aligned to help achieve this aim (Ghubaish et al., n.d.).

2.4.1 Security and privacy

While working on the MIoT security and privacy system we should consider the influence of many aspects to achieving a better balance among them. Several challenges must be addressed to achieve a better security environment.

1. *Insecure network*: Several devices and software services rely heavily on wireless networks, such as Wi-Fi, due to their convenience and low cost. However, wireless networks are known to be vulnerable to various intrusions such as unauthorized router access, man-in-the-middle attacks, spoofing, denial of service attacks, brute-force attacks, and traffic injections. Furthermore, the majority of free wireless networks in public places that have not been approved are untrusted networks.
2. *Lightweight protocols for devices:* To deliver services, low-cost devices and software applications based on sensors must adhere to strict policy and proxy requirements. At the moment, if we want to provide high-grade security for sensors, we must use expensive methods. The main task of security protection in the future will be to develop different levels of security protocols based on application scenarios, particularly lightweight security and communication networks security protocols.

3. *Data sharing*: Despite fast advancements in medical information technology, the situation of information islands is becoming more severe. The standards of data collected from different manufacturers' devices vary greatly, making management difficult to unify. However, information collaboration and sharing among heterogeneous MIoT systems is an unavoidable future development. The privatization of patient information might jeopardize the MIoT system's security. Using generic data standards to merge disparate data sets might result in more understandable information while also improving security and privacy using a hierarchical security paradigm.

2.4.2 Cost

As the COVID-19 epidemic looms, financial stress has spread to a vast number of individuals, businesses, and even organizations, restricting broad IoMT adoption. As a result, cost-effectiveness becomes a critical concern that must be addressed. The cost of developing, installing, and using an IoMT system must be reasonable. The IoMT-based system connects a huge number of medical devices and sensors. These have substantial maintenance and upgrade costs that harm both the manufacturer and the end-user. As a result, the incorporation of low-maintenance sensors with cheap initial setup costs will help in the creation of additional IoMT devices and boost their routine adoption.

2.4.3 Scalability and interoperability

Scalability refers to a healthcare device's capacity to respond to changes in the environment. As a result, a highly scalable system maintains consistency among linked devices and can perform efficiently while utilizing available resources smoothly and without delay. Continuous development and breakthroughs in IoMT technology have increased the necessity for regular device updates. This is still a struggle in today's fast-paced society. The standards that support applications created by various industries differ. Interoperability is an issue since data sharing between various IoMT systems with contrasting characteristics is difficult. As a result, the establishment of standard interfaces becomes critical, particularly in applications that allow interorganizational cross-systems. In the IoMT world, the flow of various types of information generates a large volume of data, and the procedures involved in handling the data, as well as managing the interconnected devices in an interoperable manner while considering energy limits, remain critical challenges (Baskar et al., 2020).

2.4.4 Digital Health Advisors

AI may produce significant insights when a data store has been developed from many distinct sources—EHR data, payer data, device, and IoT data, patient survey answers, consumer health data—and has been combined into a single data structure. After all, AI is all about pattern recognition, which involves comparing a specific pattern of data around a certain individual to comparable (but not necessarily identical) patterns discovered elsewhere and generating predictive predictions based on what happened in those other circumstances. These AI-derived recommendations can be useful to a new generation of Digital Health Advisors who can be trained.

When the organization transitions to MIoT-enabled infrastructure, the primary duty of Digital Health Advisors and clinicians will be to collaborate. Proper training and feedback are required for effective deployment. The conventional technique of recording a patient's data will no longer function. This is an application where on-field mobile/tablet technology may be useful since it allows for hassle-free record-keeping on the device's apps. When health data is collected electronically and security and privacy concerns are addressed, health data information will be available with a single touch. It will take some time, but we can see the path to that next generation of healthcare technology (Dimitrov, 2016).

2.5 Discussion and future directions

In this paper, we reviewed and presented some advances in artificial intelligence in IoMT applications. We discussed the challenges available in existing systems. However, we still need to consider future research directions. There is a lot of commonalities between various IoMT applications; health monitoring systems, wearables, smartphones-based solutions, and the added layer of the use of Artificial Intelligence and ML techniques and algorithms to assist in advancing the current IoMT (Chigozirim et al., 2020; Nemcova et al., 2020; Wang et al., 2018); anomaly detection, disease diagnosis, assistive living, and social/surgical robots (Loza-Matovelle et al., 2019; Vora et al., 2017). Different hardware (Babar et al., 2018) and software frameworks and methods (SVM, Naïve Bayes, CNN, Deep Learning, MLP, etc.) were proposed to build IoMT systems (Kaur et al., 2020; Martis et al., 2018; Quintana et al., 2018). All the work yields to the need for generalized architecture; sensor, edge, fog, and cloud layers as described earlier. This architecture and the interaction of the different layers is a research direction by itself. Sensor data representations, multidata fusing, bandwidth improvements, and communication with the cloud layer (Jiang et al., 2017). The need for more security and data privacy; the need for federated learning and transfer in an efficient and secure matter, our current research focus. Another future direction is how to handle multiple patients in a timely manner, how to prioritize care and the role of ML algorithms, and improvements in assisting and building such real-time systems.

In federated learning, we need to train models in the small data set and then migrate these modes to the could/edge. Yet, there is a need for more work on these ML and AI techniques to achieve better accuracy with small data sets, in other words, we move from big data to more focused and small data sets by excluding unnecessary data (Dankwa-Mullan et al., 2019). So we need to focus more on lightweight machine learning (Punithavathi et al., 2019) algorithms such as TinyML that we can use on edge/embedded devices with low capabilities and power needs.

Moreover, the integration of blockchain technologies in ensuring health data security, privacy and integrity, and user-level authorization is a fresh research direction. We hope that this work will be useful for researchers in the field, helping them to understand the huge potential of IoMT and identification of the major challenges.

2.6 Conclusion

Developments such as remote health monitoring systems and smart devices, telemedicine/teledentistry platforms, robotics, and drones have significantly aided disease prevention by enabling screening, early diagnosis, management, and facilitated living. The convenience of using these devices for healthcare monitoring has surpassed the requirement for hospital visits. However, the accompanying issues must be overcome for cost-effective, adaptable, and consistent systems appropriate for healthcare demands to gain widespread adoption.

In the case of ML and DL, AI-based systems are built on precedent, yet such algorithms might underperform in unique or uncommon situations of pharmacological side effects or treatment resistance if there is no past example to draw on. For these reasons, it is reasonable to assume that AI-based systems will supplement physicians' abilities rather than replace the conventional physician-patient interaction.

There are still significant gaps that need to be filled in future studies regarding IoT technology itself, the healthcare system and users, beneficiaries of integrated home help, and who can utilize IoMT devices. Future IoT technology research must focus on how IoMT devices can be designed with standardized protocols and interoperability with international and interstate healthcare systems. In the context of IoMT-supported healthcare delivery, more research on the efficiency of blockchain storage versus cloud-based centralized storage solutions is also required.

References

Adler-Waxman, A. (2017). *This is the biggest challenge to our health.* World Economic Forum.

Ahemd, M. M., Shah, M. A., & Wahid, A. (2017). IoT security: A layered approach for attacks & defenses. In *International conference on communication technologies, ComTech 2017* (pp. 104—110). Institute of Electrical and Electronics Engineers Inc. https://doi.org/10.1109/COMTECH.2017.8065757

Ahuja, A. S. (2019). The impact of artificial intelligence in medicine on the future role of the physician. *PeerJ, 7*, e7702. https://doi.org/10.7717/peerj.7702

Al Hayajneh, A., Bhuiyan, M. Z. A., & McAndrew, I. (2020). Improving internet of things (IoT) security with software-defined networking (SDN). *Computers, 9*(1), 8. https://doi.org/10.3390/computers9010008

Al-Turjman, F., Zahmatkesh, H., & Shahroze, R. (2019). An overview of security and privacy in smart cities' IoT communications. *Transactions on Emerging Telecommunications Technologies*. https://doi.org/10.1002/ett.3677

Aman, A. H. M., Hassan, W. H., Sameen, S., Attarbashi, Z. S., Alizadeh, M., & Latiff, L. A. (2021). IoMT amid COVID-19 pandemic: Application, architecture, technology, and security. *Journal of Network and Computer Applications, 174*, 102886. https://doi.org/10.1016/j.jnca.2020.102886.

Babar, M., Rahman, A., Arif, F., & Jeon, G. (2018). Energy-harvesting based on internet of things and big data analytics for smart health monitoring. *Sustainable Computing: Informatics and Systems, 20*, 155−164. https://doi.org/10.1016/j.suscom.2017.10.009

Baskar, S., Dhulipala, V. R., Shakeel, P. M., Sridhar, K. P., & Kumar, R. (2020). Hybrid fuzzy based spearman rank correlation for cranial nerve palsy detection in MIoT environment. *Health and Technology, 10*(1), 259−270.

Beasley, R. A. (2012). Medical robots: Current systems and research directions. *Journal of Robotics, 2012*, 1−14. https://doi.org/10.1155/2012/401613

Bohr, A., & Memarzadeh, K. (2020). *The rise of artificial intelligence in healthcare applications* (pp. 25−60). Elsevier BV. https://doi.org/10.1016/b978-0-12-818438-7.00002-2

BrookingsInst (2019). Risks and remedies for artificial intelligence in health care, https://brook.gs/350Mj9V via BrookingsInst.

Chamola, V., Hassija, V., Gupta, V., & Guizani, M. (2020). A comprehensive review of the COVID-19 pandemic and the role of IoT, drones, AI, blockchain, and 5G in managing its impact. *IEEE Access, 8*, 90225−90265. https://doi.org/10.1109/ACCESS.2020.2992341

Chatterjee, P., Tesis, A., Cymberknop, L. J., & Armentano, R. L. (2020). Internet of Things and artificial intelligence in healthcare during COVID-19 pandemic—A South American perspective. *Frontiers in Public Health, 8*. https://doi.org/10.3389/fpubh.2020.600213

Chigozirim, A., Vivian, N. O., Uchenna, N. J., & Oreoluwa, A. A. (2020). A patient monitoring system using Internet of Things technology. *Ingenierie Des Systemes d'Information, 25*(3), 351−357. https://doi.org/10.18280/isi.250309

Cho, S., & Lee, S. (2019). Survey on the application of blockchain to IoT. In *ICEIC 2019 — International conference on electronics, information, and communication*. Institute of Electrical and Electronics Engineers Inc. https://doi.org/10.23919/ELINFOCOM.2019.8706369

Collins, G. S., & Moons, K. G. M. (2019). Reporting of artificial intelligence prediction models. *The Lancet, 393*(10181), 1577−1579. https://doi.org/10.1016/S0140-6736(19)30037-6

Combi, C., Huang, Z., & Lu. (2015). *Artificial intelligence in medicine*. Elsevier B.V.

Curran, J. (2016). *Wheeler suggests ways FCC, ISPs can improve IoT cybersecurity* (Vol. 1). Cybersecurity Policy Report.

Cyber Security Report (2021). Reveals Extent of Global Cyber Pandemic and Shows How Organizations Can Develop Immunity, Check Point Research, 2021.

Dankwa-Mullan, I., Rivo, M., Sepulveda, M., Park, Y., Snowdon, J., & Rhee, K. (2019). Transforming diabetes care through artificial intelligence: The future is here. *Population Health Management, 22*(3), 229−242. https://doi.org/10.1089/pop.2018.0129

Dimitrov, D. V. (2016). Medical Internet of Things and big data in healthcare. *Healthcare Informatics Research, 22*(3), 156−163. https://doi.org/10.4258/hir.2016.22.3.156

Dwivedi, R., Mehrotra, D., & Chandra, S. (2022). Potential of internet of medical things (IoMT) applications in building a smart healthcare system: A systematic review. *Journal of Oral Biology and Craniofacial Research*. https://doi.org/10.1016/j.jobcr.2021.11.010

Ghubaish, A., Salman, T., &, Al-Ali, A. K. (n.d.). Recent advances in the internet of medical things (IoMT) systems security. IEEE Internet of Things Journal.

Hussain, A. A., Bouachir, O., Al-Turjman, F., & Aloqaily, M. (2020). *AI Techniques for COVID-19, 8*, 128776−128795. IEEE Access.

Islam, S. M. R., Kwak, D., Kabir, M. H., Hossain, M., & Kwak, K. S. (2015). The Internet of Things for health care: A comprehensive survey. *IEEE Access, 3*, 678–708. https://doi.org/10.1109/ACCESS.2015.2437951

Jara, A. J., Belchi, F. J., Alcolea, A. F., Santa, J., Zamora-Izquierdo, M. A., & Gómez-Skarmeta, A. F. (2010). A pharmaceutical intelligent information system to detect allergies and adverse drugs reactions based on Internet of Things. In *2010 8th IEEE international conference on pervasive computing and communications workshops, PERCOM workshops 2010* (pp. 809–812). https://doi.org/10.1109/PERCOMW.2010.5470547

Jiang, F., Jiang, Y., Zhi, H., Dong, Y., Li, H., Ma, S., Wang, Y., Dong, Q., Shen, H., & Wang, Y. (2017). Artificial intelligence in healthcare: Past, present and future. *Stroke and Vascular Neurology, 2*(4), 230–243. https://doi.org/10.1136/svn-2017-000101

Kaur, D., Panos, R. J., Badawi, O., Bapat, S. S., Wang, L., & Gupta, A. (2020). Evaluation of clinician interaction with alerts to enhance performance of the tele-critical care medical environment. *International Journal of Medical Informatics, 139*. https://doi.org/10.1016/j.ijmedinf.2020.104165

Khan, M. A., & Salah, K. (2018). IoT security: Review, blockchain solutions, and open challenges. *Future Generation Computer Systems, 82*, 395–411. https://doi.org/10.1016/j.future.2017.11.022

Krittanawong, C. (2018). The rise of artificial intelligence and the uncertain future for physicians. *European Journal of Internal Medicine, 48*, e13–e14. https://doi.org/10.1016/j.ejim.2017.06.017

Laavanya, M., & Vijayaraghavan, V. (2020). Residual learning of transfer-learned AlexNet for image denoising. *IEIE Transactions on Smart Processing and Computing, 9*(2), 135–141. https://doi.org/10.5573/IEIESPC.2020.9.2.135

Liu, Y., Chang, C. C., & Chang, S. C. (2017). An efficient and secure smart card based password authentication scheme. *International Journal of Network Security, 19*(1), 1–10. https://doi.org/10.6633/IJNS.201701.19(1).01

Loza-Matovelle, D., Verdugo, A., Zalama, E., & Gómez-García-Bermejo, J. (2019). An architecture for the integration of robots and sensors for the care of the elderly in an ambient assisted living environment. *Robotics, 8*(3), 76. https://doi.org/10.3390/robotics8030076

MarketWatch. https://www.marketwatch.com/press-release/medical-device-technologies-market-growth-2022-business-opportunity-industry-share-global-trends-size-dynamics-segments-and-forecast-to-2028-2022-04-21.

Martis, R. J., Gurupur, V. P., Lin, H., Islam, A., & Fernandes, S. L. (2018). Recent advances in big data analytics, Internet of Things and machine learning. *Future Generation Computer Systems, 88*, 696–698. https://doi.org/10.1016/j.future.2018.07.057

Mora, H., Gil, D., Terol, R. M., Azorín, J., & Szymanski, J. (2017). An IoT-based computational framework for healthcare monitoring in mobile environments. *Sensors, 17*(10), 2302. https://doi.org/10.3390/s17102302

Muheidat, F., Tawalbeh, L., & Tyrer, H. (2018). Context-aware, accurate, and real time fall detection system for elderly people. In *Proceedings – 12th IEEE international conference on semantic computing, ICSC 2018* (Vol. 2018, pp. 329–333). Institute of Electrical and Electronics Engineers Inc. https://doi.org/10.1109/ICSC.2018.00068

Muheidat, Fadi, & Tyrer, H. W. (2017). Counting multiple people on a floor based array sensor system. In *Accepted to HIMS'17 – The 3rd international conference on health informatics and medical systems*.

Mukherjee, M., Matam, R., Shu, L., Maglaras, L., Ferrag, M. A., Choudhury, N., & Kumar, V. (2017). Security and privacy in fog computing: challenges. *IEEE Access, 5*, 19293–19304. https://doi.org/10.1109/ACCESS.2017.2749422

Nakhla, Z., Nouira, K., & Ferchichi, A. (2019). Prescription adverse drug events system (PrescADE) based on ontology and Internet of Things. *Computer Journal, 62*(6), 801–805. https://doi.org/10.1093/comjnl/bxy076

Nazir, S., Ali, Y., Ullah, N., & García-Magariño, I. (2019). Internet of Things for healthcare using effects of mobile computing: A systematic literature review. *Wireless Communications and Mobile Computing, 2019*. https://doi.org/10.1155/2019/5931315

Nemcova, A., Jordanova, I., Varecka, M., Smisek, R., Marsanova, L., Smital, L., & Vitek, M. (2020). Monitoring of heart rate, blood oxygen saturation, and blood pressure using a smartphone. *Biomedical Signal Processing and Control, 59*, 101928. https://doi.org/10.1016/j.bspc.2020.101928

Nugroho, C., Suryo, S., & Wiseno, B. (2020). The analysis of homecare interest in pandemic covid 19 period based on disease case in Indonesia. *European Journal of Medical and Health Sciences, 2*(5). https://doi.org/10.24018/EJMED

Panch, T., Pearson-Stuttard, J., Greaves, F., & Atun, R. (2019). Artificial intelligence: Opportunities and risks for public health. *The Lancet Digital Health, 1*(1), e13–e14. https://doi.org/10.1016/S2589-7500(19)30002-0

Pavón-Pulido, N., López-Riquelme, J. A., & Feliú-Batlle, J. J. (2020). IoMT architecture for smart control of an exoskeleton robot in rehabilitation by using a natural user interface based on gestures. *Journal of Medical Systems, 44*(9), 1–10. https://doi.org/10.1007/s10916-020-01602

Pearson D. (2017). Artificial intelligence in radiology: the game-changer on everyone's mind. https://www.radiologybusiness.com/topics/technology-management/artificial-intelligence-radiology-game-changer-everyones-mind Radiology business.

Perwej, Y. (2015). An evaluation of deep learning miniature concerning in soft computing. *International Journal of Advanced Research in Computer and Communication Engineering*, 10–16. https://doi.org/10.17148/IJARCCE.2015.4203

Petrakis, E. G. M., Sotiriadis, S., Soultanopoulos, T., Renta, P. T., Buyya, R., & Bessis, N. (2018). Internet of Things as a Service (iTaaS): Challenges and solutions for management of sensor data on the cloud and the fog. *Internet of Things, 3–4*, 156–174. https://doi.org/10.1016/j.iot.2018.09.009

Punithavathi, P., Geetha, S., Karuppiah, M., Islam, S. H., Hassan, M. M., & Choo, K. K. R. (2019). A lightweight machine learning-based authentication framework for smart IoT devices. *Information Sciences, 484*, 255–268. https://doi.org/10.1016/j.ins.2019.01.073

Quintana, Y., Fahy, D., Crotty, B., Jain, R., Kaldany, E., Gorenberg, M., Lipsitz, L., Engorn, D., Rodriguez, J., Orfanos, A., Bajracharya, A., Henao, J., Adra, M., Skerry, D., Slack, W. V., & Safran, C. (2018). InfoSAGE: Supporting elders and families through online family networks. In *AMIA Annual symposium proceedings. AMIA symposium, 2018, 932–941.*

Richens, J. G., Lee, C. M., & Johri, S. (2020). Improving the accuracy of medical diagnosis with causal machine learning. *Nature Communications, 11*(1). https://doi.org/10.1038/s41467-020-17419-7

Secinaro, S., Calandra, D., Secinaro, A., et al. (2021). The role of artificial intelligence in healthcare: a structured literature review. *BMC Medical Informatics and Decision, 21*, 125. https://doi.org/10.1186/s12911-021-01488-9

Sezgin, E., Huang, Y., Ramtekkar, U., & Lin, S. (2020). Readiness for voice assistants to support healthcare delivery during a health crisis and pandemic. *Npj Digital Medicine, 3*(1). https://doi.org/10.1038/s41746-020-00332-0

Shickel, B., Tighe, P. J., Bihorac, A., & Rashidi, P. (2018). Deep EHR: A survey of recent advances in deep learning techniques for electronic health record (EHR) analysis. *IEEE Journal of Biomedical and Health Informatics, 22*(5), 1589–1604. https://doi.org/10.1109/JBHI.2017.2767063

Sun, L., Sun, L., Jiang, X., Ren, H., Ren, H., & Guo, Y. (2020). Edge-cloud computing and artificial intelligence in internet of medical things: Architecture, technology and application. *IEEE Access, 8*, 101079–101092. https://doi.org/10.1109/ACCESS.2020.2997831

Tarassoli, S. P. (2019). Artificial intelligence, regenerative surgery, robotics? What is realistic for the future of surgery? *Annals of Medicine and Surgery, 41*, 53–55. https://doi.org/10.1016/j.amsu.2019.04.001

Topol, E. (2019). *Deep medicine – how artificial intelligence can make healthcare human again*. Basic Books.

Tran, B. X., Vu, G. T., Ha, G. H., Vuong, Q. H., Ho, M. T., Vuong, T. T., La, V. P., Ho, M. T., Nghiem, K. C. P., Nguyen, H. L. T., Latkin, C. A., Tam, W. W. S., Cheung, N. M., Nguyen, H. K. T., Ho, C. S. H., & Ho, R. C. M. (2019). Global evolution of research in artificial intelligence in health and medicine: A bibliometric study. *Journal of Clinical Medicine, 8*(3). https://doi.org/10.3390/jcm8030360

US FDA. (2019). *Proposed regulatory framework for modifications to artificial intelligence/machine learning (AI/ML) – Based software as a medical device (SaMD). Discussion paper and request for feedback.*

Vora, J., Tanwar, S., Tyagi, S., Kumar, N., & Rodrigues, J. J. P. C. (2017). Faal: Fog computing-based patient monitoring system for ambient assisted living. In , *Vol. 2017. 2017 IEEE 19th international conference on e-health networking, applications and services, Healthcom 2017* (pp. 1–6). Institute of Electrical and electronics Engineers Inc. https://doi.org/10.1109/HealthCom.2017.8210825

Wang, Z., Dong, X., Li, Y., Fang, L., & Chen, P. (2018). IoT security model and performance evaluation: A blockchain approach. In *Proceedings of 2018 6th IEEE International conference on network infrastructure and digital content, IC-NIDC 2018* (pp. 260–264). Institute of Electrical and Electronics Engineers Inc. https://doi.org/10.1109/ICNIDC.2018.8525716

Waterman, J., Yang, H., & Muheidat, F. (2020). AWS IoT and the interconnected world – aging in place. In *Proceedings – 2020 international conference on computational science and computational intelligence, CSCI 2020* (pp. 1126–1129). Institute of Electrical and Electronics Engineers Inc. https://doi.org/10.1109/CSCI51800.2020.00209

Xu, L., & Pombo, N. (2019). Human behavior prediction though noninvasive and privacy-preserving Internet of Things (IOT) assisted monitoring. In *IEEE 5th world forum on Internet of Things, WF-IoT 2019 – conference proceedings* (pp. 773–777). Institute of Electrical and Electronics Engineers Inc. https://doi.org/10.1109/WF-IoT.2019.8767301

Yang, H. S., Hou, Y., Vasovic, L. V., Steel, P. A. D., Chadburn, A., Racine-Brzostek, S. E., Velu, P., Cushing, M. M., Loda, M., Kaushal, R., Zhao, Z., & Wang, F. (2020). Routine laboratory blood tests predict SARS-CoV-2 infection using machine learning. *Clinical Chemistry, 66*(11), 1396–1404. https://doi.org/10.1093/clinchem/hvaa200

CHAPTER

3

Artificial intelligence in healthcare: current situation and future possibilities

Sanskar Srivastava[1], Amit Kumar Tyagi[1,2], Sajidha S. A.[1]

[1]*School of Computer Science and Engineering, Vellore Institute of Technology, Chennai, Tamilnadu, India;* [2]*Centre for Advanced Data Science, Vellore Institute of Technology, Chennai, Tamilnadu, India*

3.1 Introduction

Healthcare changes a lot with the rise of technology and the introduction of more efficient ways. Machine Learning (ML) and Artificial Intelligence (AI) have made a big impact on the healthcare industry, and people are working hard to bridge the gap between AI and healthcare so that AI can help people. The reason for and reason for this is because there are more and more problems in the healthcare field. There aren't enough trustworthy and easily available doctors, there's more demand for better medical care because of more people living longer, and there's more general awareness. There has also been an increase in the number of long-term illnesses around the world. Any disease that is very common, like COVID 19, puts a lot of strain on the healthcare industry. The industry itself isn't easy for everyone to get into, and there are big differences and variations in the quality and practices. Recent surveys say that a lot of doctors are over the age of 55 and will be retiring in the next decade. One in three doctors are over 55. This, as well as the fact that the next generation will have different ideas, has made AI more important. AI is already being used in a lot of important areas and has had a lot of success. Fig. 3.1 explains what better heart care or healthcare 4.0 means in the smart era.

Most technical and process-based tasks that require precision and attention to detail can be easily done by AI. AI has already made a lot of things easier, and that can be seen in the healthcare field as well. AI can be used to go through a lot of data and stay up to date on the most recent methods. It can also be used to improve the effectiveness of both experienced and inexperienced doctors by giving them advice based on the data it has processed. It can be more accurate in the future if it learns from both successes and failures. It has a lot of room for improvement, but things like how it works, how safe it is, how it affects the careers of future doctors, and so on should be kept in mind.

Computational Intelligence for Medical Internet of Things (MIoT) Applications
https://doi.org/10.1016/B978-0-323-99421-7.00015-5

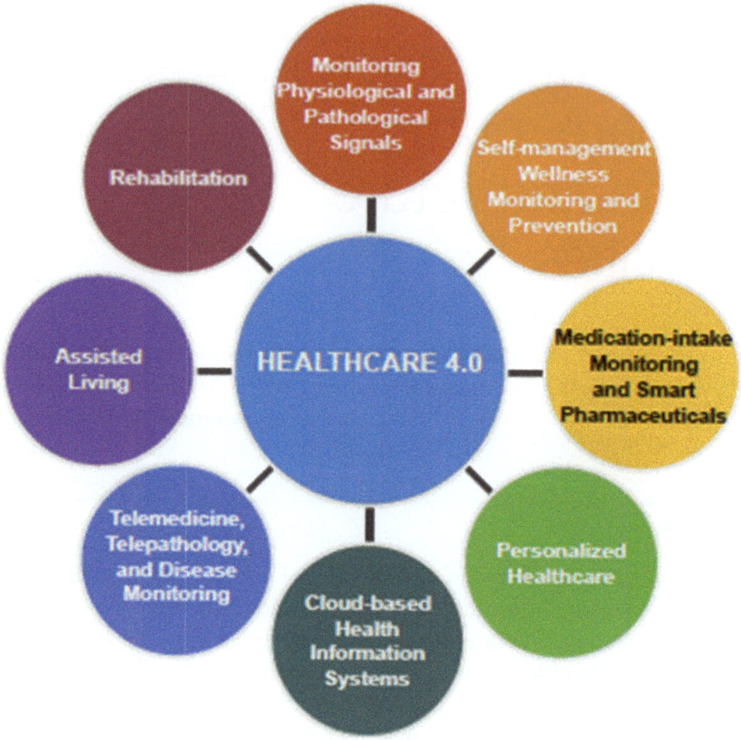

FIGURE 3.1

Healthcare application with industries 4.0.

3.1.1 Types of artificial intelligence used in healthcare

Today, there are many ways to learn that can be used to cure or predict how a disease will affect a person. A few of the ways that can learn are on this section:

Machine Learning: A part of AI that doesn't use rules, but instead learns from data, is called "data-driven AI." It is a statistical method that tells the model what to do. There are many different types of AI. This is one of them. When it comes to healthcare, precision technology and predicting treatment are two of the most common ways this can be used. Here, Fig. 3.2 shows how machine learning techniques have changed over time in great detail.

Neural Network: To predict whether a patient will have a certain disease, this is a more complicated type of machine learning that is used mostly for that. There are inputs, outputs, and how they all work together to process data and other situations with the right responses.

Deep Learning: This is the most complicated form, and it uses neural network models to try to mimic the way the brain works. It is very good at things like image recognition, language processing, and so on. It has many layers of neural network models that have different features and work together for better use. Current applications can tell if cells are cancerous. Methods for faster processing, such as better graphics processing units or cloud-based architecture, are making it more common and more useful to people. Keep in mind that Deep learning is used in clinical imaging and the analysis of Electronic Health Records (EHR) (Rajkomar et al., 2018).

Natural Language Processing: In this case, the AI is making sense of human language, and this leads to things like speech recognition and text analysis. In healthcare, NLP is used to understand, analyze, and then group a lot of medical data. It combines all the information into one place so that it can be used to make reports, give important information, and interact with patients.

3.1.2 Role of artificial intelligence in healthcare

Section 3.2 talked about how different learning methods are used in the healthcare or telemedicine field. There are a few other ways AI and IoTs can be used in healthcare (Bali et al., 2019; Han et al., 2020):

- Internet of Medical Things (IoMT)
- Internet of Health Things (IoHT)
- Internet of Nano Things (IoNT)
- Wearable Internet of Things (WIoT)
- Internet of m-health Things (m-IoT)

Keep in mind that AI in Healthcare can be used to do things like help people get better.

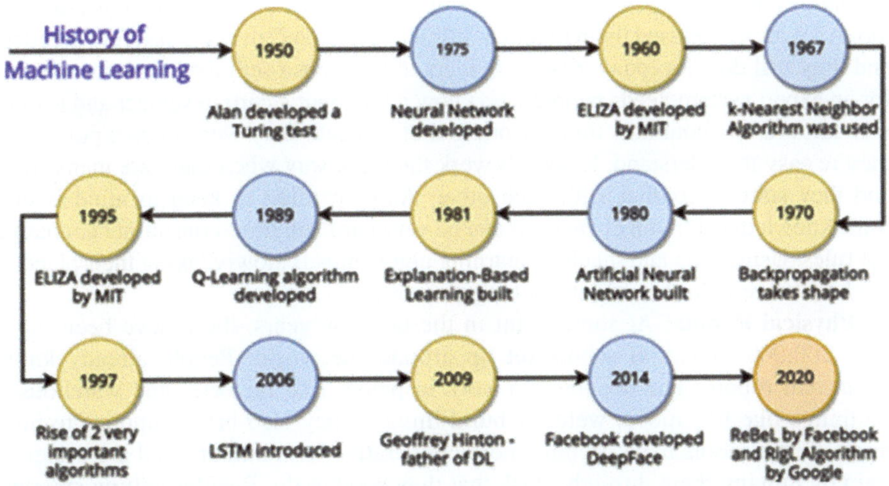

FIGURE 3.2

Progress of machine learning techniques.

- Paying attention to physiological and pathological signals.
- Self-management, monitoring health, and prevention.
- Medication intake monitoring and smart drugs
- Customized healthcare.
- Health Information Systems that are in the cloud.
- Telepathology, telemedicine, and disease monitoring
- Help People Live
- Rehabilitation.
- Prediction of bladder volume
- Prediction of epileptic seizures

3.2 Working of each application in smart era

Natural Language Processing (NLP): AI researchers have been trying to figure out how people talk since the 1950s so that they can understand their work. To know how to do things like recognize speech, read text, or translate things that are in a language, this field is called NLP. One way to do this is statistical NLP. The other way is called semantic NLP. This has helped improve the accuracy of recognition in recent years. A lot of language is important to learn from. Make, understand, and categories clinical documentation and research are the most common ways NLP can be used in the healthcare field today. The EMR stands for an electronic medical record, and the EP stands for electrophysiological records.

Fig. 3.3 shows that how clinical information, natural language processing data, machine learning data, and clinical decisions are all made.

Rule-based Expert Systems: If-then rules were the most common type of AI technology in the 1980s. They were used for business at that time and later on, too. A lot of people used them to make "clinical decisions" over the last few decades, and they still do a lot today. EHR providers today have a set of rules. A set of rules for an expert system needs people who know a lot about a certain subject and people who know a lot about how things work in that subject. They work up to a point, and they're easy to understand. It doesn't work the same way when there are many rules and they start to conflict with each other. Another thing to keep in mind is that if the knowledge domain changes, it can be very hard and time-consuming to change the rules. Using data and machine learning algorithms is slowly taking their place in the healthcare field, but it's still a long way off.

Physical Robots: At some point in the last few years, there have been more than 200,000 industrial robots set up around the world. People already know about real robots. The people who work in places like factories and warehouses do things like lift, move, weld, or build things. They also bring supplies to hospitals. Some robots have become more cooperative with humans and are easier to train by moving them through a task that they want to do. Besides getting smarter, their "brains" are also getting smarter, because other AI abilities are being added to them (really their operating systems). As AI gets better, it's likely that robots will

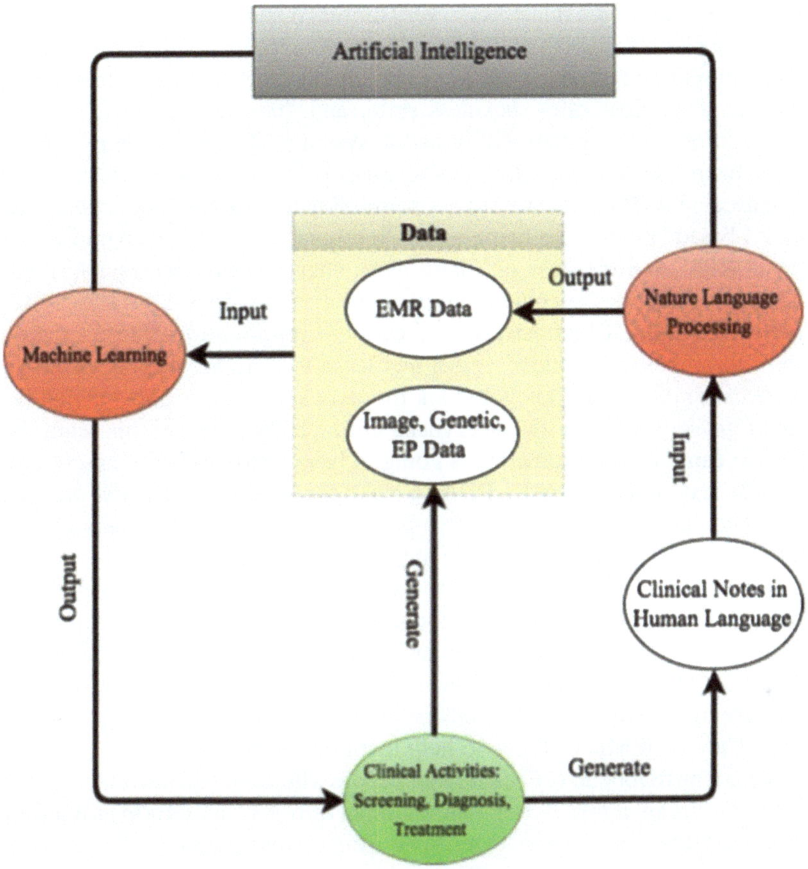

FIGURE 3.3

Procedure of clinical data generation.

Procedure of clinical data generation to natural language processing data enrichment, to machine learning data analysis, to clinical decision making.

get smarter (Khan & Anwar, 2019). They are called "superhuman" tools because they help surgeons do things that they couldn't do before 2000. Make precise and minimally invasive incisions that aren't very painful for the body to heal, stitch wounds, and so on People still have to make important decisions about surgery, but they don't have to make them all at once. Common surgeries like gynecologic surgery and prostate surgery are done with robots. The head and neck surgery is also done with robots.

Robotic Process Automation: For example, this technology can do structured digital tasks for administrative purposes, like those that involve information systems, as though they were a person who was following a script or set of rules, like they were. Compared to other types of AI, they are cheap, easy to programmed, and very clear about what they do, which makes them very useful. When it comes to Robotic Process Automation (RPA), it doesn't really have to do with robots at all. Servers are run by computer programmers, and they all work together. In this case, there are three main parts: work flow rules, business rules, and "presentation layer" integration with other information systems (information systems). There are some things that it does that make it look like a semiintelligent user of the systems. Healthcare is where they are used a lot. They are used to get permission to do something, update records, or bill. AI-based "brains" are being added to robots, and image recognition is being used with RPA. As time goes on, these technologies could become so intertwined that composite solutions become more likely or even possible.

Early Detection, Diagnosis, and Treatment Applications: 85% of the time, there is a thrombus in the blood vessel that leads to a stroke. This is called a brain injury. Because they didn't know to look for early signs of a stroke, only a few people could get help quickly (Myszczynska et al., 2020). He and his team made a gadget that can tell when someone is going to have a stroke. People used a genetic fuzzy finite state machine and a PCA to make the model, which was then used to make it. The detection process had two parts: a stage to look for signs of a stroke, and a stage to look for signs of people moving. As soon as the patient starts moving in a way that is very different from how they usually move, an alert would be raised for a stroke. They would be looked at for treatment as soon as possible. Another way to do this would be to use hidden Markov models and SVM to do it. This means that the algorithm was able to correctly place 90.5% of subjects in the right group. A few studies have tried to figure out if someone has had a stroke by looking at neuroimaging data. They used ML methods to help them figure that out.

Another way to look at CT scans from people who have had a stroke is to use ML tools. After a stroke, a free-floating intraluminal thrombus may form as a lesion on a CT scan. This lesion can be hard to tell apart from carotid plaque on the scan. It's how Thornhill et al. (Thornhill et al., 2014) used 3 ML algorithms to classify these two different kinds of shapes. linear discriminant analysis, an artificial neural network, and an SVM were used by them to find out which people were more likely to be, how good they are at getting the job done ranges from 65.2% to 76.4% of the time.

Treatment: ML has also been used to predict how well stroke treatment works and to look at how long it takes for it to work. In an emergency, intravenous thrombolysis (tPA) is a very important part of the process. How it goes has a big impact on how well people do and how long they will live. They used whole-brain images as the input for the SVM, which did better than other methods that used radiology, which did not work as well. In order to do this, they used a Bayesian thought network. In the model, there were 56 variables and three ways to look at the process of diagnosing and treating, as well as predicting what will happen next.

MYCIN was made in the 1970s, but AI has been trying to figure out how to diagnose and treat diseases for a long time, even before the 1970s (Shortliffe et al., 1975). People thought this and other rule-based systems looked good at accurately diagnosing and treating disease in the beginning, but they were never put to use. It was hard for them to figure out what was wrong with people, and they didn't work well with clinician workflows and medical record systems, either. In the last few weeks, IBM's Watson has been getting a lot of attention because of its focus on "precision medicine," especially cancer diagnosis and treatment. Watson is able to use both machine learning and natural language processing, so it can learn new things. Early enthusiasm for this use of technology has waned as customers realized how hard it was to teach Watson how to deal with different types of cancer and how to work with Watson in care processes and systems, which made them less excited about the idea. As a set of "cognitive services," Watson can be used by other programmers. Watson is not a single product, but rather a set of tools that other programmers can use. These are people who write programmers for things like speech and language, vision, and machine learning-based data analysis. A lot of people think that the Watson APIs are good at what they do. But taking on cancer treatment was too big of a goal. They have been hurt by competition from "open source" programmers, like Google's TensorFlow that can be used for free by anyone. Watson and other proprietary programmers have also been hurt by this, too.

People use rule-based systems that are part of EHR systems all the time, but they don't have the precision of more algorithmic systems that use machine learning, which are more common. It's hard to keep up with these rule-based clinical decision support systems because medical knowledge changes all of the time. There is a lot of data and information that comes from "omics-based" approaches to caring for people. They often can't keep up with all of it. In no time at all, a research lab says that it can use AI or big data to diagnose and treat a disease with the same or better accuracy as humans. Some of them use other images like retinal scans or genomic-based precision medicine to find out more about what's going on. They mostly use radiological image analysis, but some of them also use images like these. When machine learning models use statistics to make predictions, they start a new era of medicine that is based on evidence and chance. Some people think this is a good idea, but it also has a lot of problems with medical ethics and how patients and doctors work together. Some tech companies and start-ups are also putting in a lot of time and effort into the same things It can be dangerous for people to get sepsis or heart failure, so Google and health delivery networks work together to use big data to build prediction models.

To figure out how to treat certain types of cancer based on their genetic makeups, there are also a lot of companies that do this. Many types of cancer have a genetic basis, which makes it more difficult for humans to figure out how they respond to new drugs and procedures because so many of them have that. Foundation Medicine and Flatiron Health, two companies that used to be separate but are now owned by Roche, are both good at this kind of thing. There are times when these models can be good at predicting, but they don't always have all of the information that could help them, like information about a patient's socioeconomic status No matter what kind of AI-based diagnosis and treatment recommendations are, they can be hard to fit into clinical workflows and electronic health records. There are a lot of AI-based tools for diagnosis and treatment from tech companies that are stand-alone or only deal with a single part of care. A small number of people who make electronic health records (EHRs) are now adding a small amount of AI to their products, such as rule-based clinical decision support. These are still in the beginning stages. There are two options for providers. They can either do a lot of work on their own, or they can wait for EHR vendors to add more AI features.

3.2.1 Scope of artificial intelligence in present situation and in other applications

It used to be that artificial intelligence was only used in a few things like transportation and agriculture. But now it's used in almost all of these things and more. AI has a lot of different jobs in the world today and in other places, and some of them can be explained here (Esmaeilzadeh, 2020; Jiang et al., 2017; Lysaght et al., 2019):

Outcome prediction and prognosis evaluation: Many things can make it more likely that users will have a stroke and die from it. ML methods have advantages over traditional methods when it comes to making better predictions. By looking at physiological data from the first 48 h after a stroke with logistic regression, we need to come Zhou and Myrzashova (2020) up with a model for how well 3-month treatment would go for people who had a stroke. In this case, the authors used artificial neural networks and SVMs to look at the data. They came up with a prediction accuracy of more than 70%. When they looked for things that could affect the outcome of brain arteriovenous malformations that were treated with endovascular embolization, they also used ML techniques to look for them. A regression analysis model that they used could only get 43% of the time correct when they used it. Much better: Their methods worked much better and they got 97.50% of the time right!

It has been possible to figure out how treatment for a stroke will go based on brain scans. Random forest was used to automatically identify cerebrospinal fluid and look at the changes on a CT scan, which is faster and more accurate than the old method, which took longer. Ridge regression and multitask learning were used by Siegel et al. to predict how well people would be able to think after having a stroke. They used MRI and functional MRI data to figure out how the brain worked together. How did Hope et al. look at the relationship between lesions on MRI images and how well they worked after surgery? They used a Gaussian process regression model to do this. They used a model to figure out how bad cognitive impairments after a stroke would be and how long it would take to get better, like how long it would take.

AI for Drug Discovery: AI can go through a lot of healthcare data and figure out what each piece of information means. AI can be used to help find new drugs by following these steps. This helps cut down on how long it would take to find and make newer and more effective drugs.

- Bioxcel Therapeutics is a company that focuses on drug development by using AI to find and develop new medicines in the fields of neuroscience. That's what it does with this AI. It uses this AI to find new drugs or compositions that will make existing ones even better.

- Berg Health is an AI-based biotech platform that aims to improve the treatment of rare diseases. It maps and stores information about any disease so that better cures and breakthroughs can be found. It has already talked about what it learned about Parkinson's Disease. When they used this technology, they discovered connections between chemicals in the human body that had never been thought of before, but now they know about them (Zhou & Myrzashova, 2020).
- XtalPi is a unique platform because it brings together AI, cloud computing, and quantum physics. To make drugs, this company mostly uses a system to look at and predict the chemical properties of small molecules that are involved in the development of drugs. Predicting complex structures with polymorph prediction takes a lot less time than it usually does. It usually takes months to figure out what the structures look like (Bairagya et al., 2021).
- Deep Genomics (Asgari and Mofrad, 2019) focuses on drug development for neuromuscular and neurodegenerative disorders. This is what they do. It uses AI technology to look at different cell compounds to figure out which ones could be used to make drugs. This makes it more likely that a drug that has been made will pass clinical trials, while also cutting down on how long and how much work it would take to do this. It sends the feedback to the developers so that they can use it in the future.
- BenevolentAI is a platform that works with big companies to get drugs licensed from them. Using AI to get the right treatment to patents when they need it will make it more likely that they will get the treatment that they need. Doing this helps to save time and also gives new information that wasn't there before. This allows for faster and more accurate treatment.

AI for Symptom Detection and Diagnoses: AI that uses machine learning and image recognition, as well as its ability to store and analyze data, can also be used to detect symptoms in patients and make accurate diagnoses. This is because AI can also store and analyze a lot of data. *Note that* AI-enhanced microscopes are used at the Eth Israel Deaconess Medical Center in Boston. They use these microscopes to scan blood samples for harmful bacteria and viruses at a larger scale and faster than ever before. In most cases, this process is done by hand, which increases the risk of misidentifying the pathogens present, there are a lot of blood samples for the AI to compare. This increases the chances of predicting which bacteria will be bad with 95% accuracy. It is an intelligent system that receives images, scans, medical history, and blood tests. It then chooses the best findings and sends them to radiologists, who report them to the doctor. Then, these can be used to get a more accurate answer to the question. It's basically like a radiology helper. For this several available mechanisms are:

- PathAI is a machine learning technology that is being worked on in Cambridge, Massachusetts. This AI helps to make sure that the diagnoses are

correct. The main goal of this is to cut down on the chances of making mistakes or errors when diagnosing cancer in its early stages. They have also worked with a lot of other companies to get more data and information about health and medicine, as well as to spread the benefits of using this technology to more businesses.
- Buoy Health is another AI-based technology that is based in Boston and aims to cut down on the time it takes for patients to figure out their symptoms and get the help they need from the right doctor. What it does is look at the patient's medical history and symptoms to figure out who they should ask for help. It then recommends the right doctor for them. It uses algorithms to do this, and it makes the patient more satisfied and more comfortable. Besides using this tech, the Harvard Medical School also does so (Amisha et al., 2019).
- Enlitic, which is in San Francisco, has made smart medical tools that make radiology diagnoses faster. It looks at all of the unstructured data that comes from radiology, blood tests, and any medical history or data about the patients. This gives the doctor a better idea of what the patients are going through so that they can come up with better and more effective ways to help them based on the person's data (Massat, 2018).
- Freenome is another company like PathAI that is based in San Francisco and uses AI to find cancer early. This is when the artificial intelligence is used in things like screenings, diagnosis, and blood tests that could help detect cancer. The goal is to find cancer at its earliest stages and come up with new ways to treat it by looking at how it has worked in the past.
- Babylon Health is different from the other platform because it focuses more on prevention than the cure itself. It believes in preventing the disease as soon as possible to save money and avoid any unnecessary deaths, which leads to better health in the long run. It is an AI engine that was made with the help of a lot of doctors and scientists. It works like a symptom checker. It helps the doctor by giving him or her the most up-to-date medical information. People can also keep an eye on their health with the help of a health monitoring system. It also looks at the different symptoms.
- Olive is an AI platform that focuses on automating the most common tasks that are being done, which frees up time for administrators to do more important things. Because of this, the rest of the staff can then give better service to patients.

AI for Data Collection and Analysis: AI technology is used to collect all this data and information that can help healthcare providers and doctors figure out better ways to treat people and find other ways to help them get better, as well. This kind of platform focuses more on putting together all of the available information about everything from genetics sequencing to image recognition in one place so that healthcare professionals can have all of this information at their fingertips and also to help the person grow as a person. It is now focusing on cancer detection and treatment. This is not the only thing that KenSci does (Ahmad et al., 2018).

It also collects and analyses data to figure out what kinds of medical, financial, and operational risks there might be for people. It focuses on using AI to cut down on risks. This lowers the cost of healthcare. For this several available mechanisms are:

- Qventus is one of the most cutting-edge start-ups because it puts patient safety first. It uses AI technology to keep track of how long patients with critical injuries have to wait and for any procedure that needs to be done in an emergency room. The automated platform helps with managing and prioritizing patients based on how critical their injuries are. It also shows the fastest ambulance routes so that they can get to patients more quickly.
- Cloudmedx uses an AI platform to collect and manage a lot of patient data, medical history, and payment information. It then uses a predictive analysis to make the patient's journey and care better. There are some insights that healthcare providers can use so they don't have to be in a hurry or panic when they take care of patients.
- IBM's Watson: IBM's Watson is an artificial intelligence platform that helps healthcare professionals collect and use data more efficiently in order to be more effective. It does this so that it can better interact with patients and better understand and improve their care. It can be used to look at genetic tests, look for early signs of diseases, and make personalized health plans for each person. For example, there is an AI software called Google DeepMind Health. It gathers a lot of information about patients' problems, as well as their possible causes. It is being used in hospitals all over the world to help doctors treat people who are sick. The program helps doctors figure out what the illnesses are faster, and it also tells them if their health is getting worse.
- AI for clinical trials: A clinical trial is research or a study to find out how well a new medical method works on people (Angus, 2020). AI can help with this. This process has many stages and takes a long time because it needs to be tested very carefully before it can be approved. The AI is also able to make better decisions based on the tests that it has done. In terms of popularity, the most popular ones are:
- Well-planned clinical trials
- Clinical Trial cooperation and sharing of model files

3.3 AI in biomedical information processing

3.3.1 AI in biomedical research

AI as a Neural Network: For this several available mechanisms are:

AtomWise is a platform that uses AI to focus on serious diseases like Ebola, and it does this by putting a lot of attention on those diseases. There is a neural network called Atom Net that the company has made to help them with the process, and it helps. This network can look at 10 to 20 million genetic compounds every day, which allows it to deliver data a lot faster than it would normally take to do so. A computer program called Vicarious Surgical can predict how the body will work and then figure out what kind of people will need surgery. When it does this, it combines virtual reality technology with robots that can be used by doctors to do surgery more quickly and accurately. Using this technology, surgeons can see the different injuries in great detail and easily look inside the body with virtual reality (Mesko, 2017).

Auris Health has been working on a lot of different robots that are AI-enhanced to make endoscopies better, like this one. In order to study the patient's illness, this doctor can get a better and clearer view of the body while also giving all the information about the illness that he needs to do so. It is now being used to make robots that can study lung cancer and find a cure for it. When cancerous tumors are found in a patient, the Accuray Cyberknife System can help them be treated with more precision and accuracy by using robot arms that have been made with AI in mind. Tracking the tumor and its growth in real time is easier for doctors and surgeons to do because the robot can see where the tumor is and how big it is at any given time. A 6D motion detection technology is used to track the tumor very well and save all of the healthy cells that it comes across.

Initiative's Da Vinci is the first robotic surgery assistant that the FDA has given the go-ahead for (Food Drug Administration). They can do the minimally invasive surgeries with this. There is also a place that stores and updates all of the information about the surgeries, and it looks at the data to see how to make future surgeries better. As of right now, it has been used in more than five million different things. If users look at Carnegie Mellon's Heartlander, users can see that it has AI-enhanced robot technology that was made by the robotics department of the university. It is a small robot that is used to give heart therapy. The doctor controls the robot as it enters the chest through a small incision to find and treat the part of the heart that needs help.

Microsure is an AI-enhanced robot system that is designed to help surgeons perform medical procedures that can't be done with human hands. It is made to help them. They have a stabilization system that has made the job of the surgeon easier and better. Eight of these surgical procedures have been approved by the FDA so far.

People who know the most important words can explain them here:

- **Patient Care:** AI can also be used to help people. This can work on many different levels. On the most basic level, it can keep an eye on the patient and manage his data on a regular basis to see if there are any problems or ways to improve his overall health. It can also be used as a system that takes care of the patient at every step during a procedure or surgery. When it comes to childbirth and pregnancy, this is called "Maternal Care." There are a lot of childbirths that go wrong and end up with difficult deliveries that make the patient more stressed and may even harm the baby. Using AI to predict any problems with the pregnancy helps avoid any problems and mistakes that would have happened.
- **Healthcare Robotics:** This refers to medical robots that help medical workers or robots that make it easier to do hard things. When it comes to genetics, AI, and data-driven medicine, this is called "Genetics AI Data-Driven Medicine."

3.3.2 Implications for the healthcare workforce in Today's scenarios

There has been a lot of talk about how AI could lead to a lot of jobs being automated and a lot of people not having jobs. People who read other studies say that while some jobs can be automated, there are a lot more things that could keep jobs from being lost. These things include the cost of automation technologies and how much people are willing to pay for them. These things might keep the real job loss to 5% or less. AI hasn't been a big part of the industry yet, and it has been hard to get AI to work with clinical workflows and electronic health records. This has led to very few job changes. But even in jobs like being a radiologist or pathologist, AI isn't likely to spread very quickly. They won't be going out of business any time soon, even though new technologies like deep learning are making progress in being able to diagnose and categorize images. Do one thing at a time like other AI systems. People who work in labs and start-ups have to do a lot of work to train deep-learning models for certain image recognition tasks (such as nodule detection on chest-computed tomography or hemorrhage on brain magnetic resonance imaging). Many small tasks must be done to find all of the possible findings in medical images, and only a few can be done by AI right now. Other doctors can also ask radiologists for help with diagnosis and treatment, too. Interventional radiologists perform image-guided medical procedures, like cancer biopsies and stent placement, that are done with the help of images. They also define the technical parameters of imaging examinations to be done (tailored for the patient), and link findings from images to other medical records and tests. Because AI-based image work isn't ready to be used every day yet, this is the second reason.

All kinds of imaging technology and deep-learning algorithms look at things like a nodule's features and where it is, as well as its chances of having a lesion. There are a lot of different things that would make it very difficult to put deep-learning systems into current clinical practice. It's also important to have "labeled data," which is a lot of images from people who have been diagnosed with cancer or a broken bone. However, there isn't a single place where all radiology images, whether or not they are tagged, are kept together in the same place. Finally, a lot of changes will have to be made to medical regulations and health insurance in order for automated image analysis to take off in the medical field. It's the same for pathology and other parts of medicine that use computers. The idea of making new jobs for people who work with and make AI technology could also happen. The fact that AI technologies won't be able to significantly cut the costs of medical diagnosis and treatment over that time is also true, but it's also true that this is true.

Finally, there are a lot of ethical issues that arise when AI is used in healthcare as well, so it used to be that most of the decisions about healthcare were made by people. Smart machines that can make or help with things raise questions about accountability, transparency, permission, and privacy, because they can make things or help people do things. Even though technology has made it easier for people to hide things from each other, this may be the most difficult thing to deal with.

Many AI algorithms, such as deep-learning algorithms used for image analysis, are almost impossible to understand or explain, and it's hard to figure out how they work. He or she will want to know why a picture led to this. A lot of people don't know how deep-learning algorithms work. Even doctors who are familiar with them might not be able to explain how they work. In the end, AI systems are going to make mistakes when they're used to diagnose and treat patients. It may be hard to figure out who is to blame for these mistakes. When patients get medical information from AI systems, they may not want to get it from someone who cares about them, but that's not always the case. People who use machine learning in healthcare may also be biased by algorithmic bias. Then they might think that a person is more likely to get a disease because of their gender or race, even though those aren't the real reasons for it.

Healthcare institutions, as well as the government and regulatory bodies, need to have structures in place to keep an eye on important issues like security, privacy etc. They also need to respond responsibly and set up governance mechanisms to avoid malicious activities (Jones et al., 2018; Mishra & Tyagi, 2022) in such critical systems. Because this technology is so powerful and important, it will need a lot of attention for a long time from scientific community.

3.3.3 A way toward deep learning-based healthcare

Deep-learning methods are powerful tools that work well with traditional machine learning and help computers learn from the data they have. They work together to help computers learn from their data. There are more ways to make apps that are smarter this way. In the past, a lot of people have used these methods for things like computer vision and language processing. They've already been used in many different ways. It looks like deep learning can also be used to look at data from healthcare. It was actually better to use multilayer neural networks to process medical data. This led to better predictions for a number of specific applications in a number of different clinical fields. They can also be used to combine different types of data and make generalizations because of their hierarchical learning structure. They focus on representation learning instead of just classification accuracy because they don't know how to classify things.

The next generation of healthcare systems should be able to handle many millions or even billions of patients and use a single, distributed patient representation to help clinicians do their jobs better, rather than having multiple systems that use different patient representations and data to do their jobs.

As a best-case scenario, this representation would be able to show all the different types of data that an individual has, like their EHRs, their genomics, how their environment is, their wearables, and so on, in one complete picture of their health. How to describe someone's health would be to say that this would be the best way to do it. It would be installed into the EHR system at a hospital, for example. This is how it would work: When there are changes in the number of patients, the models would be updated to keep up with them. This way, they would never be out of date!

Representations of the body can be used to help with a wide range of things, such as predicting disease risk and making personalized prescriptions. For example, they can also be used for research and to look at data. They recently took first place in an online challenge to find ways to classify Parkinson's disease with a temporal deep-learning method. Instead, because Parkinson's disease progresses so quickly, it may not be the best way to figure out how the disease is progressing. Because the entries in these vectors and matrix are usually combined over time, it may not be the best way to figure out how the disease is progressing. In the end, researchers used the LSTM RNN model to look for three types of Parkinson's disease that they found to be very interesting. Each type of Parkinson's disease progresses in the same way.

Finally, deep learning can be used to organize both hypothesis-driven research and research that isn't based on a set of facts in clinical fields (e.g., clustering, visualization of patient cohorts, stratification of disease populations). It's important for people who do both statistics and medicine to work together at every step of the process, from study design to planning experiments to building models and refining them.

3.3.4 Challenges in implementing deep learning in healthcare sector

There are still a lot of things that need to be worked out before deep learning can be used in the field of healthcare. To point out these important things:

- When it comes to computer models, deep learning refers to a lot of data. This is because these models are very hard to run. Among them is a fully connected, multilayer neural network, which has a lot of information about the network that needs to be figured out. To reach this goal, the first thing users need to do is have a lot of information. Another reason why deep learning works so well in fields where a lot of data can be quickly gathered is because it can learn from a lot of different things quickly (e.g., computer vision, speech, natural language). This isn't the case with healthcare, though. In September 2016, there were about 7.5 billion people in the world. Many of them did not get the kind of basic healthcare that most people need. Trying to figure out how images or words look, or how people speak, can be even more difficult than trying to figure out how diseases and how they get better or worse. Many computers don't know how to do well and stay safe if they don't know a lot about medicine.
- The data in healthcare aren't as clean or well-structured as the data in other fields. They're also a lot more ambiguous, noisy, and incomplete than the data in other fields.
- There is a lot that can't be predicted about how the diseases move and change over time, like how they move and change over time. There are already a lot of deep-learning models out there, and some of them have already been used in the medical field. They use static vector-based inputs that can't handle time in a natural way. It's important to find new ways to make deep learning work with temporal healthcare data. This will require new ideas.

- It's more difficult to solve biomedicine and healthcare issues like image and speech analysis than to solve problems in other fields, like image and speech. People don't know how or why most of the diseases work or why they happen. Some of them are very different from each other.
- Deep-learning models have been used in many different fields, many people think of them as "black boxes." This isn't true. Even though this might not be a big deal in other, more predictable fields such as image annotation, in healthcare, not only how well an algorithm works but why it works is very important. Even more important, the predictive system must show which traits are behind its predictions, so that doctors can trust them (e.g., prescription of a specific medication, potential high risk of developing a certain disease). It's possible to do a lot of research and find new ways to make the field even better in the future.
- Many different types of data sources can be used to make these features. For example, EHRs, social media, wearable devices, environments, surveys and so on are some of them. But they aren't the only ones that can be used. This is a very important and hard question for researchers to answer. How can these very different types of data work together? People could use the hierarchical nature of deep learning to process each piece of data on its own, then put the representations together to make a more complete picture of the patient's data by putting them together (e.g., using layers of AEs or deep Bayesian networks).
- This is called a "federated inference." Each clinic has its own patients. In this case, it's hard to make a deep-learning model that can be used by people from different places without leaking their private information. It's a good thing that another research question is how to learn about deep models in this way that isn't too risky This will be used in other math fields, like cryptography, as well (e.g., homomorphic encryption and secure multiparty computation).
- With deep learning, privacy is a big deal when users want to get more people to use it (e.g., through cloud computing services). No authentication or access control systems are broken by the attack, but it gets the model's parameters or training data through APIS that are not locked down. These things could happen to both the model and the person. When it comes to privacy, there is a problem called "functional leakage." Researchers have come up with a way to make sure that individual samples in training data can't be identified through their functional outputs. People who have different privacy needs are called "differential privacy." There are, however, risks those naive approaches could make the outputs useless or not provide enough protection, which makes it hard to make practical differential privacy solutions. It was for this reason that Chaudhuri and his team came up with ways to keep the logistic regression model's parameters safe. To keep the privacy of deep-learning models safe, it's even more difficult because there are more parameters that need to be protected and there have been a lot of new works in this field. This makes it even more difficult. As a result, the use of intelligent tools for next-generation healthcare needs to think about these risks and try to set up a "differential privacy standard."

- It's very important to use the medical knowledge that other people have. So because there isn't a lot of medical data, experts can help the deep-learning process go in the right direction by giving it advice. This is an important question for researchers to look into. Examples: Online medical encyclopedias and PubMed abstracts that can be used in the deep architecture should have reliable information that can be used to make it work. This will improve the performance of the computers. There is also semisupervised learning, which is a good way to learn from a lot of unlabeled samples with only a few labeled samples. It can use both labeled and unlabeled samples to learn.
- Training a time-sensitive deep-learning model is important because time is important in all kinds of healthcare problems, especially those that involve EHRs and monitoring devices. This will help users understand the patient better and make quick clinical decisions. In terms of healthcare, temporal deep learning is very important (as already shown in some of the early studies reported in the literature review).
- It is important for healthcare problems to have models that can be understood, but they are not the same thing. If a doctor doesn't know how to use a system, he or she isn't likely to use it. In part, this is because they work so well. To understand how networks work, users should look into both algorithms and tools that can help the networks work with existing tools that explain how data-driven systems work. This means that users should look into both algorithms and tools that can help networks work with tools that explain how data-driven systems work.

To learn more about how learning techniques can be useful in Healthcare and other industries, researchers can look at the work of Mishra & Tyagi (2022).

3.3.5 Future of artificial intelligence in healthcare sector

AI is getting better and better all the time, so soon the problems that people have in these areas will also be solved. This is because speech and text recognition have already been used for simple tasks. There will be more use in all of these places, too. In the future, it's possible that some well-known surgical procedures will be automated and only need to be watched. This will make it impossible for people to make a mistake. Wearable fitness bands that record general medical data about a person are already on the market and can be bought. In the future, people will be making health bracelets that everyone can wear. This will help keep track of people's medical histories, keep track of any problems that might arise, and also help with early detection at a level that has never been seen before. This will change how diseases are identified and treated because the chances of curing a disease in its early stages are much better than in later stages. Another area that may get better is predicting new diseases and how they might affect people. Fig. 3.4 shows the evolution of healthcare 1.0 to healthcare 4.0, and Fig. 3.5 presents the characteristics healthcare 1.0 to 4.0.

People are affected by pandemics and other diseases that spread across a large area because of how these pathogens change from other diseases. Predicting this change with AI will help plan and develop cures for diseases that don't even exist yet.

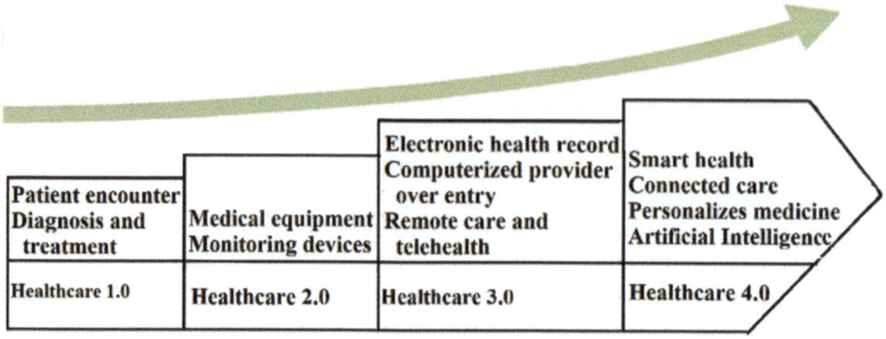

FIGURE 3.4

Evolution of healthcare 1.0 to healthcare 4.0.

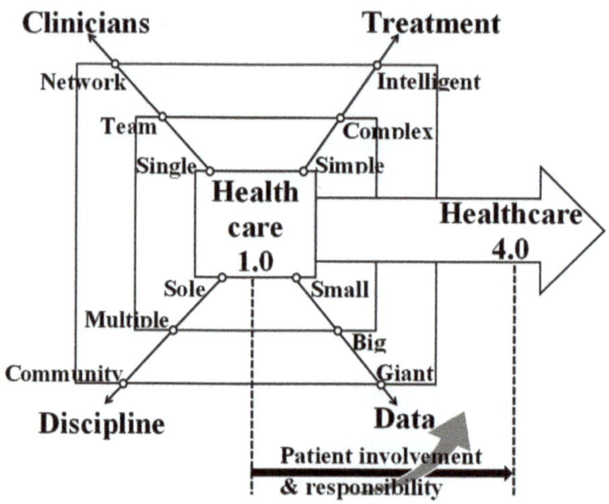

FIGURE 3.5

Evolution of healthcare 1.0 to healthcare 4.0.

AI technology used by the platforms now is very spread out and personalized. For this to happen, it will need to be approved by regulators, be standardized, be taught in a way that can be used by regular healthcare workers, and be updated on a regular basis. This will take time and effort. According to estimates, it will be at least 10 years before AI is widely used in the connected healthcare field (Fig. 3.6).

There's a good chance that most of the images from radiology and pathology will be looked at by a computer at some point. There has been a lot of progress in AI that can read images quickly. It's already common to use speech and text recognition to do things like talk to patients and write down clinical notes, and it will keep getting more common. How to use AI in real-life clinical situations is not a question of

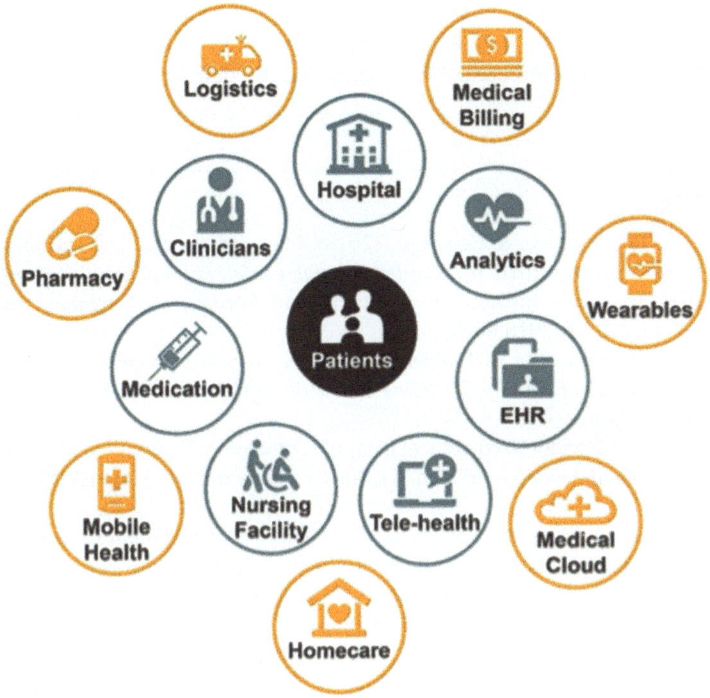

FIGURE 3.6

Connected healthcare.

whether the technologies will be good enough to be useful, but how to get them used. There are a lot of people who will use AI systems if they have been approved by regulators, are integrated with EHR systems, are standardized enough that similar products work the same way, clinicians are taught how to use them, and they are paid for by public or private payer groups over time. Another thing that is becoming more and more clear is that AI systems will not be able to completely replace human clinicians on a large scale, though. When they help them care for patients instead, they will help them out. Clinicians may move toward tasks and job designs that use their unique skills like empathy, persuasion, and big-picture integration to do their work over time. Some healthcare providers might lose their jobs in the future if they don't want to work with AI, but that might not be the case for everyone.

3.4 Conclusion

There are so many different ways and uses for AI that it's hard to keep up. People in the healthcare field can use technology to predict diseases, make new drugs or help with surgery. As new and better ways of using AI come out, the gap between AI and healthcare will keep getting smaller. This will take a long time to happen. Making this available to everyone and with enough credibility will take a lot of time and effort from both the healthcare professionals and the people who use the healthcare.

References

Ahmad, M. A., Teredesai, A., & Eckert, C. (2018). Interpretable machine learning in healthcare. In *Proceedings—2018 IEEE international conference on healthcare informatics, ICHI 2018* (p. 447). Institute of Electrical and Electronics Engineers Inc. https://doi.org/10.1109/ICHI.2018.00095

Amisha, P. M., Pathania, M., & Rathaur, V. (2019). Overview of artificial intelligence in medicine. *Journal of Family Medicine and Primary Care, 8*(7), 2328. https://doi.org/10.4103/jfmpc.jfmpc_440_19

Angus, D. C. (2020). Randomized clinical trials of artificial intelligence. *JAMA Journal of the American Medical Association, 323*(11), 1043—1045. https://doi.org/10.1001/jama.2020.1039

Asgari, E., & Mofrad, M. R. K. (2019). *Deep genomics and proteomics: Language model-based embedding of biological sequences and their applications in bioinformatics* (pp. 167—181). Elsevier BV. https://doi.org/10.1016/b978-0-12-809556-0.00012-5

Bairagya, D., Tripathy, H. K., Bhoi, A. K., & Barsocchi, P. (2021). Impact of artificial intelligence in health care: A study. *In Intelligent Systems Reference Library, 209*, 311—328. https://doi.org/10.1007/978-981-16-2972-3_15. Springer Science and Business Media Deutschland GmbH.

Bali, J., Garg, R., & Bali, R. (2019). Artificial intelligence (AI) in healthcare and biomedical research: Why a strong computational/AI bioethics framework is required? *Indian Journal of Ophthalmology, 67*(1), 3—6. https://doi.org/10.4103/ijo.IJO_1292_18

Esmaeilzadeh, P. (2020). Use of AI-based tools for healthcare purposes: A survey study from consumers' perspectives. *BMC Medical Informatics and Decision Making, 20*(1). https://doi.org/10.1186/s12911-020-01191-1

Han, C., Rundo, L., Murao, K., Nemoto, T., & Nakayama, H. (2020). Bridging the gap between AI and healthcare sides: Towards developing clinically relevant AI-powered diagnosis systems. *In IFIP Advances in Information and Communication Technology, 584*, 320—333. https://doi.org/10.1007/978-3-030-49186-4_27. Springer.

Jiang, F., Jiang, Y., Zhi, H., Dong, Y., Li, H., Ma, S., Wang, Y., Dong, Q., Shen, H., & Wang, Y. (2017). Artificial intelligence in healthcare: Past, present and future. *Stroke and Vascular Neurology, 2*(4), 230—243. https://doi.org/10.1136/svn-2017-000101

Jones, L. D., Golan, D., Hanna, S. A., & Ramachandran, M. (2018). Artificial intelligence, machine learning and the evolution of healthcare: A bright future or cause for concern? *Bone and Joint Research, 7*(3), 223—225. https://doi.org/10.1302/2046-3758.73.BJR-2017-0147.R1

Khan, A., & Anwar, Y. (2019). *Robots in healthcare: A survey* (Vol. 944, pp. 280—292). Springer Science and Business Media LLC. https://doi.org/10.1007/978-3-030-17798-0_24

Lysaght, T., Lim, H. Y., Xafis, V., & Ngiam, K. Y. (2019). AI-assisted decision-making in healthcare. *Asian Bioethics Review, 11*(3), 299—314. https://doi.org/10.1007/s41649-019-00096-0

Massat, M. B. (2018). Artificial intelligence in radiology: Hype or hope? *Applied Radiology, 47*(3), 22–26.

Mesko, B. (2017). The role of artificial intelligence in precision medicine. *Expert Review of Precision Medicine and Drug Development, 2*(5), 239–241. https://doi.org/10.1080/23808993.2017.1380516

Mishra, S., & Tyagi, A. K. (2022). The role of machine learning techniques in Internet of things-based cloud applications. In *Internet of things* (pp. 105–135). Springer Science and Business Media Deutschland GmbH. https://doi.org/10.1007/978-3-030-87059-1_4

Myszczynska, M. A., Ojamies, P. N., Lacoste, A. M. B., Neil, D., Saffari, A., Mead, R., Hautbergue, G. M., Holbrook, J. D., & Ferraiuolo, L. (2020). Applications of machine learning to diagnosis and treatment of neurodegenerative diseases. *Nature Reviews Neurology, 16*(8), 440–456. https://doi.org/10.1038/s41582-020-0377-8

Rajkomar, A., Oren, E., Chen, K., Dai, A. M., Hajaj, N., Hardt, M., Liu, P. J., Liu, X., Marcus, J., Sun, M., Sundberg, P., Yee, H., Zhang, K., Zhang, Y., Flores, G., Duggan, G. E., Irvine, J., Le, Q., Litsch, K., … Dean, J. (2018). Scalable and accurate deep learning with electronic health records. *Npj Digital Medicine, 1*(1). https://doi.org/10.1038/s41746-018-0029-1

Shortliffe, E. H., Davis, R., Axline, S. G., Buchanan, B. G., Green, C. C., & Cohen, S. N. (1975). Computer-based consultations in clinical therapeutics: Explanation and rule acquisition capabilities of the MYCIN system. *Computers and Biomedical Research, 8*(4), 303–320. https://doi.org/10.1016/0010-4809(75)90009-9

Thornhill, R. E., Lum, C., Jaberi, A., Stefanski, P., Torres, C. H., Momoli, F., Petrcich, W., & Dowlatshahi, D. (2014). Can shape analysis differentiate free-floating internal carotid artery thrombus from atherosclerotic plaque in patients evaluated with CTA for stroke or transient ischemic attack? *Academic Radiology, 21*(3), 345–354. https://doi.org/10.1016/j.acra.2013.11.011

Zhou, H., & Myrzashova, R. (2020). AI based systems for diabetes treatment: A brief overview of the past and plans for the future. *Journal of Physics: Conference Series, 1453*(1), 012063. https://doi.org/10.1088/1742-6596/1453/1/012063

CHAPTER

4 Exploring the effectiveness of cloud, Internet of Things and fog computing for healthcare monitoring systems

Said El Kafhali[1], **Iman El Mir**[2]

[1]*Hassan 1st University of Settat, Faculty of Sciences and Techniques, Computer, Networks, Modeling, and Mobility Laboratory (IR2M), Settat, Morocco;* [2]*Hassan 1st University of Settat, Institute of Sport Sciences, Computer, Networks, Mobility and Modeling Laboratory (IR2M), Settat, Morocco*

4.1 Introduction

The health of citizens is a severe area of concern for more countries around the world, as the reach of health services remains limited due to various constraints (Wei, 2021). Therefore, thc benefits of advances in medical science and related technologies are not available at all. Right now, good hospitals are only available in urban areas. Therefore, it is very difficult to get the treatment of a large number of citizens in rural areas and collect health data. For that, it is really necessary to transform healthcare with IT (El Kafhali & Lazaar, 2021). Numerous aspects of telehealthcare are needed to provide health services in the country in order to fill the gaps. They will become indispensable in rural areas where there is a shortage of doctors in hospitals. A healthcare monitoring system is an innovative system to improve healthcare services remotely using IoT. This system creates communication between patient and healthcare professionals. Healthcare professionals are available to patients only at hospitals. Monitoring patients who have undergone surgery and who have just returned home on an outpatient basis requires immediate care on a routine basis. If a patient is faced with a critical situation, they will be able to notify healthcare providers in time using IoT-enabled remote monitoring.

The Internet of Things (IoT) is seen as a rapidly evolving network paradigm that consists of billions of interconnected devices that capture and share data in real-time (Selvaraj et al., 2021). Today, IoT is used in many applications (Bang & Rao, 2021). According to (Horwitz, 2021), the number of connected devices used in IoT is expected to reach 75 billion by 2025. In addition, the economic influence of IoT will reach up to 11 trillion dollars by 2025. Moreover, an important part of these resources will reside in companies and industries (Miettinen et al., 2018). The current

Computational Intelligence for Medical Internet of Things (MIoT) Applications
https://doi.org/10.1016/B978-0-323-99421-7.00008-8

age is defined by the relationship between physical things and the internet. Integrating healthcare with IoT features through medical devices will help improve the quality of medical services. IoT offers important features to medical healthcare systems, such as scalability, mobility, and availability that provide an architectural foundation for real-time patient monitoring. This is of high significance, particularly for elderly patients with chronic diseases and people who need long-term monitoring. IoT provides interaction with billions of healthy objects across the world using the internet. All these health devices generate more and more data from patients. To process the collected data, the cloud data center is the most suitable computing resource. Cloud Computing has been touted as the next-generation architecture for IT companies and offers great capabilities that ensure improved productivity with minimal costs (El Kafhali et al., 2022). This promising technology offers an improved level of flexibility and scalability compared to traditional IT systems. Various features of cloud computing such as on-demand self-service, resource pooling, fast elasticity, a pay-as-you-go pricing model, etc. have prompted more and more companies to embrace the different cloud deployment models, especially healthcare companies. High scalability and flexibility as well as low infrastructure cost enable cloud technology to be widely used in public and different companies. This growing adoption has highlighted the need to improve the computing, storage, and network resources of the cloud environment (Salah & El Kafhali, 2017). Since everything in the cloud is defined as an on-demand service, availability and delay are critical requirements in the cloud environment.

This leads to major problems related to the ability of the cloud to process MIoT-collected data in real-time. To overcome such issues, localized storage and processing need to be done close to the MIoT devices. A very important premise for today's computer systems is the use of fog and edge computing to reduce server load and low latency responses, especially when used in healthcare applications (Kumari et al., 2018). Deploying architectures and models closer to the end devices (fog-based applications) allows low latency and independence from network failures. This chapter aims to provide a rapid review introducing, discussing state-of-the-art, and future perspectives on IoT, cloud, and FC in healthcare. In particular, it will mainly focus on the convergence and utilization of IoT-Fog-Cloud technologies for healthcare monitoring.

The rest of this chapter is structured as follows: Section 4.2 presents a healthcare monitoring system cluster architecture. A detailed description of a healthcare patient monitoring system, using fog and cloud, is described in Section 4.3. Section 4.4 presents the artificial intelligence techniques for healthcare services on the cloud and IoT, and we compare and discuss the different reviewed techniques. Finally, Section 4.5 provides concluding remarks.

4.2 A healthcare monitoring system components

Healthcare monitoring systems are dominating the market of new technologies due to their valuable help to patients, families, and medical staff. They are conceptually a

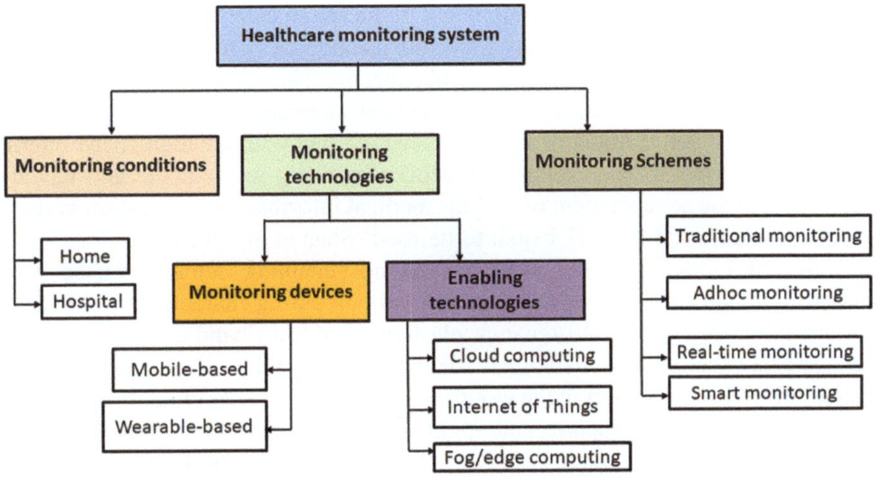

FIGURE 4.1

Healthcare monitoring system components.

series of actions of remote communication over the internet by physicians to predict medical services of higher quality to their patients. They offer ubiquitous health services to patients with specific conditions and can render ubiquitous communication between patients and caregivers. Fig. 4.1 shows healthcare monitoring system components.

4.2.1 Monitoring conditions

Hospitals are the primary battlefield where health employees are directly in contact with infected patients and render treatment. To avoid physical contact, home health care is used to reduce the infection of health workers. In a home health care monitoring system, it is necessary to continuously monitor the patient's health conditions.

4.2.2 Monitoring technologies

Several health care hospitals located in rural areas have no digital systems and keep paper-based systems to function, resulting in patient records being preserved by the patients themselves. The disadvantage of using numerous systems is that it is hard and expensive to develop a national survey of patient statistics. At a more fundamental level, it is highly difficult for single institutions in the health area to share data with each other. With the options available to the health authority to enhance the efficacy and effectiveness of its basic health care delivery process, mobile and wearable technologies offer exciting opportunities for low-cost and high-reaching services. There is strong evidence that mobile and wireless technologies could help address the slow response rates of the existing health system for rural sectors (Gupta & Hasija, 2022).

During the last decade, the development of the health care monitoring system has been mainly characterized by many experiments attempting to apply different computer technologies to solve several medical concerns. The appearance coincides with the advent of modems allowing various medical information to be transmitted via the internet. The replacement of the low-speed internet with the high-speed internet has led to attempts to use corporate videoconferencing in medicine and has also contributed to the advancement of various medical information digitization systems. Cloud computing and the IoT began to be used (Shah et al., 2021).

Today, the cloud-computing system is the most enabling technology used by the healthcare monitoring system. Due to the cloud-computing characteristics including on-demand self-service, multi-tenancy, elasticity, and broadband network access, IT managers face the greatest challenges. Availability of healthcare services is seen as a critical security requirement in the cloud since everything in the cloud is defined as a service. As cloud infrastructure and applications are distributed around the world, this leads to much-anticipated resource scalability challenges. Due to the growth of cloud systems, the health service provider needs to create a large and distributed number of data centers around the world to ensure rapid access to global health customers. This places an increasing demand and usage of the cloud-networking infrastructure. Currently, with the sensitive delay in healthcare applications, the use of small data centers close to customers is needed to respond to the request of this type of application. For this reason, some healthcare systems use fog/edge computing to handle health request applications (Awotunde et al., 2021).

For real-time monitoring, IoT technology is used to collect health data from patients in hospitals over the internet (Kavitha & Ravikumar, 2021). In addition, a wireless sensor network plays a crucial role with IoT in health monitoring systems by deploying sensors that are automatically connected inside and outside of a human body for the health monitoring system. The interconnected sensor network system is known as wireless body area network (WBAN) where the small battery has implanted biomedical sensor nodes that monitor and collect health data. Some advantages and disadvantages of using IoT for remote patient monitoring are presented in Table 4.1.

4.2.3 Monitoring schemes

Using a traditional monitoring scheme, the healthcare monitoring system has complex equipment technology, unstable monitoring operation, and a high cost. High costs make it impossible for large-scale healthcare monitoring system installation. This system can only be installed in key monitoring locations of some key enterprises, thus system data is unavailable to predict the overall health service situation. To overcome defects of traditional monitoring systems and reduce cost, currently, some healthcare enterprises use real-time, smart, or ad hoc monitoring schemes. These new systems have received great consideration in the field of research today because the favors and benefits are not only for the patient but also for the sportsmen, the elderly, the homemakers, and the driving community.

Table 4.1 Advantages and disadvantages of IoT in Healthcare

Advantages	Disadvantages
- With IoT devices, the patient can get remote consultation, which saves the patient's time and the doctor's workload. - The IoT in healthcare provides long-term innovation for researchers. - Wearable devices such as IoT-enabled watches, wristbands, and bracelets are used to transmit health information such as heart rate, blood pressure, pulse rate, sugar level, etc. directly to the doctor. - The IoT simplifies patient engagement to reduce folk remedies and enable remote monitoring of their medication adherence. - The IoT overcomes the problem of the lack of staff to monitor patients with connected technology that oversees patient admission, staff work and predicts patient influx. - IoT in healthcare is an efficient autonomous system that reduces long-term maintenance costs. - With IoT, the healthcare authorities can construct enhanced healthcare management that comprises valuable information about equipment and the effectiveness of staff that helps in innovation. - Flexible availability of medical records allows patients to feel quality care and make the proper decision by the health cloud providers.	- It is required to do essential attention to the privacy portion of the patient's content. - The private health data of the patient needs to be accessed only with an earlier permit from the patient. - Healthcare monitoring system security becomes a challenge in transferring and safeguarding health data. - The patient's information in the healthcare system is centralized to speed up the treatment process. There are opportunities for fraud in accessing the patient's data. - The risk of power failure can have an important effect on the sensor's performance.

4.3 A healthcare patient monitoring system using fog and cloud

Fig. 4.2 shows a typical architecture of a patient monitoring system within a fog-cloudy environment. Wearable devices using wireless body sensors such as smart health watches, electrocardiogram (ECG), fitness bracelets, blood pressure (BLE), electrooculography (EOG), pulse oximeter oxygen saturation (SpO2), temperature, electroencephalography (EEG), electromyography (EMG), location and humidity are designed for the patient to monitor patient health. These wearable MIoT devices are capable of adjusting a person's calorie count, exercise control, drinking water reminder, body mass index, bone density, blood pressure variation,

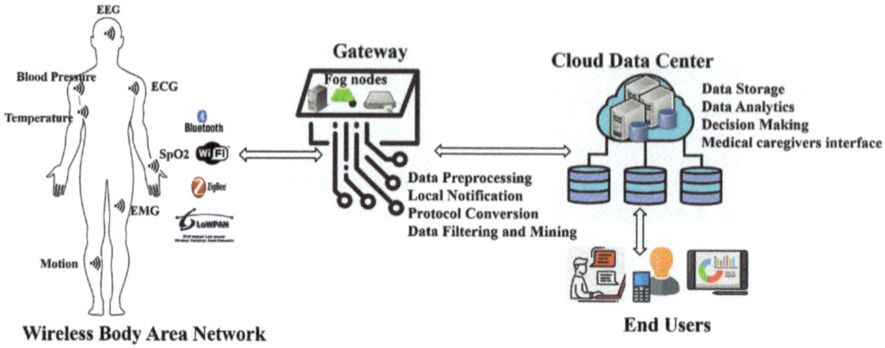

FIGURE 4.2

Typical architecture of patient monitoring system within a fog-cloud environment.

etc. (El Kafhali & Salah, 2019). The health-related data collected by the MIoT devices is transmitted to a fog gateway through a wireless communication protocol such as Wi-Fi, Bluetooth, 6LoWPAN, or ZigBee. The fog gateway is used for communication between the wearable MIoT devices and cloud data center, particularly for sophisticated health data. Fog nodes deployed between MIoT devices and the cloud data center are also used to carry out localized storage and processing to further reduce the response time of the cloud data center. The health data processing by cloud and fog node is permanently visible for any doctor or medical staff from any platform to provide the right treatment to the patient (El Kafhali et al., 2018).

MIoT devices address new healthcare challenges to create excellent support systems for physicians, surgeons, and patients. The different process steps are identified in Fig. 4.2 for effective MIoT implementation in the healthcare monitoring system. Body sensors are used to detect and capture health information regarding a patient's health and receive needed data. All devices are networked and display continuous patient health monitoring. The required health data is well provided to specified physicians as per their requirements via computers, tablets, and mobile devices.

4.3.1 Wireless Body Area Network

The wireless body network (WBAN) can use biometric sensors to monitor a patient's health within the medical facility or remotely. The collected data can be stored either on the patient's mobile and viewed in real-time or periodically by the doctors. This allows patients to live at home while benefiting from remote medical services. Health monitoring systems can simultaneously monitor multiple physiological signals, providing important and comprehensive data for doctors. Another benefit of remote health monitoring is that it dramatically reduces the cost of a hospital bed. The WBAN is used to monitor the patient continuously without strain on the patient's daily activities. Various types of technologies have been developed to assist

WBAN in patient monitoring applications such as remote monitoring, biofeedback, and assisted living to meet their high-quality services (Abdullah and Ur Rehman, 2018). WBAN is made up of different biological sensors. The sensors are attached to various parts of the human body and can be wearable or implanted under the patient's skin. These types of patterns are used to measure various changes in patients' vital signs as well as to determine patient emotions like happiness, fear of stress, etc. The WBAN device can communicate using coordination nodes, which generally consume little energy and have high processing capacities. The WBAN is responsible for sending the patient's biological signals to the caretakers or doctor's clinic for taking the necessary actions (Akkaş et al., 2020).

The WBAN devices convert the analog signal to digital data and the communication between the different WBAN devices and other technologies is accomplished by using different technologies like Bluetooth Low Power, ZigBee, IEEE 802.15.6, 6LoWPAN, and Wi-Fi. WBAN devices communicate with each other using the master node and other particular devices such as home service robots and notebooks. The WBAN can diagnose various diseases and monitor different physiological characteristics of a patient, for example, temperature, humidity, pulse, location, and blood pressure.

WBAN is widely used for healthcare applications as shown in Fig. 4.3. The first WBAN application is the remote control of medical devices such as patient monitoring, remote surgeons, telemedicine, ambient assisted living, and so forth (Taleb et al., 2021). Patient monitoring is the important part that is more and more popular and has previously witnessed attention from the current healthcare monitoring system (Rajagopal et al., 2021). Robotic surgery is another revolutionary trend that

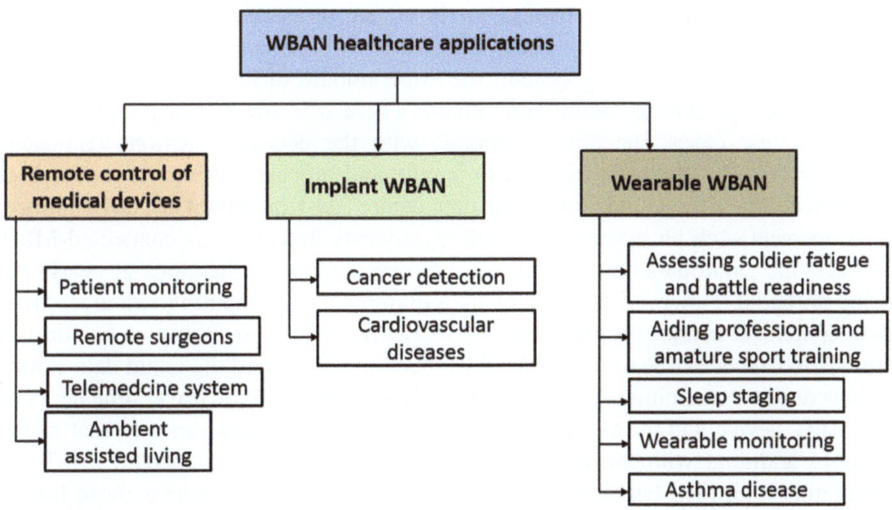

FIGURE 4.3

WBAN healthcare applications.

permits remote surgeons to carry out minimally invasive surgery (Taleb et al., 2021). Ambient assisted living is another field that provides help to older people in living a confident and independent life by developing advanced and original Information and Communication Technology (ICT) based systems, products, and services (Patro et al., 2021).

The second application is the implant WBAN, which includes cancer detection and cardiovascular diseases (Cai et al., 2019). Wearable WBAN is another application that is a concern. For example, assisting soldier fatigue and battle readiness, aiding professional and amateur sports training, sleep staging, wearable monitoring, asthma disease, and so forth (Gupta et al., 2020).

4.3.2 Cloud data center

Along with the development of technology with big data, cloud computing, and artificial intelligence, the use of cloud-computing data centers for processing the collected health data of remote medicine has been considered more important in recent days. In these times, the use of the cloud in the health area is at the center of the scene, since it permits us to store, access, and process enormous volumes of data in real-time, remotely, and diagnose some types of conditions in patients who otherwise would not have received timely medical attention. On the other hand, its impact is increasing on the economies of countries and renders savings to the public and private health sectors (Raghavan et al., 2021).

4.3.3 Fog nodes

Currently, the use of IoT in the healthcare system is increasing in our daily life, which means that the MIoT devices involved are producing massive amounts of health data every second from patients in hospitals (Hassan et al., 2020). Usually, in the healthcare monitoring system, the huge amount of health data collected by MIoT devices is sent to cloud data centers where it is stored and processed and, in certain use cases, the cloud responds with the necessary actions (Elhoseny et al., 2021). The current way used to handle and process these great amounts of generated data is the cloud computing data center (Al-Khafajiy et al., 2018). Moreover, to meet such an immense amount of requests from various connected MIoT devices, the cloud data centers will need to operate around the clock at nearly the same potential. However, because of its requirement of computing resources from data centers, it cannot become possible to easily do the processing of health data from MIoT devices due to the distance between the MIoT and the cloud data center. This is due to the minimal delay required by health data, and the travel time between the MIoT device and the cloud data center could affect the relevance of that health data. In addition, with the ever-increasing number of cloud-connected MIoT devices, this issue will become more prominent. Therefore, to address these issues, the FC paradigm is placed closer to MIoT terminals. If introduced successfully, FC can lead to quality of service (QoS) improvements offered to systems that require the processing of delay-sensitive health data that could benefit from the rapid processing of patient data to allow patient monitoring.

4.4 Artificial intelligence for healthcare services on cloud and Internet of Things

4.4.1 Artificial intelligence for healthcare on cloud and Internet of Things

To date, the cloud-computing paradigm plays a significant role in healthcare services due to its capability to enhance healthcare request performance. However, finding the optimal selection of virtual machines (VMs) in a cloud data center to process a healthcare request is a big issue. Optimal VMs selection maximizes the utilization of cloud resources and makes an important enhancement of the cloud performance that reduces the execution time of healthcare requests coming from patients, medical staff, doctors, and so forth (Hanini et al., 2019). Traditional and static algorithms for VMs selection and consolidation do not give important performance, especially for healthcare requests, which are very sensitive to delay (El Kafhali & Salah, 2018). Accordingly, it is critical for the healthcare service providers to determine automatically the optimal number of VMs required for handling the healthcare requests automatically at a very reasonable time. Therefore, the artificial intelligence approach can solve this problem by providing real-time monitoring of the daily health activities of patients, especially for elderly citizens (El Kafhali & El Mir, 2022). Several papers in the literature use machine-learning models for improving healthcare services in the cloud-computing environment. For instance, the authors (Abdelaziz et al., 2018) proposed a machine-learning model for healthcare services based on the cloud to optimize the VMs selection. They also proposed a model for chronic kidney disease diagnosis and prediction based on linear regression and neural networks to measure the performance of the proposed algorithm. The results obtained showed that the proposed model outperforms the existing models in total execution time at a rate of 50%.

Hassan et al. (2018) proposed an intelligent hybrid architecture for patient monitoring that adopts a model with both local and cloud-based components. The cloud part of the architecture is used to monitor patients suffering from chronic diseases at home, especially the elderly. The local part monitors the patients in the case of internet disconnection or other cloud system failure. A case study on patients suffering from blood pressure disorders is provided to demonstrate the effectiveness of the proposed model. The authors (Abdelaziz et al., 2018) predicted chronic kidney diseases in a cloud-computing environment. For that, they proposed a hybrid intelligent model-based IoT and Cloud Computing in Smart Cities using two machine-learning techniques, which are linear regression and neural network. The obtained results showed that the accuracy of the model in predicting chronic kidney diseases is 97.8%. During the SARS-CoV-2 pandemic, cloud-based machine learning-assisted services were used to identify the cases of SARS-CoV-2 virus coronavirus. For instance, the authors (Whitelaw et al., 2020) used cloud-based tools for screening and alerting the authorities if quarantine is breached. IoT technology offers a very good way to detect the infected patient and helps to maintain proper supervision with real-time data (El Kafhali & Salah, 2017).

Thanks to this technology, all medical devices are connected to the internet and provide timely information to health providers that allow them to easily treat infected cases remotely (Otoom et al., 2020). Today, IoT technology is used in many situations to help patients, doctors, healthcare providers, and hospital management to recognize the symptoms of the COVID-19 virus and manage infected cases around the world. IoT also helps to minimize the time and complexity required to manage effectively the COVID-19 virus during this pandemic. Besides, IoT technology provides a diversity of health applications such as telehealth, digital digitization, digital workforce, and many more. IoT-based telemedicine is an important way for healthcare providers during this pandemic time to provide treatment for patients infected with COVID-19. The authors in Singh et al. (2020) proposed an IoT-based framework to minimize the impact of the communicable COVID-19 virus. The records of confirmed cases of COVID-19 are used to develop a machine-learning-based predictive model of infection as well as provide and monitor the treatment responses. Many other cloud-IoT-based artificial Intelligence-assisted healthcare applications (Abdelaziz et al., 2018; Alghamdi et al., 2020; Arjun & Anto, 2015; Azghadi et al., 2020; Bhatia et al., 2020; El-Rashidy et al., 2020; Hossain et al., 2020; Patro et al., 2021; Prerana et al., 2015; Rahman et al., 2020; Sharma, 2016; Tintu & Paulin, 2013), which can be summarized in Table 4.2.

4.4.2 Artificial intelligence technology for clinical diagnosis

Many artificial intelligence methods have been used for disease detection and diagnosis. Some have been more effective than others, principally depending on the type of disease. Deep learning is a suitable method for diagnosing pathology by imaging tissue slides. To handle complex biological data, including omics (transcriptomics and genomics data), medical and clinical data; Bayesian probabilistic modeling has proven to be a suitable method. For general multimodal issues, such as prediction of clinical outcomes, patient assessments, and risk prediction, artificial intelligence methods based on domain knowledge are greater appropriate choices. Methods based on natural language processing can help clinicians to predict Alzheimer's disease within healthy people before it develops for early intervention to preserve cognitive ability and quality of life. However, there are many issues with artificial intelligence techniques to consider when applying them clinically for disease diagnosis.

The serious issue is overfitting, which is a real problem with every artificial intelligence prediction algorithm. Overfitting takes place when the prediction

Table 4.2 Summary of existing cloud-IoT-based machine learning-assisted healthcare applications.

Authors	Applications	Intelligent algorithms
Abdelaziz et al. (2018)	Application to find the optimal choice of VM consolidation in a cloud environment to set up patients' records, disease diagnosis, and other medical areas in less time and lower cost.	Genetic algorithm (GA), particle swarm optimization (PSO), and parallel particle swarm optimization (PPSO).
Sharma (2016)	Model to predict cervical cancer disease of the patients.	Decision tree.
Alghamdi et al. (2020)	Medical IIoT based model for smart urban healthcare centers.	Convolution neural network.
Arjun and Anto (2015)	Method for diagnosis of diabetes disease.	Support vector machine.
Prerana et al. (2015)	Model to predict patient's disease on Google App Engine.	Naive Bayes.
Tintu and Paulin (2013)	A framework to detect breast cancer.	Fuzzy logic.
Azghadi et al. (2020)	Medical IIoT based model for biomedical and healthcare practitioners.	Spiking neural network.
Rahman et al. (2020)	COVID-19 diagnosis-based framework to meaningful visualization of the principal decision-making activities that exploit the low-latency and high-bandwidth features provided by 5G at the edge of the network.	Deep learning.
Hossain et al. (2020)	5G-enabled health care framework to control and manage the COVID-19 epidemic.	ResNet50, deep tree, and Inception v3.
Patro et al. (2021)	IoT based framework for predicting heart disease using key risk factors.	K-nearest neighbors, support vector machine, Lasso, Naive Bayes, and ridge regression.
El-Rashidy et al. (2020)	Fog-cloud-based framework for COVID-19 detection and monitoring.	Convolutional neural network
Bhatia et al. (2020)	Fog-cloud computing-based framework for domestic animal healthcare.	Data mining technique

algorithm works unusually well on the training data, but very poorly on testing clinical data. In this case, the physician may not have a correct diagnosis; this may therefore affect the treatment performance of the patient. There are various ways to recognize and solve the issue of overfitting. First, if the diagnosis accuracy changes dramatically when the artificial intelligence algorithm is applied to the new clinical data set, we need to stop training. Second, the quality of the fit test can estimates how well the predicted values of the algorithm return the observed true values. Third, when we have the choice between diverse comparable algorithms, we can favor the simpler ones among others to avoid any complexity of the model. Finally, we can further reduce the issue of overfitting by a sampling method including cross-validation that repeatedly partitions the sample clinical data to validate the prediction of the model internally. The important result to overcome the disadvantages of a single method is the combination of different approaches based on artificial intelligence algorithms. For example, where data knowledge is lacking, the use of Bayesian reasoning networks in combination with deep learning that forms Bayesian deep learning is believed to have great potential.

4.5 Conclusion

Current developments in information and communication technologies, such as the IoT and FC, allow us to develop emerging health solutions with greater intelligent capabilities and prediction both for daily life at home and in hospitals. In the case of the healthcare system, we talk about MIoT devices that are usually equipped with body sensors, which sense and generate data for several health applications, such as hospital management, medical imaging, and patient healthcare monitoring. MIoT consists of cloud data centers and cloud extended FC nodes, delivering distributed IoT-based services to healthcare applications. However, due to the computation and storage constraints of IoT devices, the cloud platform has become the preferred solution to process the generated health data. In this chapter, we have explored the effectiveness of IoT-Fog-Cloud architecture for the healthcare monitoring system. Some existing approaches in the literature that used the IoT-Fog-Cloud system to evaluate patient healthcare monitoring systems are reviewed and presented. We have identified the role and advantage of MIoT and FC from the perspective of IoT-Fog-Cloud models for the healthcare monitoring system. This chapter concludes by presenting some advantages of using artificial intelligence technology for clinical diagnosis in healthcare.

References

Abdelaziz, A., Elhoseny, M., Salama, A. S., & Riad, A. M. (2018). A machine learning model for improving healthcare services on cloud computing environment. *Measurement, 119*, 117–128. https://doi.org/10.1016/j.measurement.2018.01.022

Abdelaziz, A., Elhoseny, M., Salama, A. S., Riad, A. M., & Hassanien, A. E. (2018). Intelligent algorithms for optimal selection of virtual machine in cloud environment, towards enhance healthcare services. *Advances in Intelligent Systems and Computing, 639*, 289–298. https://doi.org/10.1007/978-3-319-64861-3_27

Abdelaziz, A., Salama, A. S., Riad, A. M., & Mahmoud, A. N. (2018). *A machine learning model for predicting of chronic kidney disease based internet of things and cloud computing in smart cities* (pp. 93−114). Springer Science and Business Media LLC. https://doi.org/10.1007/978-3-030-01560-2_5

Akkaş, M. A., Sokullu, R., & Ertürk Çetin, H. (2020). Healthcare and patient monitoring using IoT. *Internet of Things, 11*, 100173. https://doi.org/10.1016/j.iot.2020.100173

Al-Khafajiy, M., Webster, L., Baker, T., & Waraich, A. (2018). Towards fog driven IoT healthcare: Challenges and framework of fog computing in healthcare. *ACM International Conference Proceeding Series*, 1−7. https://doi.org/10.1145/3231053.3231062

Alghamdi, A., Hammad, M., Ugail, H., Abdel-Raheem, A., Muhammad, K., Khalifa, H. S., & Abd El-Latif, A. A. (2020). Detection of myocardial infarction based on novel deep transfer learning methods for urban healthcare in smart cities. *Multimedia Tools and Applications*, 1−22. https://doi.org/10.1007/s11042-020-08769-x

Abdullah, I., & Ur Rehman, S. (2018). Wireless body area networks for child healthcare monitoring: A review. In *Proceedings of the 21st international multi topic conference, INMIC 2018, 1−8*. https://doi.org/10.1109/INMIC.2018.8595655

Arjun, C., & Anto, M. (2015). Diagnosis of diabetes using support vector machine and ensemble learning approach. *International Journal of Engineering and Applied Sciences, 2*(11), 68−72.

Awotunde, J. B., Bhoi, A. K., & Barsocchi, P. (2021). Hybrid cloud/fog environment for healthcare: An exploratory study, opportunities, challenges, and future prospects. *In Intelligent Systems Reference Library, 209*, 1−20. https://doi.org/10.1007/978-981-16-2972-3_1. Springer Science and Business Media Deutschland GmbH.

Azghadi, M. R., Lammie, C., Eshraghian, J. K., Payvand, M., Donati, E., Linares-Barranco, B., & Indiveri, G. (2020). Hardware implementation of deep network accelerators towards healthcare and biomedical applications. *IEEE Transactions on Biomedical Circuits and Systems, 14*(6), 1138−1159. https://doi.org/10.1109/TBCAS.2020.3036081

Bang, A. O., & Rao, U. P. (2021). *Context-aware computing for IoT: History, applications and research challenges*. Springer Science and Business Media LLC. https://doi.org/10.1007/978-981-15-6707-0_70

Bhatia, M., Sood, S. K., & Manocha, A. (2020). Fog-inspired smart home environment for domestic animal healthcare. *Computer Communications, 160*, 521−533. https://doi.org/10.1016/j.comcom.2020.07.004

Cai, G., Fang, Y., Wen, J., Han, G., & Yang, X. (2019). QoS-Aware buffer-aided relaying implant WBAN for healthcare IoT: Opportunities and challenges. *IEEE Network, 33*(4), 96−103. https://doi.org/10.1109/MNET.2019.1800405

El Kafhali, S., El Mir, I., & Hanini, M. (2022). Security threats, defense mechanisms, challenges, and future directions in cloud computing. *Archives of Computational Methods in Engineering, 29*(1), 223−246. https://doi.org/10.1007/s11831-021-09573-y

El Kafhali, S., & El Mir, I. (2022). Artificial intelligence-based diseases detection and diagnosis. In *Healthcare monitoring and data Analysis using IoT: Technologies and applications* (pp. 371−387). United Kingdom: IET Press.

El Kafhali, S., & Lazaar, M. (2021). *Artificial intelligence for healthcare: Roles, challenges, and applications* (pp. 141−156). Springer Science and Business Media LLC. https://doi.org/10.1007/978-3-030-72588-4_10

El Kafhali, S., & Salah, K. (2017). Efficient and dynamic scaling of fog nodes for IoT devices. *The Journal of Supercomputing, 73*(12), 5261−5284. https://doi.org/10.1007/s11227-017-2083-x

El Kafhali, S., Salah, K., & Ben Alla, S. (2018). Performance evaluation of IoT-fog-cloud deployment for healthcare services. In *4th international conference on cloud computing technologies and applications (cloudtech), 1–6*. https://doi.org/10.1109/CloudTech.2018.8713355

El Kafhali, S., & Salah, K. (2018). Modeling and analysis of performance and energy consumption in cloud data centers. *Arabian Journal for Science and Engineering, 43*(12), 7789–7802. https://doi.org/10.1007/s13369-018-3196-0

El Kafhali, S., & Salah, K. (2019). Performance modelling and analysis of Internet of Things enabled healthcare monitoring systems. *IET Networks, 8*(1), 48–58. https://doi.org/10.1049/iet-net.2018.5067

El-Rashidy, N., El-Sappagh, S., Islam, S. M. R., El-Bakry, H. M., & Abdelrazek, S. (2020). End-to-end deep learning framework for coronavirus (COVID-19) detection and monitoring. *Electronics, 9*(9), 1439. https://doi.org/10.3390/electronics9091439

Elhoseny, M., Thilakarathne, N. N., Alghamdi, M. I., Mahendran, R. K., Gardezi, A. A., Weerasinghe, H., & Welhenge, A. (2021). Security and privacy issues in medical internet of things: Overview, countermeasures, challenges and future directions. *Sustainability (Switzerland), 13*(21). https://doi.org/10.3390/su132111645

Gupta, A., & Hasija, Y. (2022). Next generation 5G wireless technologies in healthcare. *In Smart Innovation, Systems and Technologies, 248*, 393–402. https://doi.org/10.1007/978-981-16-4177-0_40. Springer Science and Business Media Deutschland GmbH.

Gupta, A., Tripathi, M., & Sharma, A. (2020). A provably secure and efficient anonymous mutual authentication and key agreement protocol for wearable devices in WBAN. *Computer Communications, 160*, 311–325. https://doi.org/10.1016/j.comcom.2020.06.010

Hanini, M., El Kafhali, S., & Salah, K. (2019). Dynamic VM allocation and traffic control to manage QoS and energy consumption in cloud computing environment. *International Journal of Computer Applications in Technology, 60*(4), 307–316. https://doi.org/10.1504/IJCAT.2019.101168

Hassan, S. R., Ahmad, I., Ahmad, S., Alfaify, A., & Shafiq, M. (2020). Remote pain monitoring using fog computing for e-healthcare: An efficient architecture. *Sensors, 20*(22), 6574. https://doi.org/10.3390/s20226574

Hassan, M. K., El Desouky, A. I., Elghamrawy, S. M., & Sarhan, A. M. (2018). Intelligent hybrid remote patient-monitoring model with cloud-based framework for knowledge discovery. *Computers and Electrical Engineering, 70*, 1034–1048. https://doi.org/10.1016/j.compeleceng.2018.02.032

Horwitz, L. (2021). Internet of things (IoT). *The future of IoT miniguide: The burgeoning IoT market continues*. https://www.cisco.com/c/en/us/solutions/internet-of-things/future-of-iot.html.

Hossain, M. S., Muhammad, G., & Guizani, N. (2020). Explainable AI and mass surveillance system-based healthcare framework to combat COVID-I9 like pandemics. *IEEE Network, 34*(4), 126–132. https://doi.org/10.1109/mnet.011.2000458

Kavitha, D., & Ravikumar, S. (2021). IOT and context-aware learning-based optimal neural network model for real-time health monitoring. *Transactions on Emerging Telecommunications Technologies, 32*(1). https://doi.org/10.1002/ett.4132

Kumari, A., Tanwar, S., Tyagi, S., & Kumar, N. (2018). Fog computing for Healthcare 4.0 environment: Opportunities and challenges. *Computers and Electrical Engineering, 72*, 1–13. https://doi.org/10.1016/j.compeleceng.2018.08.015

Miettinen, M., Nguyen, T. D., Sadeghi, A. R., & Asokan, N. (2018). Revisiting context-based authentication in IoT. In *Proceedings—design automation conference, 137710*. https://doi.org/10.1145/3195970.3196106

Otoom, M., Otoum, N., Alzubaidi, M. A., Etoom, Y., & Banihani, R. (2020). An IoT-based framework for early identification and monitoring of COVID-19 cases. *Biomedical Signal Processing and Control, 62*, 102149. https://doi.org/10.1016/j.bspc.2020.102149

Patro, S. P., Padhy, N., & Chiranjevi, D. (2021). Ambient assisted living predictive model for cardiovascular disease prediction using supervised learning. *Evolutionary Intelligence, 14*(2), 941—969. https://doi.org/10.1007/s12065-020-00484-8

Prerana, T. H. M., Shivaprakash, N. C., & Swetha, N. (2015). Prediction of heart disease using machine learning algorithms-Naïve Bayes, introduction to PAC algorithm, comparison of algorithms and HDPS. *International Journal of Science and Engineering, 3*(2), 90—99.

Raghavan, A., Demircioglu, M. A., & Taeihagh, A. (2021). Public health innovation through cloud adoption: A comparative analysis of drivers and barriers in Japan, South Korea, and Singapore. *International Journal of Environmental Research and Public Health, 18*(1), 1—30. https://doi.org/10.3390/ijerph18010334

Rahman, M. A., Hossain, M. S., Alrajeh, N. A., & Guizani, N. (2020). B5G and explainable deep learning assisted healthcare vertical at the edge: COVID-I9 perspective. *IEEE Network, 34*(4), 98—105. https://doi.org/10.1109/MNET.011.2000353

Rajagopal, A., Geetha, N. A. P. D. K., & Swathi, J. (2021). *Remote health monitoring system for multiple patients using WSN and NFC. Design engineering* (pp. 14370—14380).

Salah, K., & El Kafhali, S. (2017). Performance modeling and analysis of hypoexponential network servers. *Telecommunication Systems, 65*(4), 717—728. https://doi.org/10.1007/s11235-016-0262-3

Selvaraj, R., Kuthadi, V. M., Baskar, S., Shakeel, P. M., & Ranjan, A. (2021). Creating security modelling framework analysing in internet of things using EC-GSM-IoT. *Arabian Journal for Science and Engineering*, 1—13. https://doi.org/10.1007/s13369-021-05887-y

Shah, J. L., Bhat, H. F., & Khan, A. I. (2021). *Integration of cloud and IoT for smart e-healthcare* (pp. 101—136). Elsevier BV. https://doi.org/10.1016/b978-0-12-819664-9.00006-5

Sharma, S. (2016). Cervical cancer stage prediction using decision tree approach of machine learning. *International Journal of Advanced Research in Computer and Communication Engineering, 5*(4), 345—348.

Singh, R. P., Javaid, M., Haleem, A., & Suman, R. (2020). Internet of things (IoT) applications to fight against COVID-19 pandemic. *Diabetes and Metabolic Syndrome: Clinical Research and Reviews, 14*(4), 521—524. https://doi.org/10.1016/j.dsx.2020.04.041

Taleb, H., Nasser, A., Andrieux, G., Charara, N., & Motta Cruz, E. (2021). Wireless technologies, medical applications and future challenges in WBAN: A survey. *Wireless Networks, 27*(8), 5271—5295. https://doi.org/10.1007/s11276-021-02780-2

Tintu, P. B., & Paulin, R. (2013). Detect breast cancer using fuzzy C means techniques in Wisconsin prognostic breast cancer (WPBC) data sets. *International Journal of Computer Applications Technology and Research*, 614—617. https://doi.org/10.7753/IJCATR0205.1017

Wei, X. (2021). Research on the health of senior citizens from an interdisciplinary perspective: Framework, core topics, and prospects. *China Population and Development Studies, 5*(4), 345—362. https://doi.org/10.1007/s42379-021-00098-2

Whitelaw, S., Mamas, M. A., Topol, E., & Van Spall, H. G. C. (2020). Applications of digital technology in COVID-19 pandemic planning and response. *The Lancet Digital Health, 2*(8), e435—e440. https://doi.org/10.1016/S2589-7500(20)30142-4

CHAPTER

Patients using real-time remote health monitoring applications: a review

5

Shariq Aziz Butt[1], Arshad Ali[2], Abbas Khalid[1], Qaisar Shaheen[3], Paola Ariza-Colpas[4], Muhammad Shiraz[5]

[1]*Department of Computer Science, The University of Lahore, Lahore, Pakistan;* [2]*Department of Computer Science, FAST University, Lahore, Pakistan;* [3]*Department of Computer Science, University of South Asia, Lahore, Pakistan;* [4]*Universidad De la Costa, CUC Barranquilla, Colombia;* [5]*Department of Computer Science, Federal Urdu University of Arts, Sciences and Technology, Islamabad, Pakistan*

5.1 Introduction

Due to telemedicine's many advantages, including the ability to provide patients with health-related knowledge and provide remote medical services, telemedicine is being employed more and more in the healthcare industry. The practice of medicine known as telemedicine involves several healthcare professionals working together remotely to diagnose or cure patients. Patients receiving treatment and support from doctors or experts who travel to see them can benefit from remote healthcare services if they reside in remote areas or rural areas. Through the use of information technology and connectivity, telemedicine enables collaboration between many people and facilitates their collaborative efforts to diagnose or treat an illness. Therefore, multidisciplinary advancements are required in this field, especially in the application of mobile health monitoring and hardware for the sharing and monitoring of health data.

Since mHealth is important from both social and economic perspectives, in this study, we discuss the existing frameworks that have been developed for patient monitoring. This study thoroughly analyzes such frameworks and mentions their limitations for the research community to propose novel health models. This study also scrutinizes the existing mobile health applications that are developed per guidelines of such frameworks. The main goal of this study is to conduct a review analysis of existing frameworks and highlight factors that must be kept in mind before suggesting any new contribution to mobile health monitoring. Patient prioritizing difficulties and open issues in remote health monitoring system (RHMS) applications need to be investigated further, as shown in Fig. 5.1.

Computational Intelligence for Medical Internet of Things (MIoT) Applications
https://doi.org/10.1016/B978-0-323-99421-7.00016-7

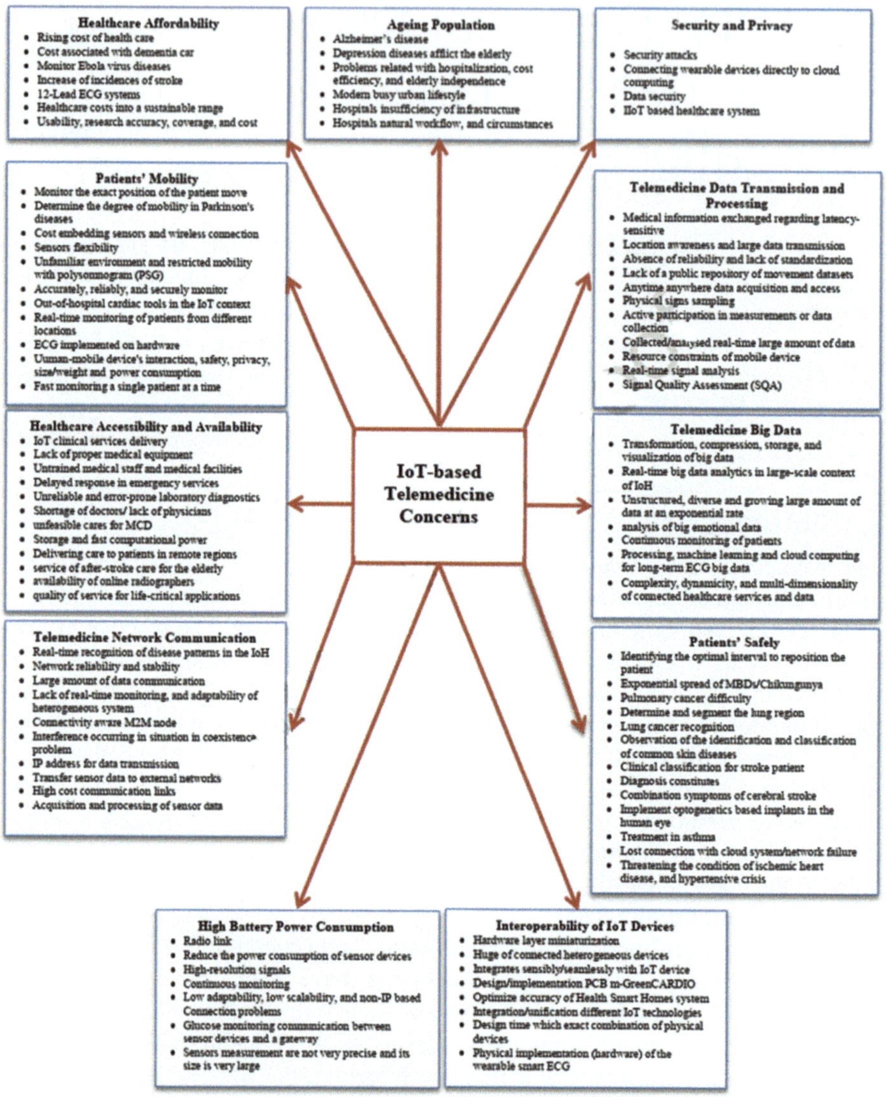

FIGURE 5.1

Overall background of telemedicine (Ali et al., 2021).

5.2 Significance of study

Medical research is now moving from conventional health monitoring trends to advanced technologic health monitoring. Medical research needs more advanced and smart health monitoring ways to monitor the patients and enhance their life span. One of the ways is telemedicine that enables the patient and doctor to be connected for health monitoring. In telemedicine, a doctor can remotely monitor any chronic disease patient such as a heart patient. Currently, the revolutions in the mobile industry have boosted telemedicine due to the easy availability of mobile and wearable devices at a nominal cost. These revolutions made the medical domain smarter and more technical. In this study, we have scrutinized these technical frameworks suggested by the research community in medical research. We have comprehensively studied and analyzed such frameworks. Moreover, we have analyzed the mobile health applications developed by the researchers according to their frameworks. This study highlights the limitations of the existing frameworks in medical research. The findings of the review provide numerous open challenges to researchers to propose new novel frameworks. These frameworks would be more advanced with novel, unique features.

5.3 Comprehensive study of remote health monitoring

The internet of things (IoT) has grown exponentially during the past few years due to rapid growth in wireless sensor network (WSN) technology. It enables remote connectivity of smart devices (i.e., mobiles, sensors) and smart applications to the internet. Smart devices are defined as electronic gadgets that can connect, share, and interact with their users and other devices. The connectivity of smart devices is growing exponentially due to low cost as well as the easy availability of the internet. The availability of smart devices plays a remarkable role in the new era of mobile health (mHealth) monitoring, which has evolved from eHealth monitoring (Sega et al., 2022; Salazar et al., 2021).

Due to advancements in mobile health (mHealth) and awareness of the patients with the technologies, the health domain is introducing different innovative technologies. These technologies include sensors, wearable devices, and smart health applications. The main reason for the development of such technologies is a direct link with human life. Currently, remote health monitoring is growing under the umbrella of digital health monitoring. Digital health is defined as disease monitoring with the use of technologies, e.g., wearable devices and smart applications (Calvillo-Arbizu et al., 2021; Dang et al., 2019). mHealth is facilitating the monitoring of different diseases remotely. mHealth needs different kinds of smart mobile-based applications for monitoring of disease and should take appropriate actions during any abnormality (Ali et al., 2021; Butt, Jamal, et al., 2019).

The phrase "telemedicine" is not clearly defined. Several researchers use the term "telemedicine" purely in the meaning deriving from the syllable "tele," referring to the practice of medical care "remotely," which frequently entails a conversation among a patient and a doctor who is located elsewhere through using a teleconference connection. Conversely, several others define telemedicine as "quick accessibility of distributed and distant healthcare knowledge using telecommunications and data technology," regardless of where the patients or relevant data are located: (1) the Science Direct database, which provides access to scientific knowledge, future technologies, and articles from highly reputable journals; (2) the IEEE Xplore Library, which contains scientific papers in health monitoring and technologies for remote patient monitoring; and (3) the Web of Science (WoS). The objective of this collection is to include scientific and technical publications and to provide a comprehensive view of researchers' work throughout a broad yet significant variety of disciplines (Sarker, 2019a, 2019b; Temdee & Prasad, 2018). Looking for existing literature, followed by three phases of screening and filtering, is how studies are chosen. Using the Mendeley software, a first iteration eliminates duplicated publications and gathers only publications from the recent 6 years (2017–21). The second iteration removes items from our domain by filtering the reading titles and abstracts. Finally, as shown in Fig. 5.2, the third phase includes the complete paper reading and excludes papers that are not in our domain or do not meet our criteria. The same qualifying criteria are applied in all rounds, followed by filtering and assessing. A study is performed using the search boxes in the Science Direct, IEEE Xplore, and WoS databases. We used a set of words that included "medical system," "telemonitoring," "e-health," "telemedicine," "tele-health," "healthcare services," "remote monitoring," and "mobile medical physicians" in various combinations linked by

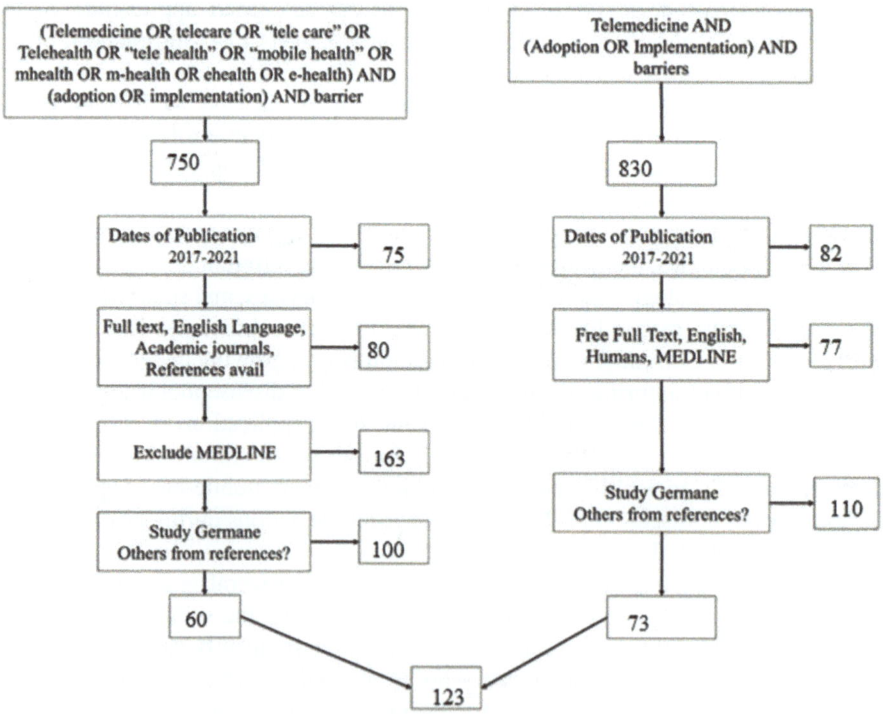

FIGURE 5.2

Methodology applied with inclusion and exclusion criteria.

the operators "OR" and "AND", followed by "triage"; and "priority" in various combinations linked by the operators "OR" and "AND." Fig. 5.2 shows the precise query text at the top (Asam et al., 2019; Hilbert et al., 2021).

5.3.1 IoT in healthcare

In the field of supply management, Ashton (2009) provided the first definition of the term IoT in 1999. Today, different IoT concepts can be addressed, such as a complex network of uniquely addressable and identifiable objects. These devices establish connections with computers to transport data and extract priceless information that effectively delivers the necessary services. In other words, the IoT is made up of countless items and devices, including a variety of sensors and actuators, that connect to and communicate with each other online.

The term "internet of things" refers to an idea that connects everyone, everything, everywhere, at any time, with any service, over any network. The IoT is a huge phenomenon in next-generation advanced technology that has the potential to have a significant impact on all business sectors. It can be conceptualized as the linkage of individually identifiable intelligent devices and objects with improvements within the current internet infrastructure. Advantages frequently have included sophisticated machine-to-machine (M2M) scenarios with explicit connectivity of various devices, platforms, and applications.

The IoT paradigm now encompasses a wide range of applications, including those in transportation, smart cities, tracking, healthcare, etc. The data in IoT applications like smart cities or smart homes are easily connected, aggregated, and analyzed to be customized to people's requirements despite the heterogeneity of IoT devices. For instance, the IoT paradigm's introduction in the healthcare sector has the potential to improve sanitary systems. It can be crucial in telemonitoring at the hospital, particularly for elderly people with chronic illnesses who live at home. The use of this technology will have a significant impact on healthcare systems in the future, resulting in high-quality care, affordable hospitalization, and increased life expectancy. Furthermore, adding automation is feasible in almost every industry. Smart cities, traffic congestion, environmental services, architectural health, security, emergency personnel, logistics, retailing, industrial equipment, and medical services are just a few of the sectors for which the IoT offers adequate solutions. For a more comprehensive explanation of the IoT, the interested reader is directed to the literature (Alavi et al., 2018; Bajaj et al., 2021; Dang et al., 2019; Sarker, 2019a, 2019b).

One of the most alluring IoT application domains is the medical and healthcare sector (Moore & Pham, 2019). Numerous medical technologies, including remote health monitoring, fitness initiatives, chronic illnesses, and elder care, have the potential to emerge as a result of the IoT. Another significant potential use is ensuring that patients follow their healthcare providers' instructions regarding treatment and medication. As a result, different medical gadgets, sensors, and diagnostics and imaging equipment can be seen as smart objects or gadgets that form a crucial component of the IoT. Healthcare services powered by the IoT are anticipated to lower costs, improve quality of life, and improve user experience. The IoT has the potential to decrease device availability by remote provision, according to healthcare professionals.

Additionally, the IoT can accurately pinpoint the best times to replace supplies for different devices to maintain continuous and efficient performance. The IoT also makes it possible to schedule scarce resources effectively by ensuring that they are used to serve more patients. Emerging changes in healthcare are seen in Pimenidis et al. (2019). A significant trend is the ease of cost-effective exchanges between patients, hospitals, and healthcare providers using continuous and secure communication. Modern healthcare networks powered by wireless technology are anticipated to enable medical emergencies, early identification of chronic diseases, and ongoing real-time monitoring. To create healthcare data and provide on-demand healthcare services to approved stakeholders, portals, medical servers, and health systems are essential tools.

Researchers have been paying close attention to this area in recent years as they attempt to understand the possibilities of the IoT within the healthcare industry by taking into account a variety of practical issues. As a result, there are currently many apps, services, and prototypes available. Architectures, interfaces, and new applications development are just a few of the existing researches in IoT-based healthcare. In addition, several nations and organizations across the globe have set standards for the use of IoT technologies throughout the medical profession. Furthermore, the IoT is still in its early stages in the healthcare industry. Different stakeholders with an interest in the healthcare IoT are likely to benefit at this stage from having a comprehensive awareness of the current research on this subject (Amft et al., 2020; de Matos et al., 2020; Hecht et al., 2019).

Several experts and companies are focusing on the creation of IoT-based solutions for healthcare uses in an effort to maximize the potential of IoT in medical systems. The purpose of this study is to give a systematic overview of technologic solutions and smart health monitoring devices as well as a summary of the development and history of cutting-edge studies in IoT-based medical systems. Specifically, the concepts and effective implementation include data planning, knowledge management, and ontology-based resource planning (Bagdasaryan et al., 2019; Dagadu & Li, 2018; Elleithy, 2021; Hecht et al., 2019; Thanigaivelan et al., 2018).

Furthermore, IoT-based smart treatment has been launched to help with the issue of limited resources forced by an aging population. It can be seen as a component of the smart city. To accomplish medical tasks like diagnostics, tracking, and distant procedures over the internet, an IoT-based medical system combines all of the resources available as a system.

The integration of monitoring devices, the public interface of which is handled as a system administrator, has seen extensive use of wireless technology. The system links patients with all of the community-based healthcare resources (such as hospitals, medical clinics, physicians, nurses, ambulances, devices, etc.). There is a consolidated database on the server. An intermediate processing proxy is in charge of data analysis, aggregation, the identification of major events, and the development of recovery plans (Al-Sharhan et al., 2019; Asam & Ajaz, 2019; Babalola et al., 2021; Kakria et al., 2015).

The IoT healthcare concept has been developing over time. The paradigm is divided into three sections: things, server, and master (García-Magariño et al., 2018). Doctors, nurses, and patients who have been granted access to the system specifically via end-user devices are considered master (e.g., smartphone, PC, or tablet). The focal point of the entire healthcare system is sever. It is responsibility of creating prescriptions, managing knowledge bases, managing databases, analyzing data, and building subsystems. Things are any physical items linked to a WAN, using multimedia technologies, or using Short Message Service (SMS), involving patients and human resources.

5.3.2 IoT healthcare services

These consist of internet services, cross-connectivity interfaces for embedded systems, sharing of resources facilities, notification services, and connection technologies for significant connectivity. This listing can be expanded to include the simple, quick, secure, and low-power identification of devices and services.

- **Ambient assisted living (AAL)**

Neither a standard IoT-based medical service nor a smart home is generally intended to provide specialized services to elderly people. In other words, a unique IoT service is required. AAL is an IoT platform that uses intelligent technology to handle the healthcare needs of elderly and disabled people.

AAL is designed to give older people in their homes a comfortable, safe extension of their independent lives. Solutions offered by AAL services can boost elderly people's confidence by enabling better autonomy and providing them with help similar to that of a human servant in the case of an emergency.

AAL depending on the IoT has been discussed in several papers. For IoT-based AAL, a modular design for automation, safety, management, and communication is suggested in Babalola et al. (2021). This infrastructure essentially acts as a foundation for giving older and disabled people access to healthcare services. Radio frequency identification and near-field communications are required for active connectivity, whereas 6LoWPAN is the enabling infrastructure for executing this system.

- **Internet of mhealth things (m-IoT)**

Mobile computers, medical sensors, and communication systems are all that constitute mhealth in terms of healthcare services. Theoretically, the m-IoT introduces a revolutionary healthcare networking model that links the upcoming web-based mobile devices with health services. Although the m-IoT typically represents the IoT for medical care, it is important to note that some particular features are inherent to the users' worldwide mobility.

The installation, programming, testing and screening, and release are the four fundamental processes in creating an android application (app). On other platforms, generally speaking, similar strategies are used. To ensure an app of acceptable quality, an approved body or association of medical specialists is often necessary to participate in the development of mHealth apps. Regular improvements to healthcare apps that take into account the most recent developments in medical science are also essential. The IoT-based healthcare network must be able to accommodate patient mobility so that they can interact at any time and any place. The connection between various patient surroundings is finally made possible by this mobility feature.

- **Community health**

The idea of health service monitoring is to build a network that surrounds a local community. This might be an IoT network centered on a local hospital, a community, or a small town. A collaborative network model can be created by combining many such networks. To achieve all of the technical specifications as a whole, a specialized service known as community healthcare (CH) is necessary. To implement CH, this network combines several wireless body area networks (WBANs). It is possible to think of a hospital and medical network's organizational architecture as a "virtual hospital." An approach to data sharing among health providers and the platform as a service for getting healthcare data and receiving remote medical assistance has been taken into consideration.

- **Wearable device access**

For a variety of biomedical applications (Chenthara et al., 2019), particularly for WSN-based healthcare services, different nonintrusive sensors have been produced. These sensors have the potential to offer the same services via the IoT. On the other hand, wearable technology may have a number of attractive characteristics that are compatible with IoT architecture. Therefore, it is clear that the foregoing sensors will be included in wearable items. For researchers and programmers aiming to achieve the stated connectivity, the varied design of wearable items and medical devices reveals a number of difficulties. In this situation, a special service known as wearable device access is necessary.

5.3.3 Analyze the classification

For literature purposes, we have searched the reputed digital libraries such as IEEE, Springer, Elsevier, ACM, Sage, and so on. We have also searched the medical databases such as Pubmed and MEDLINE. PubMed primarily accesses the MEDLINE database, which contains references and abstracts on subjects related to the life sciences and biomedicine. The database is maintained by the United States National Library of Medicine at the National Institutes of Health as part of the Entrez information retrieval system. The goal of PubMed is to promote the free search and retrieving of biomedical and health sciences publications with the goal of enhancing both individual and global health. The PubMed database contains more than 34 million citations and abstracts of biomedical literature (Bajaj et al., 2021). Most of the papers we have found in the PubMed because it has all health-related articles with a huge repository.

The original query search yielded 3064 publications published between 2007 and 2017 (91 articles from Science Direct, 1496 articles from IEEE Xplore, and 657 articles from WoS). However, due to accessibility concerns, we are now only able to collect two scientific papers from WoS. The papers screened using the following order are adopted with three categories. There were 62 duplicate papers among the 1612 papers gathered throughout the last 6 years (2017–22). Table 5.1 depicts the occurrence in literature (Moore & Pham, 2019; Pimenidis et al., 2019).

5.3.4 Wearable based

The problems and sensor technologies that enable continuous monitoring of healthcare are highlighted in this area. Smaller wireless sensors receive and transmit vital sign data within WBANs (Amft et al., 2020; de Matos et al., 2020; Hecht et al., 2019). Sensor-based RHMS technologies have been considered in seven fields in the research. The first field is an ontology that emphasizes extended topological principles that describe wearable platforms in depth. The second area, which has three sections in the research, is reliability. The first is overload management; some works aim to detect congested and control protocols for WBANs for remotely monitoring patients' healthcare problems. Several works' main contribution is the traffic control protocol, which is frequently used in medical applications. Packet latency and link quality are the second topics (Bagdasaryan et al., 2019; Dagadu & Li, 2018).

In healthcare applications, "real-time publish-subscribe middleware functions" are introduced in Thanigaivelan et al. (2018). Others (Asam & Ajaz, 2019; Elleithy, 2021) looked at strategies for multiple feature decision processing and decision schemes. Another research (Babalola et al., 2021) described a healthcare system layout that handles WBAN's dynamic behavior and congestion. Some other research projects centered on a health-tracking method and sensor architecture, with simulated outcomes. Some other researches aimed to improve the tele-health system's efficiency by proposing architecture. However, in the third category, electromagnetic interference (EMI), the number of patients is lowered by maintaining an acceptable frequency of EMI on medical sensors. Energy effectiveness is the third domain. Some research aimed to improve energy effectiveness and data transfer reliability by lowering energy usage and extending the lifetime of the network by boosting system prediction. On WBANs, the previous research presented green-cloud-assisted health services. The fourth area is quality of service (QoS). Some research addressed QoS for WBANs and presented factors for determining the performance of the application (Al-Sharhan et al., 2019).

Table 5.1 Frequency, weightage, ranking, and preference of various elements.

Elements	Occurrence in literature
E1. mHealth survey	(Ali et al., 2021; Butt, Jamal, et al., 2019; Calvillo-Arbizu et al., 2021; Dang et al., 2019; Nazir et al., 2019)
E2. mHealth surveys	(Asam et al., 2019; Hilbert et al., 2021; Nusairat et al., 2021; Patel et al., 2021; Sarker, 2019a, 2019b; Temdee & Prasad, 2018)
E3. mHealth review	(Alavi et al., 2018; Bajaj et al., 2021; Dang et al., 2019; de Matos et al., 2020; Moore & Pham, 2019; Pimenidis et al., 2019; Sarker, 2019a, 2019b)
E4. mHealth literatures	(Amft et al., 2020; Asam & Ajaz, 2019; Babalola et al., 2021; Bagdasaryan et al., 2019; Dagadu & Li, 2018; Elleithy, 2021; Hecht et al., 2019; Thanigaivelan et al., 2018)
E5. mHealth applications	(Al-Sharhan et al., 2019; García-Magariño et al., 2018; González et al., 2014; Hassan et al., 2018; Kakria et al., 2015; Signorini et al., 2018; Venkatesan et al., 2018)
E6. mHealth frameworks	(Kim et al., 2020; Nifakos et al., 2021; Offner et al., 2020; Platt et al., 2020; Raikhelkar & Raikhelkar, 2019; Ratcliff et al., 2021; Yaacoub et al., 2019)
E7. mHealth limitations	(Abou Allaban et al., 2020; Butt, Diaz-Martinez, et al., 2019; De Michele & Furini, 2019; Liu & Park, 2012; Ministry of Health, 2015)
E8. mHealth remote study	(Alsswey & Al-Samarraie, 2019; Ayani et al., 2021; Azeez & Van der Vyver, 2018; Biduski, 2019; Harrington et al., 2019; Jamshed, 2021; Khan & Reyad, 2020; Kristina et al., 2019; Sadeniemi et al., 2018; Sadiq et al., 2018; Sammoud et al., 2020; Shaikh et al., 2018)
E9. mHealth remote monitoring	(Alhejazi et al., 2019; Alzubi, 2021; Berrouiguet et al., 2018; Chenthara et al., 2019; Comulada et al., 2019; Geddes et al., 2019; Hofmaier et al., 2019; Kibiwott, Zhang, et al., 2019; Kibiwott et al., 2019, 2019; Krithika & Rohini, 2020; Mathew et al., 2020; Rafique et al., 2020; Signorini et al., 2018; Sun, 2020; Uzair et al., 2018; Weber & Kuziemsky, 2019; Williams et al., 2019; Zachlund & Kallin, 2019)
E10. mHealth telemedicine	(Lv et al., 2021; Misbhauddin et al., 2019; Nguyen et al., 2020; Saba et al., 2020; Sani, 2021; Sefa-Yeboah et al., 2021; Thilakarathne et al., 2020; Yang et al., 2020)
E11. mHealth scope and future work	(Alsswey & Al-Samarraie, 2019; Biduski, 2019; Brown et al., 2020; Cornet & Holden, 2018; Giudice et al., 2020; Otoom et al., 2020; Thaduri et al., 2017; Vianna & Barbosa, 2020)

5.3.5 Mobile health (mHealth)

Ambulatory patients are defined as "those patients who are suffering from any kind of disease but discharged from the hospital and need the care to monitor their health" (Asam & Ajaz, 2019; Signorini et al., 2018). These patients in the current era are also known as remote/mobile patients. In the medical research, such a patient needs remote monitoring now. Thus, mHealth is facilitating ambulatory patients by providing continuous monitoring using wireless devices such as cell phones under telemedicine. mHealth also has a significant impact socially because it connects people through continuous monitoring. mHealth continuously provides satisfaction to patients as well as their relatives and reduces their stress level. On other hand, mHealth is economically less costly than the traditional health monitoring ways. It does not need a massive infrastructure to monitor the patient's health. It only needs a smartphone and a low-cost wearable sensor to connect to the mobile application to enable the monitoring. Due to this reason, mHealth is increasingly adopted by different countries (Khan & Reyad, 2020; Raikhelkar & Raikhelkar, 2019; Sadeniemi et al., 2018; Thanigaivelan et al., 2018).

RHMS is becoming a more widely adopted domain of research in healthcare due to its numerous advantages, including the ability to provide health-related data and provide remote health services. RHMS is a type of remote practice of medicine in which multiple healthcare experts work together to diagnose or treat a disease. Patients in remote areas and far places can take benefits such as patients can get medical help from doctors. In RHMS, assessment describes the process of classifying patients in a large-scale emergency for their medical treatment priority order. It is the process of evaluating and scheduling healthcare for all patients and fatalities (Hofmaier et al., 2019; Ministry of Health, 2015). The quality and accuracy of medical services need the earlier detection of patients and their categorization into priority categorization upon admission to the emergency department (ED). As a result, a patient seeks to determine which patient can adequately wait and which cannot for receiving of medical facilities (González et al., 2014). Because it efficiently allocates available services within a location, patient prioritizing enhances fairness and reduces critical patients' waiting times from different locations. The abnormality case of a patient should be the primary consideration for determining priority for medical facilities. Due to their importance in people's lives, remote health prioritizing methods have gotten a lot of attention (Ayani et al., 2021). After evaluating their vital signs, remote prioritizing entails categorizing patients and determining their priority for treatments and taking them into hospitals.

A continuous monitoring from a hospital at a distance is extremely desirable for remote patients since it assures optimal treatment and gives appropriate health instructions (Lv et al., 2021). Additionally, the distanced-based patient monitoring is now become the most interesting domain of research in the healthcare sector. Patients who have numerous serious illnesses (such as heart disease, blood pressure, and diabetes) are at a higher risk to do their daily normal activities due to multiple chronic diseases (MCDs) (Nguyen et al., 2020; Sani, 2021). Patients at distant locations are known as the patients who are aged and having the MCDs, so they are at a higher threat of health conditions. As a result, MCD prioritizing methods are critical for the continuing care of remote patients in complex and dynamic environments. For analyzing the procedure of patient prioritizing in RHMS applications, a comprehensive literature analysis is required (Sefa-Yeboah et al., 2021).

The health monitoring sensors are producing a large amount of data. Surroundings of the patient play a vital role in managing the patient's data and are gaining popularity due to unique features, such as dealing with the current environment, timely reaction to the current situation, tracking patient's location, and data collection from sensors (Biduski, 2019; Lv et al., 2021; Sani, 2021). It is also used to examine the temperature, body movement, environment sensing, and monitoring (Khodadad-Saryazdi, 2021; Mansouri-Rad, 2012; Samonte et al., 2019). The doctor can continuously monitor the patient's health and can take action on any abnormal event. Figs. 5.3 and 5.4 depict scenarios about ambulatory patient scenarios in mobile health monitoring under the telemedicine umbrella. Fig. 5.3 explains the normal care monitoring scenario of a patient who suffers from a chronic disease without any physical disability. The alert goes to the specified location like a hospital, doctors, and ambulance services. Fig. 5.4 explains the extensive care health scenario where the patient has a chronic disease as well as physical challenges and cannot use technology by himself. In both cases, the mobile health application is the main support for health monitoring and medication.

The availability of smart devices plays a remarkable role in the new era of mobile health (mHealth) monitoring, which evolved from eHealth monitoring. Due to advancements in mobile health (mHealth) and awareness of the patients with the technologies, the health domain is introducing different innovative technologies. These technologies include sensors, wearable devices, and smart health applications. The main reason for the development of such technologies is a direct link with human life. Currently, remote health monitoring is growing under the umbrella of smart health monitoring. Smart health is defined as disease monitoring with the use of

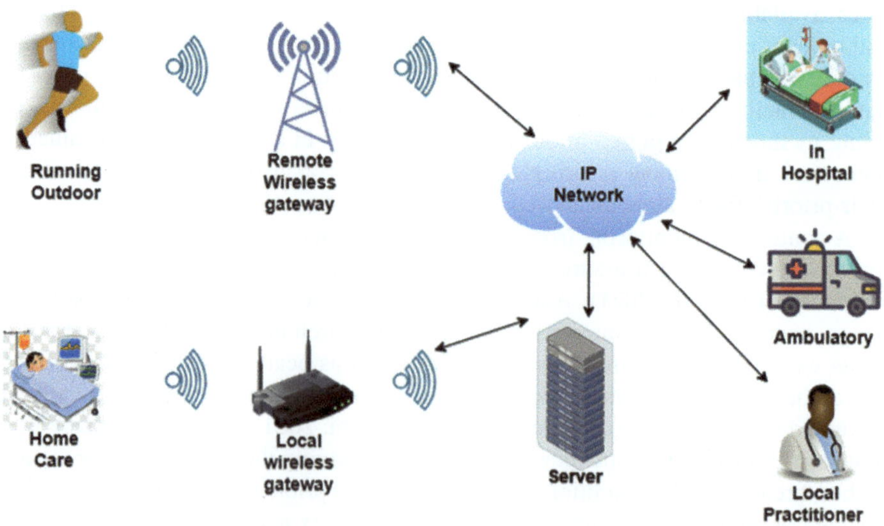

FIGURE 5.3

Normal health care (simple scenario) (Butt, Jamal, et al., 2019).

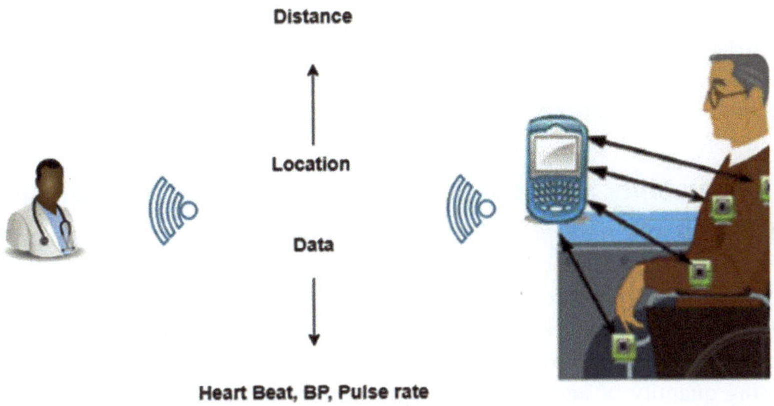

FIGURE 5.4

Intensive care (technical scenario) (Butt, Jamal, et al., 2019).

technologies, e.g., wearable devices and smart applications (Kristina et al., 2019; Williams et al., 2019). mHealth is facilitating the monitoring of different diseases remotely.

Smartphones are regarded as cutting-edge IoT medical equipment. Despite the fact that there are a lot of healthcare applications and more are being added to the list every day, the tendency has only affected a select few types of ailments. It is crucial to engage in R&D for novel diseases and disorders, and it has consistently been a priority to find ways to make the earlier diagnosis of rare diseases accessible.

5.3.6 Remote monitoring under telemonitoring

In remote monitoring, a healthcare physician remotely examines a patient's urgent situation and also provides real-time data evaluation and immediate feedback to the patients. Telemonitoring research is divided into three categories: patient screening, patient service delivery, and patient prioritizing. The first is patient assessment, which entails classifying patients based on their emergencies (Comulada et al., 2019; Hofmaier et al., 2019). Some research looked at treatment inside the ED that is described, while others looked at treatment outside the ED that is also described (Berrouiguet et al., 2018).

The second category refers to the supply of distant healthcare services. Many researchers have emphasized an alert emergency service that notifies a physician, so that they can respond quickly if vital signs become abnormal. Several researches offered services including suggestions, recommendations, medicine prescription, and remote consulting (Alhejazi et al., 2019). Several types of research suggest choosing neighboring and appropriate hospitals or doctors per patients' situations. The goal of this project is to provide health treatment services while traveling in cars on the go. In another investigation, the presence of medical facilities in an ambulance is established (Chenthara et al., 2019).

Another research provided a novel aged monitoring concept that links a remote psychiatrist's clinic with an elderly person's home. Lastly, he developed a method for patients to manage their prescription medication by telling them about substances and doses (Weber & Kuziemsky, 2019).

5.3.7 Scalability issues with patient's prioritizing in medical care

Scalability, notably in the procedures of patient prioritizing, is one of the main concerns in delivering healthcare services. Healthcare treatments that are extremely effective and accessible are desperately needed to meet the growing desire for medical care. Many studies have been performed to improve patient prioritizing in RHMS to address scalability difficulties. In the literature, the challenge of an increasing quantity of aged patients requiring fast and efficient telemedicine facilities has been highlighted (Saba et al., 2020). Discussed in the following subsections, growth in the number of patients is expected to occur under a variety of situations, including disasters and population aging. Regarding increasing patient numbers, as the population ages, healthcare services face significant obstacles. To fulfill the growing system demand, healthcare practitioners must be able to efficiently use any modern system. Current demographic shifts, which produce chronic and serious difficulties including the incidence of aging diseases and social and economic costs, are the main causes for the continued expansion of older generation sets. According to a survey, the population aged 45 and up increased by 11% in the previous contract, while the consultations by doctors for similar age of patients in the same period rose by 26% (Misbhauddin et al., 2019). Table 5.2 provides a comparison with other existing review studies in telemedicine.

5.4 Communication and location technologies in remote health

The transmission of data over a short distance is supported by all of the aforementioned methods. The properties of such technologies also range in respect of transmission capacity, working distances, the variety of nodes that are permitted, the degree of energy usage, and the price of installation and maintenance due to differences in functioning radio frequency and privacy standards.

- **Location-based services**

Object tracking and position identification are done using real-time location systems (RTLS). In healthcare applications, RTLS safely monitors the therapeutic process and aids in rearranging the healthcare system in accordance with the allocation of resources. The global positioning system (GPS), the most significant RTLS, is a navigation system that can detect objects of all kinds. A satellite-based navigation system is able to find ambulances, patients, doctors, and other objects in a healthcare system.

Table 5.2 Comparison of this study with existing review studies.

References	Scope of study	Year	Existing frameworks	Mobile health applications
(Khodadad-Saryazdi, 2021)	Study describes the multiple chronic diseases; discusses the telemedicine benefits and wearable devices	2019	×	×
(Sega et al., 2022)	Describe the IoT applications in health, telemedicine, security of health data, and security protocols	2019	×	×
(Salazar et al., 2021)	Explains the concept of remote health monitoring; moreover describes the patient prioritization in telemedicine for medical support	2018	×	×
(Mahajan & Kaur, 2020)	This study explains the ECG monitoring technologies and system; mentions the limitations with the system to get the ECG values of remote patients	2021	×	×
(Wang et al., 2019)	Review study describes the number of studies for hospital location selection	2021	Does not explain the limitations with these studies included in survey; only gives an overview of studies	×
(Beitelspacher et al., 2020)	Discusses the remote health monitoring and analyzes the device types	2022	×	×
(Ariza-Colpas et al., 2022)	Describes the tele-health with benefits and discusses use of tele-health in rural areas and developed systems	2021	×	×

It is significant that interior availability to systems including GPS or China's Beidou System is typically subpar because building structures limit the transmission of satellite signals. Since GPS is insufficient to establish a functional healthcare system, real-time locating systems (LPSs) must be used to compensate GPS and improve location accuracy. Based on the analysis of radio signals passing between the objects and a variety of the predeployed receivers, an LPS identifies the location of an object. In the research, LPSs are covered in great detail (Ministry of Health, 2015).

- **Sensing technologies**

Sensing technology is essential to the collection of a patient's physiologic data in order for a doctor to properly diagnose the ailment and suggest the appropriate course of therapy. Additionally, new developments in sensing technology enable ongoing data collection from patients, which helps to improve treatment outcomes and lower healthcare costs.

The pulse oximeter was invented in the early 1970s and has since grown to be one of the commonly utilized diagnostic tools (Harrington et al., 2019). A pulse oximeter can accurately measure the heart rate (HR) and blood oxygen saturation (SpO2), two medical parameters that are especially significant for the emerging service. In Comulada et al. (2019), a pulse oximeter depending on a mote was introduced. From the waveforms of transmitted light, the usual digital signal processing method can be used to determine HR and SpO2.

All information gathered about patients' health issues can be promptly translated to digital form and sent across the network. The use of wireless sensors has dramatically streamlined the data collecting procedures and allowed patients to wear mobile sensors for longer periods of time without having to carry around a big data logger.

- **Resource management**

The problems of tracking, detecting, identifying, and authenticity are part of resource management. Information gathering is frequently the initial step in the operation of medical systems and is crucial since it serves as the foundation for further diagnosis and treatment.

- **Tracking**

Since the visibility issue raises the uncertainty of present healthcare systems, tracking attempts to address the absence of "visibility" on the positions, the situations of patients, clinicians, medical devices, or other helpful resources. A medical smartphone's regular maintenance may go undiscovered if its status is not tracked in real time. Additionally, a disorganized patient flow would cause emergency health procedures to be delayed. Despite all of these issues, a tracking system's main purpose is to locate patients or things in real time.

The device would immediately notify the caregivers whenever a patient is in a place where falling is very likely to happen to him or her. To enhance the medical services provided to the elderly, Bowser and Woodworth (Otoom et al., 2020) merged location technologies with video analytics and wireless communications technology. For mobile applications, a research work presents an ultrasound-based locating system with multicell coverage. To aid in the development of public health services and policy, a web-based environment health-related data system has also been created. It suggests a brand-new tracking system to take the place of the largely separate and disjointed information systems at the level of each particular enterprise. the thorough comparison of the tracking technologies experiments.

- **Sensing**

Detection systems are patient-focused and function in healthcare systems as both essential and introducing new technologies. The devices were created to make diagnoses and to offer real-time data on patients' health indicators (Brown et al., 2020; Giudice et al., 2020). A variety of telecommunication service systems, monitoring equipment, and alerting systems for medical conditions are among the application areas. Innovative research has been done in this area. One of the first efforts to connect wearable technology with smart devices like watches and mobile phones is MobiHealth. AlarmNet is a remote medical sensor network experiment. It offers both location monitoring and medical monitoring capabilities. A mobile phone serves as the access point for the Mobile ECG system, which measures and analyses ECGs for users.

- **Authenticity and identification**

Identifying and authenticity are essential to lowering the likelihood of mistakes that could be harmful to patients, such as using the incorrect drug, dose, timing, or treatment, etc. Identification and authorization are widely used among clinical staff to allow private data to be accessed and to boost morale by resolving patient privacy concerns. Identification and authenticity are mostly utilized for medical facilities to comply with security protocol needs and prevent the loss of expensive tools and supplies.

- **Knowledge management**

The acquisition, growth, collection, and reuse of medical information in the intelligent system is essential to the success of rehabilitation since modern healthcare is fueled by advanced information and expertise. Ontology may be the most promising way of knowledge management since it makes it simple to share and reuse previously acquired knowledge (De Michele & Furini, 2019). This idea offers the rehabilitation engineering field with well-structured domain information, which makes it possible to execute data mining with minimal to no ambiguity and unambiguous hierarchic relationships. Thus, ontology helps medical professionals reach a consensus regarding the best therapies and matching resources. Additionally, the usage of ontologies makes it easier to share knowledge because information with the same or comparable structures greatly enhances the potential for reuse. For the lower-limb treatment system, there are two local ontologies: one for diseases and one for resources. The disease ontology offers a benchmark for comparability and facilitates finding one or more related instances in the database. To deal with the new patient, one can employ the same or a related treatment technique as in previous circumstances. Healthcare resources, comprising both material and human resources as Control pulse management (CPM) and rehabilitation robots, etc., are formalized by the resource ontology. It facilitates the system's rapid selection of the best resources in accordance with the treatment needs inferred from the disease ontology.

Ontology therefore serves two goals when applied to a treatment strategy. First, ontological data structures make it possible to reason more accurately and quickly. Ontology also offers well-organized domain knowledge on rehabilitation engineering, making it simple to share and reuse knowledge. The relationships between distinct terms in the rehabilitation lexicon are defined by a well-organized ontology and are crucial for identifying, comprehending, and diagnosing disorders.

5.4.1 Impact of mHealth

Smart health has different impacts on the health of the patients and the environment. Smart health facilitates the patient to get medical facilities including the patient's rescue from location, continuous monitoring, and medical support in any abnormal situation. Further, smart health has different benefits and limitations, as follows (Amft et al., 2020; Hecht et al., 2019).

5.4.1.1 Benefits

5.4.1.1.1 There is no time nor cost for traveling

- It provides the continuous monitoring of patients remotely by the specified doctor.
- It enables the rescue of a patient from their location whenever there is any abnormality.
- The patient can save money on travel by being examined by their doctor over the smartphone. Additionally, the patient will not waste traveling time or risk getting stuck in road traffic, which will cause the patient to be late for their appointment.
- Patients with different kinds of diseases get medical facilities from home, which ultimately increases the quality of care.

5.4.1.2 There's no need to take off from work

- When it comes to working, video conferences largely reduce the need for time off. Simply make your appointment throughout a break at work or before or after work. Rather than skipping a day of work or spending their valuable paid time off, patients may follow their doctor's recommendations and manage overall health (Hecht et al., 2019).

5.4.1.3 Remove all difficulties with child or elder care

- Most of us are responsible for the care of children or elders. It is very difficult and expensive to seek alternative solutions. That is why sometimes it becomes stressful or impractical to bring them along. Fortunately, smart health addresses this problem by enabling people to consult their doctors online (Bagdasaryan et al., 2019).

5.4.1.4 Improved health

- Patients can effectively manage their medicines, lifestyle, and other health activities (Dagadu & Li, 2018).

5.4.1.5 Services of specialists

- It includes an expert often helping a medical professional make a diagnosis. It might include sending medical images, videos, and medical data to a professional for later review or a patient "seeing" a professional via a live, remote appointment. All healthcare specialties that rely primarily or partially on visual information, including such radiology, pathology, dermatology, ophthalmology, and cardiology, are routinely referred to specialists.

5.4.1.6 Remote patient monitoring

- With applying (miniature) equipment, remote patient monitoring gathers and sends information for monitoring and analysis. Applications for "home telehealth" may monitor a particular critical symptom, including blood sugar levels or the heart's ECG, or a range of symptoms for patients who are housebound. The support of visiting doctors is also provided by such services.

5.4.1.7 Medical education

- Healthcare education provides specific medical training sessions for specialized populations in remote places as well as continuing healthcare education courses for medical practitioners.

5.4.2 Drawbacks

5.4.2.1 Care delays

- When a patient requires emergency care using smart health primarily may cause treatment to be delayed, especially when a doctor cannot deliver life-saving treatments over the internet.

5.4.2.2 Technological concerns

- It can be difficult to choose the correct digital platform to deploy health solutions. Poor connectivity can also make it extremely difficult to provide high-quality care. Doctors should also assure that the smart health application they deploy is safe and follow all applicable privacy regulations (Thanigaivelan et al., 2018).

5.4.2.3 Send the ambulance

This approach is to send medical support to the patient's location when there is any abnormality and has the following limitations (Al-Sharhan et al., 2019; Babalola et al., 2021):

- a long geographic distance between doctor and patient that causes late receiving of medical facilities
- availability of an ambulance at the doctor's end to send for patient's rescue from his/her location
- patient surviving condition in the case of any delay of medical services

5.4.2.4 Scalability of application

- When the number of patients is increased with single or multiple doctors then the scalability of health applications is a critical issue. As whenever the number of patients is increased, the possibility of false alerts sent to the doctor is also increased (Elleithy, 2021).

5.4.2.5 False generation of alerts

- When there is any abnormality, then the existing systems generate alerts to medical services providers, e.g., doctors, hospitals, and medical staff. But the issue with the existing alert concept is that due to some environmental factors, the heartbeat can fluctuate and generate wrong emergency alerts to those providers (Asam & Ajaz, 2019).

5.5 Conclusion

Telemedicine technologies are already becoming extremely prevalent, particularly in terms of patient prioritizing. mHealth application's development is a very trendy topic among the research community due to its direct involvement with human life. Remote patient monitoring is getting fame due to advanced innovations. In this chapter, we have investigated different mHealth frameworks with the analysis of their major features for mobile applications development. We have provided comprehensive comparisons of such frameworks. Furthermore, we investigated the health applications and their open research issues. We have highlighted mHealth frameworks and applications with their limitations and conclude the study with new open research directions in mobile health monitoring.

References

Abou Allaban, A., Wang, M., & Padır, T. (2020). A systematic review of robotics research in support of in-home care for older adults. *Information, 11*(2), 75.

Al-Sharhan, S., Omran, E., & Lari, K. (2019). An integrated holistic model for an eHealth system: A national implementation approach and a new cloud-based security model. *International Journal of Information Management, 47*, 121–130.

Alavi, A. H., Jiao, P., Buttlar, W. G., & Lajnef, N. (2018). Internet of Things-enabled smart cities: State-of-the-art and future trends. *Measurement, 129*, 589–606.

Alhejazi, M. M., AL-Dahasi, E. M., & Saqib, N. A. (May 2019). A new remote user authentication scheme for E-health-care applications using steganography. In *2019 2nd international con*ference on computer applications & information security (ICCAIS) (pp. 1–10). IEEE.

Ali, M. R., Sen, T., Li, Q., Langevin, R., Myers, T., Dorsey, E. R., … Hoque, E. (2021). Analyzing head pose in remotely collected videos of people with Parkinson's disease. *ACM Transactions on Computing for Healthcare, 2*(4), 1–13.

Alsswey, A., & Al-Samarraie, H. (2019). Elderly users' acceptance of mHealth user interface (UI) design-based culture: The moderator role of age. *Journal on Multimodal User Interfaces*, 1–11.

Alzubi, J. A. (2021). Blockchain-based Lamport Merkle digital signature: Authentication tool in IoT healthcare. *Computer Communications, 170*, 200–208.

Amft, O., Favela, J., Intille, S., Musolesi, M., & Kostakos, V. (2020). Personalized pervasive health. *IEEE Pervasive Computing, 19*(3), 11–13.

Ariza-Colpas, P. P., Vicario, E., Butt, S. A., De-la Hoz-Franco, E., Piñeres-Melo, M. A., Oviedo-Carrascal, A. I., … Patara, F. (2022). *Machine learning applied to datasets of human activity recognition-an applications of data analysis in HealthCare. Current medical imaging*.

Asam, M., & Ajaz, A. (2019). Challenges in wireless body area network. In *Proceedings of international journal of advanced computer science and applications* (Vol. 10).

Asam, M., Ghuman, K., Ajaz, A., & Jamal, T. (2019). *Ubiquity of healthcare system.*

Ayani, S., Mirzaei, M., Abbasi, N., & Moulaei, K. (2021). Enterprise resource planning in the health industry: Problems of its usage based on the extent of the countries' development. *Applied Medical Informatics, 43*(1), 1–13.

Azeez, N. A., & Van der Vyver, C. (2018). Security and privacy issues in e-health cloud-based system: A comprehensive content analysis. *Egyptian Informatics Journal, 20*, 97–108.

Babalola, D., Anayo, M., & Itoya, D. A. (2021). Telehealth during COVID-19: Why Sub-Saharan Africa is yet to log-in to virtual healthcare? *AIMS Medical Science, 8*(1), 46–55.

Bagdasaryan, E., Berlstein, G., Waterman, J., Birrell, E., Foster, N., Schneider, F. B., & Estrin, D. (November 2019). Ancile: Enhancing privacy for ubiquitous computing with use-based privacy. In *Proceedings of the 18th ACM wor*kshop on Privacy in the electronic Society (pp. 111–124).

Bajaj, A., Bhatnagar, M., & Chauhan, A. (2021). Recent trends in internet of medical things: A review. *Advances in Machine Learning and Computational Intelligence*, 645–656.

Beitelspacher, S., Mubashir, M., Besher, K. M., & Ali, M. Z. (2020). Prioritizing health care data traffic in a congested IoT cloud network. In *2020 IEEE wireless communications and networking conference workshops (WCNCW)*. https://doi.org/10.1109/WCNCW48565.2020.9124867

Berrouiguet, S., Perez-Rodriguez, M. M., Larsen, M., Baca-García, E., Courtet, P., & Oquendo, M. (2018). From eHealth to iHealth: Transition to participatory and personalized medicine in mental health. *Journal of Medical Internet Research, 20*(1), e2.

Biduski, D. (2019). *Avaliando a experiência do usuário de longo prazo em aplicações m-Health.*

Brown, S. A., Rhee, J. W., Guha, A., & Rao, V. U. (2020). Innovation in precision cardio-oncology during the coronavirus pandemic and into a post-pandemic world. *Frontiers in Cardiovascular Medicine, 7*, 145.

Butt, S. A., Diaz-Martinez, J. L., Jamal, T., Ali, A., De-La-Hoz-Franco, E., & Shoaib, M. (July 2019). IoT smart health security threats. In *2019, 19th international conference on computational science and its applications (ICCSA)* (pp. 26–31). IEEE.

Butt, S. A., Jamal, T., Azad, M. A., Ali, A., & Safa, N. S. (2019). A Multivariant secure framework for smart mobile health applications. *Transactions on Emerging Telecommunications Technologies*, e3684.

Calvillo-Arbizu, J., Román-Martínez, I., & Reina-Tosina, J. (2021). Internet of things in health: Requirements, issues, and gaps. *Computer Methods and Programs in Biomedicine*, 106231.

Chenthara, S., Ahmed, K., Wang, H., & Whittaker, F. (2019). *Security and privacy-preserving challenges of e-health solutions in cloud computing*. IEEE Access.

Comulada, W. S., Wynn, A., van Rooyen, H., Barnabas, R. V., Eashwari, R., & van Heerden, A. (2019). Using mHealth to deliver a home-based testing and counseling program to improve linkage to care and ART adherence in rural South Africa. *Prevention Science, 20*(1), 126–136.

Cornet, V. P., & Holden, R. J. (2018). Systematic review of smartphone-based passive sensing for health and wellbeing. *Journal of Biomedical Informatics, 77*, 120–132.

Dagadu, J. C., & Li, J. (2018). Context-based watermarking cum chaotic encryption for medical images in RHMS applications. *Multimedia Tools and Applications, 77*(18), 24289–24312.

Dang, L. M., Piran, M., Han, D., Min, K., & Moon, H. (2019). A survey on internet of things and cloud computing for healthcare. *Electronics, 8*(7), 768.

De Michele, R., & Furini, M. (September 2019). IoT healthcare: Benefits, issues and challenges. In *Proceedings of the 5th EAI inter*national conference on smart objects and technologies for social good (pp. 160–164). ACM.

Elleithy, A. (April 2021). Privacy and security in pervasive and ubiquitous computing. In *2021 ASEE st. Lawrence sect*ion conference.

García-Magariño, I., Bedia, M. G., & Palacios-Navarro, G. (March 2018). Famap: A framework for developing m-health apps. In *World conference on informat*ion systems and technologies (pp. 850–859). Cham: Springer.

Geddes, N., Gupta, G. S., & Hasan, F. (May 2019). An energy efficient protocol for wireless body area network of health sensors. In *2019 IEEE international instrumentation and measurement technology conference (I2MTC)* (pp. 1–6). IEEE.

Giudice, A., Barone, S., Muraca, D., Averta, F., Diodati, F., Antonelli, A., & Fortunato, L. (2020). Can teledentistry improve the monitoring of patients during the covid-19 dissemination? A descriptive pilot study. *International Journal of Environmental Research and Public Health, 17*(10), 3399.

González, F. C. J., Villegas, O. O. V., Ramírez, D. E. T., Sánchez, V. G. C., & Domínguez, H. O. (2014). Smart multi-level tool for remote patient monitoring based on a wireless sensor network and mobile augmented reality. *Sensors, 14*(9), 17212–17234.

Harrington, E. K., Drake, A. L., Matemo, D., Ronen, K., Osoti, A. O., John-Stewart, G., … Unger, J. A. (2019). An mHealth SMS intervention on postpartum contraceptive use among women and couples in Kenya: A randomized controlled trial. *American Journal of Public Health, 109*(6), 934–941.

Hassan, M. K., El Desouky, A. I., Elghamrawy, S. M., & Sarhan, A. M. (2018). Intelligent hybrid remote patient-monitoring model with cloud-based framework for knowledge discovery. *Computers & Electrical Engineering, 70*, 1034–1048.

Hecht, H. S., Shaw, L., Chandrashekhar, Y. S., Bax, J. J., & Narula, J. (2019). Should NICE guidelines be universally accepted for the evaluation of stable coronary disease? A debate. *European Heart Journal, 40*(18), 1440–1453.

Hilbert, A., Zenger, M., Luck-Sikorski, C., & Brähler, E. (2021). Weight stigma and disease and disability concepts of obesity: A survey of the German population. *Obesity Facts*, 1–8.

Hofmaier, S., Huang, X., & Matricardi, P. M. (2019). RHMS and mobile health technology in the diagnosis, monitoring and treatment of respiratory allergies. In *Implementing precision medicine in best practices of chronic airway diseases* (pp. 117–124). Academic Press.

Jamshed, R. (2021). *A comprehensive ontology of information disruption attacks for IoT based health care systems (doctoral dissertation, Capital University).*

Kakria, P., Tripathi, N. K., & Kitipawang, P. (2015). A real-time health monitoring system for remote cardiac patients using smartphone and wearable sensors. *International Journal of RHMS and Applications*, 2015.

Khan, F., & Reyad, O. (2020). *Application of intelligent multi agent based systems for E-healthcare security. arXiv preprint arXiv:2004.01256.*

Khodadad-Saryazdi, A. (2021). Exploring the RHMS implementation challenges through the process innovation approach: A case study research in the French healthcare sector. *Technovation, 107*(February), 102273. https://doi.org/10.1016/j.technovation.2021.102273

Kibiwott, K. P., Zhang, F., Kimeli Victor, K., Omala, A. A., & Opoku-Mensah, E. (2019). Privacy preservation for eHealth big data in cloud accessed using resource-constrained devices: Survey. *IJ Network Security, 21*(2), 312–325.

Kibiwott, K. P., Zhao, Y., Kogo, J., & Zhang, F. (2019). Verifiable fully outsourced attribute-based signcryption system for IoT eHealth big data in cloud computing. *Mathematical Biosciences and Engineering, 16*(5), 3561–3594.

Kim, J., Kassels, A. C., Costin, N. I., & Schmidt, H. (2020). Remote monitoring of medication adherence and patient and industry responsibilities in a learning health system. *Journal of Medical Ethics, 46*(6), 386–391.

Kristina, S. A., Ekasari, M. P., & Wati, M. R. (2019). Internet use for searching information on Health and Medicine: An Exploratory study among Indonesian customers. *Research Journal of Pharmacy and Technology, 12*(12), 5927–5931.

Krithika, D. R., & Rohini, K. (2020). A survey on challenging capabilities of big data analytics in healthcare. *International Journal of Innovative Research in Applied Sciences and Engineering, 4*, 593–597.

Liu, W., & Park, E. K. (July 2012). E-healthcare security solution framework. In *2012 21st international con*ference on computer communications and networks (ICCCN) (pp. 1–6). IEEE.

Lv, Y., Ma, C., Li, X., & Wu, M. (2021). Big data driven COVID-19 pandemic crisis management: Potential approach for global health. *Archives of Medical Science: AMS, 17*(3), 829.

Mahajan, M., & Kaur, S. (2020). Congestion control protocols in wireless sensor networks: A comprehensive survey. In *Proceedings of the international conference of intelligent engineering and management ICIEM 2020* (pp. 160–164). https://doi.org/10.1109/ICIEM48762.2020.9160268

Mansouri-Rad, P. (2012). *Factors affecting the adoption of RHMS : A three-country empirical investigation*.

Mathew, O. C., Dhanapal, R., Visalakshi, P., Parthiban, K. G., & Karthik, S. (2020). Distributed security model for remote healthcare (dsm-rh) services in internet of things environment. *Journal of Medical Imaging and Health Informatics, 10*(1), 185–193.

de Matos, E., Tiburski, R. T., Moratelli, C. R., Johann Filho, S., Amaral, L. A., Ramachandran, G., … Hessel, F. (2020). Context information sharing for the internet of things: A survey. *Computer Networks, 166*, 106988.

Ministry of Health. (2015). *HISO 10029:2015 health information security framework* [cited 2017 May 3]. Available from: http://www.health.govt.nz/publication/hiso100292015-health-information-security-framework.

Misbhauddin, M., Malik, M. A., & Mohiuddin, A. H. (December 2019). An initial framework for mobile healthcare systems using deep neural networks. In *2019 IEEE 9th international conference on advanced computing (IACC)* (pp. 205–210). IEEE.

Moore, P., & Pham, H. V. (2019). A fog computing model for pervasive connected healthcare in smart environments. *International Journal of Grid and Utility Computing, 10*(4), 375–391.

Nazir, S., Ali, Y., Ullah, N., & García-Magariño, I. (2019). Internet of things for healthcare using effects of mobile computing: A systematic literature review. *Wireless Communications and Mobile Computing*, 2019.

Nguyen, T. H., Nguyen, T. N., & Nguyen, T. T. (2020). A deep learning framework for heart disease classification in an IoTs-based system. In *A handbook of internet of things in biomedical and cyber physical system* (pp. 217–244). Cham: Springer.

Nifakos, S., Chandramouli, K., Nikolaou, C. K., Papachristou, P., Koch, S., Panaousis, E., & Bonacina, S. (2021). Influence of human factors on cyber security within healthcare organisations: A systematic review. *Sensors, 21*(15), 5119.

Nusairat, N., Abdellatif, H., Al-Gasawneh, J., Akhorshaideh, A., Aloqool, A., Rabah, S., & Ahmad, A. (2021). Determinants of behavioral intentions to use mobile healthcare applications in Jordan. *International Journal of Data and Network Science, 5*(4), 547–556.

Offner, K. L., Sitnikova, E., Joiner, K., & MacIntyre, C. R. (2020). Towards understanding cybersecurity capability in Australian healthcare organisations: A systematic review of recent trends, threats and mitigation. *Intelligence and National Security, 35*(4), 556–585.

Otoom, M., Otoum, N., Alzubaidi, M. A., Etoom, Y., & Banihani, R. (2020). An IoT-based framework for early identification and monitoring of COVID-19 cases. *Biomedical Signal Processing and Control, 62*, 102149.

Patel, S. A., Patel, S. P., Adhyaru, Y. B. K., Maheshwari, S., Kumar, P., & Soni, M. (2021). Developing smart devices with automated machine learning approach: A review. *Materials Today: Proceedings*.

Pimenidis, E., Polatidis, N., & Mouratidis, H. (2019). Mobile recommender systems: Identifying the major concepts. *Journal of Information Science, 45*(3), 387–397.

Platt, J. E., Raj, M., & Wienroth, M. (2020). An analysis of the learning health system in its first decade in practice: Scoping review. *Journal of Medical Internet Research, 22*(3), e17026.

Rafique, W., Qi, L., Yaqoob, I., Imran, M., Rasool, R. U., & Dou, W. (2020). Complementing IoT services through software defined networking and edge computing: A comprehensive survey. *IEEE Communications Surveys & Tutorials, 22*(3), 1761–1804.

Raikhelkar, J., & Raikhelkar, J. K. (2019). Advances in tele-cardiology. In *RHMS in the ICU* (pp. 225–242). Cham: Springer.

Ratcliff, C. L., Wong, B., Jensen, J. D., & Kaphingst, K. A. (2021). The impact of communicating uncertainty on public responses to precision Medicine research. *Annals of Behavioral Medicine, 55*, 1048–1061.

Saba, T., Haseeb, K., Ahmed, I., & Rehman, A. (2020). Secure and energy-efficient framework using Internet of Medical Things for e-healthcare. *Journal of Infection and Public Health, 13*(10), 1567–1575.

Sadeniemi, M., Almeda, N., Salinas-Pérez, J. A., Gutiérrez-Colosía, M. R., García-Alonso, C., Ala-Nikkola, T., … Salvador-Carulla, L. (2018). A comparison of mental health care systems in Northern and Southern Europe: A service mapping study. *International Journal of Environmental Research and Public Health, 15*(6), 1133.

Sadiq, F. I., Selamat, A., & Ibrahim, R. (2018). A systematic literature review on activity recognition with context-awareness techniques for mitigation of disasters. *International Journal of Digital Enterprise Technology, 1*(1–2), 177–217.

Salazar, L. H. A., Leithardt, V. R., Parreira, W. D., da Rocha Fernandes, A. M., Barbosa, J. L. V., & Correia, S. D. (2021). Application of machine learning techniques to predict a patient's no–show in the healthcare sector. Future Internet, *14*(1), 3.

Sammoud, A., Chalouf, M. A., Hamdi, O., Montavont, N., & Bouallegue, A. (2020). A new biometrics-based key establishment protocol in WBAN: Energy efficiency and security robustness analysis. *Computers & Security, 96*, 101838.

Samonte, M. J. C., Aguilar, V., Marino, A. K., & Tolentino, R. (2019). InTelect: Interactive RHMS communication technologies mobile app. *IOP Conference of Series: Materials Science and Engineering, 482*(1). https://doi.org/10.1088/1757-899X/482/1/012022

Sani, S. (January 2021). Design and implementation of A low-cost ECG monitoring system using ARM Cortex-M4 Family Microcontroller. In *2021 IEEE international confer*ence on consumer electronics (ICCE) (pp. 1–2). IEEE.

Sarker, I. H. (2019a). Research issues in mining user behavioral rules for context-aware intelligent mobile applications. *Iran Journal of Computer Science, 2*(1), 41–51.

Sarker, I. H. (2019b). Context-aware rule learning from smartphone data: Survey, challenges, and future directions. *Journal of Big Data, 6*(1), 1–25.

Sefa-Yeboah, S. M., Osei Annor, K., Koomson, V. J., Saalia, F. K., Steiner-Asiedu, M., & Mills, G. A. (2021). Development of a mobile application platform for self-management of obesity using Artificial intelligence techniques. *International Journal of RHMS and Applications*, 6624057, 2021.

Sega, C. L., Rossetto, A. G. D. M., Correia, S. D., & Leithardt, V. R. (2022, June). An architectural proposal to protect the privacy of health data stored in the Blockchain. In 2022 17th Iberian Conference on Information Systems and Technologies (CISTI) (pp. 1–6). IEEE.

Shaikh, Y., Parvati, V. K., & Biradar, S. R. (February 2018). Survey of smart healthcare systems using internet of things (IoT). In *2018 international conference on communication, computing and internet of things (IC3IoT)* (pp. 508–513). IEEE.

Signorini, M. G., Lanzola, G., Torti, E., Fanelli, A., & Magenes, G. (2018). Antepartum fetal monitoring through a wearable system and a mobile application. *Technologies, 6*(2), 44.

Sun, P. (2020). Security and privacy protection in cloud computing: Discussions and challenges. *Journal of Network and Computer Applications, 160*, 102642.

Temdee, P., & Prasad, R. (2018). Introduction to context-aware computing. In *Context-aware communication and computing: Applications for smart environment* (pp. 1−13). Cham: Springer.

Thaduri, A., Kumar, U., & Verma, A. K. (2017). Computational intelligence framework for context-aware decision making. *International Journal of System Assurance Engineering and Management, 8*(4), 2146−2157.

Thanigaivelan, N. K., Nigussie, E., Hakkala, A., Virtanen, S., & Isoaho, J. (2018). CoDRA: Context-based dynamically reconfigurable access control system for android. *Journal of Network and Computer Applications, 101*, 1−17.

Thilakarathne, N. N., Kagita, M. K., & Gadekallu, T. R. (2020). The role of the internet of things in health care: A systematic and comprehensive study. *International Journal of Engineering and Management Research (IJEMR), 10*(4), 145−159.

Uzair, M., Khan, M. A., Mann, S., & Imran, M. (November 2018). A review: Ubiquitous healthcare monitoring with mobile phone. In *2018 9th IEEE annual ubiquitous computing, electronics & mobile communication conference (UEMCON)* (pp. 988−996). IEEE.

Venkatesan, C., Karthigaikumar, P., Paul, A., Satheeskumaran, S., & Kumar, R. J. I. A. (2018). ECG signal preprocessing and SVM classifier-based abnormality detection in remote healthcare applications. *IEEE Access, 6*, 9767−9773.

Vianna, H. D., & Barbosa, J. L. V. (2020). Pompilos, a model for augmenting health assistant applications with social media content. *Journal of Universal Computer Science, 26*(1), 4−32.

Wang, X., Zhang, Z., Zhao, J., & Shi, Y. (2019). Impact of RHMS on healthcare service system considering patients' choice. *Discrete Dynamics in Nature Society, 2019*. https://doi.org/10.1155/2019/7642176

Weber, J. H., & Kuziemsky, C. (May 2019). Pragmatic interoperability for ehealth systems: The fallback workflow patterns. In *Proceedings of the 1st int*ernational workshop on software engineering for healthcare (pp. 29−36). IEEE Press.

Williams, S., Hardy, C., & Nitschke, P. (January 2019). Configuring the internet of things (IoT): A review and implications for big data analytics. In *Proceedings of the 52nd Hawaii* international conference on system sciences.

Yaacoub, E., Abualsaud, K., Khattab, T., Guizani, M., & Chehab, A. (2019). Secure mHealth IoT data transfer from the patient to the hospital: A three-tier approach. *IEEE Wireless Communications, 26*(5), 70−76.

Yang, S., Guo, B., Ao, L., Yang, C., Zhang, L., Zhou, J., & Jia, P. (2020). Obesity and activity patterns before and during COVID-19 lockdown among youths in China. *Clinical Obesity, 10*(6), e12416.

Zachlund, P., & Kallin, M. (2019). *"Technology can always crash; pen and paper will always work": The Internet of Things in the Swedish Hockey League.*

Further reading

Asam, M., & Jamal, T. (November 2019). Security issues in WBANs. In *Proceedings of the Arxiv, Volume arXiv:1911.04330 [cs.NI]*.

Baba, E., & Hammouch, A. (2018). *A health remote monitoring application based on wireless body area networks* (pp. 3–6).

Bernardini, S., Cianfrocca, C., Maioni, M., Pennacchini, M., Tartaglini, D., & Vollero, L. (2018). A mobile app for the remote monitoring and assistance of patients with Parkinson's disease and their caregivers. In *2018 40th annual international conference of the IEEE engineering in medicine and biology society (EMBC)* (pp. 2909–2912). https://doi.org/10.1109/EMBC.2018.8512989

Blüher, M. (2020). Metabolically healthy obesity. *Endocrine Reviews, 41*(3), 405–420.

Brauchli, K. (2006). RHMS for improving access to health care in resource-constrained areas: From individual diagnosis to strengthening health systems *(doctoral dissertation, University_of_Basel)*.

Butt, S. A., Anjum, M. W., Hassan, S. A., Garai, A., & Onyema, E. M. (2022). Smart health application for remote tracking of ambulatory patients. *Smart Healthcare System Design: Security and Privacy Aspects*, 33–55.

Butt, S. A., Gochhait, S., Andleeb, S., & Adeel, M. (2021). Games features for health disciplines for patient learning as entertainment. In *Digital entertainment* (pp. 65–86). Singapore: Palgrave Macmillan.

Chand, R. D., Kumar, A., Kumar, A., Tiwari, P., Rajnish, R., & Mishra, S. K. (2019). Advanced communication technologies for collaborative learning in RHMS and telecare. In *2019 9th international conference on cloud computing, data science & engineering* (pp. 601–605).

Dissertation: Toward a model RHMS program for the delivery of psychological services to developmentally delayed children ages 3 to 11 in a rural environment with a Focus on autism, Fragile X and Down Syndrome. DOI:10.13140/RG.2.1.1520.4320.

Fengou, M. A. (2014). A new framework for structuring and deploying advanced personalized and ubiquitous healthcare services *(Doctoral dissertation)*.

Gochhait, S., Butt, S., De-La-Hoz-Franco, E., Shaheen, Q., Luis, D. M., Piñeres-Espitia, G., & Mercado-Polo, D. (2021). A machine learning solution for bed occupancy issue for smart healthcare sector. *Automatic Control and Computer Sciences, 55*(6), 546–556.

Guffey, T. (2017). Smartphone application self-tracking use and health *(Doctoral dissertation)*.

Hollander, J. E., & Carr, B. G. (2020). Virtually perfect? RHMS for COVID-19. *New England Journal of Medicine, 382*(18), 1679–1681.

Holmen, Heidi (2017). *Mobile health for diabetes self-management* (Doctoral Thesis).

Jamal, T., & Butt, S. A. (2018). Malicious node analysis in MANETS. *International Journal of Information Technology*, 1–9.

Johanna, G. R., Patricia, A. C. P., Agustín, O. B. A., del Carmen, S. B. E., Miguel, U. T., Luis, D. M. J., … Diego, M. (2021). Predictive model for the identification of activities of daily living (ADL) in indoor environments using classification techniques based on Machine Learning. *Procedia Computer Science, 191*, 361–366.

Liau, J. C., & Ho, C. Y. (2019). Intelligence IoT(Internal of things) RHMS health care space system for the elderly living alone. In *Proceedings of the 2019 IEEE Eurasia conference biomedical engineering healthcare and sustainability ECBIOS 2019* (pp. 13–14). https://doi.org/10.1109/ECBIOS.2019.8807821

Nasiri, S., Sadoughi, F., Tadayolln, M. H., & Dehnad, A. (2019). Security requirements of internet of things-based healthcare system: A survey study. *Acta Informatica Medica, 27*(4), 253.

Ndlovu, K., Mars, M., & Scott, R. E. (2021). Interoperability frameworks linking mHealth applications to electronic record systems. *BMC Health Services Research, 21*(1), 1–10.

Otto, C. M. (2020). Heartbeat: Weather, air pollution and cardiac arrest. *Heart, 106*(16), 1193–1195.

Portnoy, J., Waller, M., & Elliott, T. (2020). RHMS in the era of COVID-19. *Journal of Allergy and Clinical Immunology: In Practice, 8*(5), 1489–1491. https://doi.org/10.1016/j.jaip.2020.03.008

Riffat, S. A., Harun, F., & Hassan, T. (2020). An interactive tele-medicine system via android application. In *Proceedings of the advanced computing and communication technologies for high performance applications (ACCTHPA)* (pp. 148–152). https://doi.org/10.1109/ACCTHPA49271.2020.9213200

Taiwo, O., & Ezugwu, A. E. (2020). Smart healthcare support for remote patient monitoring during covid-19 quarantine. *Informatics in Medicine Unlocked, 20*, 100428.

Tariq, M. I., Diaz-Martinez, J., Butt, S. A., Adeel, M., De-la-Hoz-Franco, E., & Dicu, A. M. (2018). A learners experience with the games education in software engineering. In *International workshop soft computing applications* (pp. 379–395). Cham: Springer.

Wang, X., Lei, S. M., Le, S., Yang, Y., Zhang, B., Yao, W., ... Cheng, S. (2020). Bidirectional influence of the COVID-19 pandemic lockdowns on health behaviors and quality of life among Chinese adults. *International Journal of Environmental Research and Public Health, 17*(15), 5575.

SECTION 2

Computational Intelligence for Medical Internet of Things (MIoT): Applications

CHAPTER

A review on the application of the Internet of Things in monitoring autism and assisting parents and caregivers

6

Fatima Ez Zahra El Arbaoui, Kaoutar El Hari, Rajaa Saidi
SI2M Laboratory, National Institute of Statistics and Applied Economics (INSEA), Rabat, Morocco

6.1 Introduction

Autism Spectrum Disorder (ASD) is a set of neurodevelopmental disorders called Pervasive Developmental Disorders (PDD). In Faras et al. (2010), the authors mentioned that these disorders lead to three main troubles: deficit in communication, limited social interaction, and stereotyped patterns of movements or interests which are usually repetitive. However, these troubles are irregular in range, symptoms, and severity.

Autism is challenging for parents and caregivers (Shattnawi et al., 2021), especially in countries where health services are restricted. According to Papadopoulos (2021), mothers of children with ASD revealed that they have issues in managing their child's problems because of a lack of knowledge. Consequently, the care provided to the child may be negatively impacted. Autism has a significant impact not only on the affected child but on the entire family dynamics. In Shattnawi et al. (2021), mothers demonstrated their concerns about their children's future. These concerns included autonomy in doing movements and daily living without assistance, the probability of marriage, and the influence on their siblings. In addition, worries about dangerous repetitive movement raise the stress of parents (Li & Lo, 2016).

Monitoring the health state of ASD children is a major concern. Parents need to keep an eye on their children affected by ASD and supervise their activities to prevent crises and be able to intervene at the correct moment. Meanwhile, IoT health applications are already deployed in the health care field. The main features of IoT applications are performance and real-time monitoring. Indeed, recent research in both IoT and sensing technology is demonstrated to be promising in the development of monitoring solutions for autism. In particular, IoT applications can monitor the health status of people with autism in real-time which provides an early intervention if an emergency (Ortolan-Soto et al., 2021).

Computational Intelligence for Medical Internet of Things (MIoT) Applications
https://doi.org/10.1016/B978-0-323-99421-7.00011-8

In this review, we explore numerous papers that show how IoT can be used to monitor people with autism and help parents and caregivers in assisting them. For this purpose, we apply the Systematic Literature Review (SLR) process introduced in (Kitchenham et al., n.d., p. 51). The main contributions of this review are:

- Presenting a review and evaluating how IoT can help parents and caregivers in supporting ASD people;
- Presenting a classification of papers based on IoT monitoring areas to monitor people with autism; and
- Analyzing and discussing the results of SLR.

This survey is organized as follows: Section 6.2 presents the literature study. Section 6.3 introduces the research methodology. Section 6.4 introduces the proposed classification of selected papers. Section 6.5 presents a discussion by answering technical research questions. Finally, Section 6.6 concludes this paper.

6.2 Related work

Investigations concerning the application of sensing technologies for monitoring biological signs for screening and therapy were presented in Cabibihan et al. (2017). The authors of this work demonstrated the potential of technological innovations in sensors and networks in assisting clinicians and therapists to screen autism and support the affected people. The taxonomy of the reviewed studies was based on what the smart device can track. The main categories were: eye trackers, movement trackers, electrodermal activity monitors, prosody and speech detection, and sleep quality assessment detection. The study did not consider devices that track environmental parameters. Autism is characterized by variable sensory sensitivities. For example, some individuals with autism may be frustrated and react in an excessive way to environmental stimuli such as fluorescent lights and sounds (Benssassi et al., 2018). Therefore, environmental trackers are necessary for monitoring and interventions. The study does not demonstrate how tracking parameters can help parents and caregivers. Closely related to this study, the authors of Ahmed et al. (2017) presented a review on studies that use sensing technologies to support autism. This review distinguishes between technologies used for assessment, intervention systems, and monitoring approaches. It introduces studies that use IoT for processing data concerning facial expressions, voices, body movement, cognition, social behavior, multimodal information, etc. The authors demonstrated the potential of this information in assessment. However, some limitations should be noted. The review relies on a few studies for each category. Only four studies were presented in the monitoring category while this field is promising for IoT applications.

On the other hand, the authors of Zwaigenbaum and Penner (2018, p. 361) reported that the progress of mechatronic devices promises a useful solution for ASD detection and rehabilitation. Mechatronic devices were categorized into screening and therapeutic groups. This review indicated that nonwearable devices are applied for recording behavioral data more than the wearable ones in the screening field. Furthermore, therapeutic devices can help in the therapy process and provide a great opportunity for parents to implement rehabilitation even at home. However, this categorization is insufficient since mechatronic devices can assume a key role in many other fields such as education and developing social skills. In addition to this review, a study presented by El Arbaoui et al. (2022) highlights the use of IoT wearables and mobiles technologies to address issues related to ASD intervention. The authors of this study presented a SLR to help researchers develop practical and convenient products. They identified 77 relevant papers to show the latest trends in wearable and mobile devices and investigations using these technologies in the field of ASD. Additionally, this work revealed that only 5.7% of projects target parents, and 2.6% target caregivers, which reflects the limited number of contributions to these targeted groups. Another SLR was introduced in Francese and Yang (2021) to specify how IoT-based systems apply machine learning in screening autism and improving the Quality of Life (QoL) of ASD people. The authors identified a total of 28 pertinent papers that committed to using IoT-based devices and approaches for ASD. They divided the collected papers into two main categories: IoT-based systems for autism diagnosis and IoT-based systems for improving the QoL.

6.3 Research methodology

This section presents the use of SLR. In Kitchenham et al. (n.d.), the authors designated SLR as a methodology widely used in literature. Following this methodology means identifying, detecting, gathering, and examining relevant papers that meet our research purposes.

Formulating the Goal-Question-Metric approach (GQM) (Solingen et al., 2002) is the first step in defining the scope of the review. Hence, to identify pertinent papers that explore how IoT and sensing technology are used in monitoring children with autism and helping parents and caregivers, we proposed research questions depicted in Table 6.1:

The next two sections describe the remaining steps of SLR to answer research questions based on SLR guidelines as depicted in Solingen et al. (2002). First, the section "Search Strategy" presents the search terms and the source of resources. The section "Papers selection process" describes the search criteria, the quality assessment, and data collection steps.

6.3.1 Search Strategy

6.3.1.1 Search terms

We follow five steps provided in Keele (2007):

1. The identification of population, intervention, and the outcome is as follows:
   - Population: children with autism and their parents and caregivers;

Table 6.1 Research questions.

N	Research question	Motivation
RQ1	What are the results acquired by the use of the proposed IoT approaches?	To analyze the outcomes obtained by applying the selected approaches.
RQ2	What IoT approaches have been used in assisting parents of children with autism?	To provide the different IoT approaches in the selected papers (e.g., Monitoring vital signs, etc.).
RQ3	What types of sensors have been utilized?	To specify what devices are used to monitor children with autism (wearable/nonwearable devices).
RQ4	What Techniques (e.g., algorithms) have been used to analyze data for early intervention?	To define techniques that support IoT for ASD monitoring
RQ5	What metrics have been used for evaluation?	To study the efficiency of the selected papers in ASD monitoring.

- Intervention: IoT;
- Outcome: Kind of action.

2. Synonyms recognition
   - Autism (“autism” OR “Autism Spectrum Disorder” OR “ASD” OR “autistic people” OR “Children affected by autism” OR “individuals on the spectrum disorder”);
   - IoT (“Internet of Things” OR “IoT” OR “Sensing technology” OR “sensors”);
   - Parents OR caregivers.
3. Keywords analysis
4. The formulation of search queries using “OR” and “AND” operators. The operator “AND” is for concatenation. For example:

```
(“Autism” OR “Autism Spectrum Disorder” OR “ASD” OR “autistic people” OR
“Children affected by autism” OR “individuals on the spectrum disorder”) AND
(“Internet of Things” OR “IoT” OR “Sensing technology” OR “sensors”) AND
(“Parents” OR “Caregivers”)
```

5. The formulation of a search query with a limited number of Boolean operators. For example:

```
(“Autism” OR “Autism Spectrum Disorder”) AND (“Internet of Things” OR
“Sensing technology”) AND (“Parents” OR “Caregivers”)
```

6.3.1.2 Search resources

Most of the papers were published in journals, conferences, and books. We used Google Scholar, Springer, IEEE, ACM, Science Direct, SCOPUS, PubMed, and Research Gate as main libraries.

The next section "Papers selection process" presents steps of selecting relevant papers. This section is divided into three parts: the search criteria, the quality assessment, and data collection.

6.3.2 Papers selection process

The process of retrieving related studies is presented in Fig. 6.1:

More than 60 articles were retrieved from the initial selection using the selected databases. Meanwhile, some papers (for example papers that are referenced in a retrieved paper from a database) were searched manually.

In the succeeding stage, we applied inclusion and inclusions factors. We detail this part in the "Search Criteria" paragraph. The result of this selection was 52.

The Quality of the rest of the papers was evaluated using the criteria specified in the paragraph: "Quality assessment."

Search Criteria.

Following SLR, we apply two types of criteria:

6.3.2.1 Inclusion criteria

- Research is not concerned with autism;
- Research is not concerned with IoT or sensing technology;
- Research is not in English and it is written in a different language;
- Research doesn't in peer-reviewed journals or conferences, books, and lecture notes;
- Research has written before 2012.

6.3.2.2 Exclusion criteria

1. Research is published between 2012 and 2021.
2. The research uses keywords.

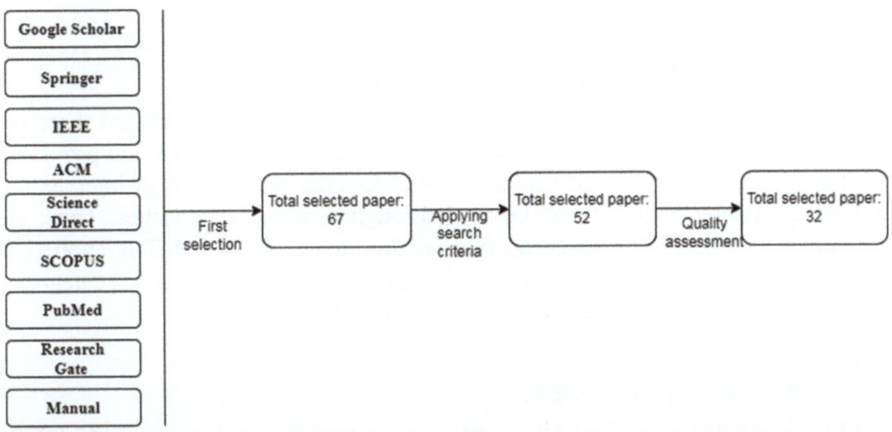

FIGURE 6.1

The adopted paper selection process.

3. The research exploits IoT to monitor children with autism and assist parents and caregivers.
4. Full version (not abstract) research.

As mentioned in Fig. 6.1. The final result of the "Search Criteria" step gathered 52 research papers.

6.3.2.3 Quality assessment

In this phase, we verify in detail the collected papers from the previous step. According to SLR, we conducted this phase with a set of questions. Each research answers the following questions:

- Q1: Is the approach presented?
- Q2: Is the proposed solution specified in detail?
- Q3: Is the IoT applied?
- Q4: Are the validation strategies and performance measures explicitly detailed?
- Q5: Does the approach have been tested in a real environment?

Each selected paper has a score that corresponds to the quality. According to the scoring procedure specified by SLR, each question is scored as: "YES" = 1, "Partially" = 0.5, "NO" = 0, or Unknown. The score of the paper is the sum of the five questions score. Then, we categorized the research quality as "High (score $\geq$ 4)", "Medium (3$\leq$ score < 4)", and "Low (score < 3)".

Only papers having medium or high scores were selected.

6.3.2.4 Data collection

The final papers which passed all selection phases were examined to answer the research questions. For this purpose, we propose in the next section a categorization of papers that explore the use of IoT in autism monitoring. Then, we answer the research aspects in the "Results" sections.

6.4 The use of IoT in autism monitoring

The result of the paper selection was 32 pertinent studies. We analyzed these researches to demonstrate the role of IoT in monitoring ASD children and providing solutions used by parents and caregivers. We detected many areas of intervention and we considered that IoT can be used through different approaches. Then, we developed a classification based on intervention areas and how IoT is applied in our research aspects. The remaining of this section presents our proposed categories to classify the IoT approaches in autism monitoring.

6.4.1 Monitoring vital signs

AutiLife is a healthcare monitoring system conceived for autism centers to handle medical emergencies. The authors of Mamun et al. (2019) proposed the integration of the 5G technology to send alerts faster. The system continuously records data through sensors. Several vital signs are tracked: heart rate, body temperature, motions, speech signals, and blood pressure. Data is analyzed through a support vector machine (SVM) algorithm to identify the health status. The system sends alerts when an emergency is detected. AutiLife combines 5G and IoT technology. 5G was proposed to provide low-latency and secure exchange and reliable data. IoT was the appropriate technology according to the authors to allow the massive connection between different devices. Detecting emergency situations was also a purpose for. The authors of Alwakeel et al. (2016) presented a system for monitoring patients that did not act only in an autism center. Regardless of the place, the system records data about motions and behaviors and detects if the person with autism is in danger. Indeed, autism is associated with numerous repetitive behaviors; sometimes they can be harmful, for example, when an affected person beats himself. The system is named Autistic Child Sensor and Assistant system (ACSA) and it is based on a wireless sensor network. The ACSA system involves three components: an ACSA wearable sensor for motion and location detection, an ACSA parent mobile application to receive alerts and notifications, and machine learning algorithms used to process data gathered by the ACSA sensor. A similar study was conducted by Amiri et al. (2017). But, the authors of Amiri et al. (2017) analyzed only gestures to identify stereotyped behaviors and introduced an IoT-based using a smartwatch called "WearSense." This system is based on three components: smartwatch, smartphone app, and cloud computing. The smartwatch is equipped with an accelerometer to detect motions. One hundred and two features were extracted and behaviors were classified using the decision tree (DT) method. Motions were classified into three types of stereotyped behaviors: sobbing, hand flapping, and painting. The system is connected to the cloud and sends notifications to parents and caregivers to let them know about negative situations. The accuracy of the system was calculated and estimated at around 94.6%. Another research was developed in Srinivasa et al. (2016) to deal with medical emergencies. The authors proposed a software framework constructed by four modules: (1) a module for data collection that requires sensors (2) Rest services that provide the communication between components, (3) client applications, and (4) a data storage and analysis module. The client applications send calls to the cloud to get real-time data to display results and alert if there is an emergency. Real-time data is collected from the learner using on-body sensors inspired by Shimmer's work (Shimmer Sensor Kit, n.d.), and then it is analyzed through a statistical program that deduces alert situations by comparing real-time with training data. When the system detects an alert, it sent notifications to the connected Android device.

In Alwakeel et al. (2016), Amiri et al. (2017), Mamun et al. (2019), the researchers used many sensors to collect different vital signs data using different sources. We noticed that the authors of Krishna and Sampath (2017) used only two measures: oxygen saturation and skin temperature. They designed an IoT-based system was designed to monitor the health of patients (Krishna & Sampath, 2017). The system sends real-time vital signs data to parents or caregivers. The authors proposed connecting the Arduino UNO board and Raspberry Pi board to sensors and using the Message Queuing Telemetry Transport (MQTT) protocol for data transfer. Two main sensors were involved: pulse oximeter to measure the oxygen saturation percentage and a temperature sensor. A cloud server (Amazon EC2) is installed to process data and send information to a mobile or a laptop. A Wi-Fi module was implemented for data transmission between computing boards and the server. To present results, measurements, and dashboards, "MQTT Lens" was used for laptops and "MQTT Dashboard" for smartphones.

All wearable devices mentioned in the studies of this section (Monitoring vital signs) can be worn in many contexts. The research conducted by Sundhara Kumar and Bairavi (2016) is different; the proposed wearable device is designed only for the medical environment. The proposed system provides a methodology for continuous monitoring and alerting caregivers. A head-gear wearable sensor is implemented to gather the electroencephalogram (EEG) signals, then, this data is transferred to a monitoring server where it is processed. When an anomaly is detected, an email is sent to the caregiver, but in case of the situation is critical the system involves the medical specialist as well. The wearable device consists of several electrodes that require special positions to receive brain readings.

Parents and caregivers accompany children with ASD in their daily activities including learning, playing, etc. They should supervise their health status and provide them with the appropriate assistance. To help parents and caregivers in their tasks, the authors of Rahman and Bhuiyan (2015) proposed an open computing platform for autistic children; the system is based on a wearable system with an array of sensors. It collects and analyzes physiological signs. Data is sent to medical servers to recognize the healthcare status of children with ASD. The multimodal intelligent mode supports the daily activities of patients. The system applied a modular approach to make prototyping and creation easier. The most important sensors are the temperature sensor and heart rate sensor. The system contains several tiers to make the platform ubiquitous. These tiers are the wearable computing platform, a server for data storage, and mi-children.org which is an artificial intelligence (AI) platform used for processing sensor data with advanced machine learning techniques.

The next section presents the second category (social safety monitoring), in which, we detailed selected papers that alert parents and caregivers about safety concerns.

6.4.2 Social safety monitoring

Social safety skills are both verbal and nonverbal behaviors that the individual should do when an emergency occurs Clees and Gast (1994). Unfortunately, children with ASD may have deficits in social safety skills. According to Bergstrom et al. (2012), it is necessary to teach children how to look for help around them when they are lost. In addition to that, parents and caregivers need to be informed constantly about their children's location and if they face any problems. To supervise activities and locations The Alzimio app for dementia, autism, and Alzheimer's was developed Helmy and Helmy (2016). It is a mobile application for patients with autism, Alzheimer's, and dementia. The Alzimio app allows parents and caregivers to set safe zones and activities for their patients on how to carry a smartphone with the application. Then they receive alerts if the safe zones or activities are violated. The application is based on four modules: Sensors, detection algorithms, notification subsystem, and the user interface. The Alzimio app provides both activity-based alarms and location recognition. It introduces three different algorithms for activity recognition: "threshold-based," "max-in-window," and "direct Android API output." In Madhuri et al. (2020), the authors addressed also safety issues as the previous research, but they proposed an application that tracks only the location in public events to ensure the protection of children in these events. Therefore, the authors developed a tracking system to deal with this concern. The system depends on an IoT-based cloud platform (Salesforce cloud) for data storage, an Android mobile application owned by parents or caregivers, and GPS (Global Positioning System) technology. The child wears a GPS tracking band. Based on the identified safe zone, alerts are sent to the Android application if the child is outside the safe zone. Location recognition is also a feature provided in a system designed by Goel and Kumar (2015). The authors consider safety as a serious problem for individuals affected by Alzheimer's, dementia, and autism. They conceive a smart locator band connected with the mobile of parents and caregivers to keep tracking their location. When the wearer is in an emergency, he can click on the emergency button to call the configured emergency contact. When the emergency contact is called, he also receives the current location displayed in Google Map. According to the authors, existing commercial devices that provide location are expensive and do not contain the emergency press button. The test stage and experiments demonstrate the efficiency of the custom device and the developed Android-based application.

In Bouras et al. (2021), the authors indicated that people with ASD are at risk of being missed when they are in unfamiliar environments. The proposed system by the authors aimed to search and save these people in dangerous situations. The system is called WeSAR (Wearable Based Search and Rescue system) and it is based on a wearable device that considers energy efficiency and battery life, and a Narrow Band Internet of Things (NB-IoT) system. WeSAR's architecture consists of five layers: user device, network transponders, network management servers, IoT cloud platform, and application service layer. WeSAR allows real-time location tracking, device monitoring, danger detection, and emergency notifications.

In addition to the location tracking, controlling the health status of children with autism continuously is challenging for parents. According to Ahmed et al. (2017), body temperature, heart rate, location, and pulse are the main parameters that require continual observation. The issue that faces most tracking devices is the restriction of battery life. To overcome this issue, a wearable device was developed based on solar power. The proposed system of Ahmed et al. (2017) is built upon a power generation component and data processing component. The first component is responsible for charging. The second component has two modules: A sensor module and a data transfer module. A temperature sensor and pulse sensor construct the sensor module. GPS technology and SMS will be used for transferring data and calling emergency contact directly. In addition to this project, the authors of Khullar et al. (2019) designed a real-time monitoring and alerting prototype called "ACHI" (Assistive Companion for Hypersensitive Individuals). It is based on three modules: a module for recording data and decision-making, a monitoring and analyzing module, and a module for feedback and alerts. A Fuzzy Inference System (FIS) process and analyze data collected via sensors that are installed in a toy bag. These sensors are connected via Arduino and Raspberry Pi. Whenever something goes wrong, an email is sent to the caregiver. If the caregiver takes too much time to respond, ACHI activates the automatic calm-down mode to relax the child via auditory video. ACHI was tested in different environments for validation. 93% of caregivers and individuals affected by ASD who participated in the testing stage were satisfied with the performance of the system.

Rather than monitoring a few elements to ensure safety. The authors of Lebedev et al. (2019) identified the prerequisites to construct a telemedicine monitoring system at home for children with ASD. The proposed system explores the use of digital technologies. The authors developed a hardware-software system (HSS) to keep tracking the biological signs. In addition, the system required an automated workplace (AW) to allow the supervision by doctors, a video surveillance system to dynamically detect the child's reactions, a virtual reality (VR) system for remote learning, and many other subsystems. IoT technology is needed to maintain the connection between health mobile devices. To assist the medical decision-making, a set of methods for data processing will be implemented to analyze data recorded from mobile medical devices and questionnaires.

The authors of Al Banna et al. (2020) underlined the negative impact of Covid 19 not only on children affected by ASD but parents and caregivers as well. The lockdown makes finding doctors and therapists a tough task. Therefore, the authors propose regulating the learning approach by monitoring the health status and concentration. The system is based on AI and sensors to track emotion and facial expressions. The system sends alerts to parents and caregivers when detecting abnormal situations while studying. To achieve this purpose, the authors used a camera attached to an interactive monitor and a smart wristband containing a set of sensors. All of the devices are connected to a mobile application designed for parents and caregivers. For emotion detection, an inception-ResNetV2 model was used to process pictures captured by the camera. On the other hand, a data set named CK+48 was used for facial expression recognition. In addition to this study, the authors of Abdullah and Al-Allaf (2021) aimed also to design a prototype system based on IoT to protect autistic children from any abnormal situation. Their solution suggested the usage of several sensors connected via "Particle Photon" which is an integrated Wi-Fi and a fully cloud-based IoT prototyping platform. The system sends a notification or an email to parents and caregivers when dangerous behavior is identified. The authors proposed also the Blynk platform for allowing parents and caregivers to monitor and control the system sensors by their mobile devices. Blynk provides the possibility of designing apps for controlling IoT devices. Furthermore, the system supervises continuously the location of the child by a GPS unit. The system integrates also a calming unit that plays music until the intervention of parents.

The category presented in the next section is stereotypical movement monitoring. The selected papers of this category underline the importance of intervening when stereotypical movement occurs because it can be dangerous.

6.4.3 Stereotypical movement monitoring

Self-injurious behaviors (SIB) were observed in children with autism. Usually, they hit themselves in one single location, which can be dangerous and harmful. To address this issue, Min and Tewfik (2010) develop an IoT-based system using a custom accelerometer as the main sensor for data acquisition and linear predictive coding (LPC) model for classifying behavioral events. A user interface was designed to receive sensor data and allow doctors and therapists to tag events instantaneously. Particularly, behaviors that were observed in this work are hand flapping, body rocking, punching one's face, and hitting. The distinction between stereotypical movements and SIB was an important requirement of the system. In addition, the system learns new SIB patterns rapidly. As a future evolution, the authors consider the prediction of events before happening. A similar study was conducted by Bansode et al. (2019), the authors of this work focused only on hand flapping as a common stereotypical movement in children with autism and it can lead to SIB. To detect hand flapping, the authors proposed a wearable device that consists of a smart bracelet, a smartphone for alerting parents and caregivers, and a component that responds to the behavior by calming the child. This response can be a configured audio of parents, music, or simply a vibration. The primary aim of the system is to identify abnormal behavior and to inform parents and caregivers about the child's activities. The experiments of this prototype were conducted in a laboratory where hand flapping was simulated. The results show that audio is automatically activated once significant hand flapping is detected. The identification of stereotypical motor movement (SMM) was the purpose of Rad et al. (2015). The authors proposed the usage of conventional neural networks (CNN) and wireless sensing technology to expose SMM in real-time. The deep learning model was implemented to detect all of the properties of atypical motions. The advantage of CNN is its ability to convert many accelerometer signs from different resources into a group of features. A classifier based on SVM affects the behavior of SMM classes or no-SMM classes. Six children affected by ASD have participated in experiments in the classroom and laboratory. Each child wore three accelerometer sensors, which are three axes and wireless. Data was gathered through these sensors and was analyzed, the classification was done by learned features and handcrafted features to compare between approaches. The results of the experiments show the outperformance of CNN over the traditional classification methods.

According to Manocha and Bhatia (n.d.), different SMM is recognized to be a serious hurdle for autistic individuals and can negatively affect their QoL. Therefore, the study presented in Manocha and Bhatia (n.d.) proposed a framework to detect SMM in real-time. Using intelligent wearable sensors for activity recognition and CNN + long short-term memory (LSTM), the framework can monitor SMM and improve assistive care by sending notifications in real-time. The framework is based on two modules to predict Stereotypic Movement Disorder (SMD): the cloud module and the IoT fog module. The collected data is analyzed on the fog layer using CNN and LSTM. A cloud database is used to store all predicted SMM. The authors of Coronato et al. (2014) tried to identify SMM by using the eZ430-Chronos as a wireless smartwatch to acquire SMM signals, then data was analyzed via a statistical approach to detect and classify SMM. The smartwatch contains a three-axis accelerometer. The test of the proposed system was conducted in a classroom with the participation of five ASD children. An application based on LabVIEW was developed to get and analyze the smartwatch data. It was observed that sometimes the child tried to throw off the bracelet. Despite this constraint, the system detected 75% of SMM. In Coronato et al. (2014), the identification of SMD relied on a template matching technique, accelerometers, the Situation-Awareness paradigm, and classifiers. The proposed system consists of a software unit named "Data Acquirer," a preprocessor unit, and ANN classifier. The "Data Acquirer" gathers the eZ430-Chronos accelerometer's sensors. The preprocessor unit is for extracting features and generating events for four types of behavior: hand rotation down (HRD), hand rotation up (HRU), hand hitting against the ear (HE), and arm flapping (AF). The system implements an intelligent situation-aware component that receives the generated events of the detected SMD. This prototype is already deployed in a hospital room and allows caregivers to observe the child's behavior in real-time.

The next section presents the category of papers that address emotion recognition issues. On one how the child can be aware of his emotions, on the other side how parents and caregivers should read the child's emotions.

6.4.4 Emotion recognition

In Tang (2016), the authors conceived a play environment embedded with sensors that identify facial expressions and body movements. This environment lets NT individuals recognize autistic children's emotions by reading emotion labels exposed by an emotion APIs. The authors relied on three main measures to qualify the behavior pattern: vital signs, behavioral data, and sociometer. An Arduino unit captures data, and with the Wi-Fi technology, data is transferred to a local server where it is stored, then numerous computers can read and analyze the stored data. The authors used Emoncms as an open-source web application for data analysis and visualization. Emoncms is connected to the local database. In this work, each sensor is tested separately; the authors expect the integration of all sensors in testing in future contributions. In the same category(emotion recognition), the authors of Bondy and Frost (1994) aimed to deduce the emotional state of children with autism and communicate it to others, they suggested the development of a smart bracelet that helps also the child to enhance his self-knowledge and his social interaction. The authors used Photo-PlethysmoGraphy (PPG) and electrodermal activity (EDA) since they are helpful to determine the emotional status of patients as mentioned in medical research. Therefore, the bracelet aims to measure EDA and PPG signals in children with ASD. Because of COVID-19 conditions, the authors didn't test the bracelet with volunteers but they used an existing database to evaluate the device. It has been deduced that when children with autism react nervously to a stimulus, their sweating and heart rate rise.

According to Lavanya (2019), the recent autistic therapy involves a bimodel system for human emotion recognition. This existing system combines facial expressions and speech signals data. The authors suggested enhancing emotion recognition by using both thermal infrared pictures and visible images. The advantage of thermal images is that they are insensitive to light conditions. Least square support vector-machines (LSSVM) is a kernel-based learning method that was used for data processing. Then, an LCD shows the state of the child. For long-term monitoring, emotion recognitions are stored in an "IoT think speak" account accessible by doctors. For the same aim, another study conducted by Kashanian et al. (2017) considered the application of cloud technology and smart wearable devices to communicate with people with autism and understand their emotional status. This approach was built on three modules: the collection of data via smart clothes, emotional analysis, and the control of emotional interaction. The approach includes processing images, audio, social and physiological dimensions. Time-space tags were used to gather data from videos, and speeches. To process all collected data, the authors used the cloud-based method. They included also the possibility to send the emotional status to a phone or a server.

In this category, we found also an IoT-based system presented in Fadhil and Mandeel (2018) that proposes remote monitoring using a galvanic skin response (GSR) sensor to measure the electrical conductivity of the skin while the patient faces different emotions. Experiments were performed with two groups of children: neurotypical and autistic children. The results show that children with autism do have not have a notable variation in the GSR sensor signal values. The authors achieve their work by processing three phases: (1) the hardware setup; (2) the code of NodeMCU, and the preparation of the server; and (3) data analysis. Fourteen children participated in the experiment of this system; seven of them were affected by ASD. Data was collected from GSR sensors that they wear and was analyzed using different models. Relaxation, happiness, nervousness, and many other emotions were observed and inspected. Furthermore, the authors compared the reaction of children to their emotions. They noticed that children with autism have irregular patterns of emotional response.

The next section presents the category of papers that support parents and caregivers in facing communication deficits in children with autism.

6.4.5 Communication

Augmentative and Alternative Communication (AAC) is an area of research that assists people who have communication difficulties and understandable speaking in their social interaction and communication (Beukelman & Light, n.d.). Deploying AAC solutions for people with autism is essential because they can also suffer from communication disturbances. A study conducted by Fazana et al. (2017) considers combining AAC and assistive technologies to assist children with ASD. In this work, a framework was developed to improve communication skills, health monitoring, and behaviors. The proposed solution enhances children's communication, allows parents and caregivers to track the child's location, and provides data about physiological signs for medical professionals. The system has many functionalities including the identification of stress prompt, monitoring the physiological level of stress and sending notifications, supervising activities, etc. To achieve these functionalities, the authors suggested a wearable device that contains a GPS sensor, EDA sensor, heart rate sensor, etc. Secured cloud infrastructure was used for data processing and clustering. The Picture Exchange Communication System (PECS) technology is a training program associated with AAC (Bondy & Frost, 1994). This program aims to teach children with autism how to use picture cards to ask for anything or any activity. However, only a few software applications were designed for PECS. The authors of Tang and Winoto (2018) aimed to propose a system that extends and customizes PECS by adding three main features: location, event sensing, and on-demand request via WeChat, which is a popular communication tool in China. For example, when the child is in a restaurant, the system enables location and event sensing to propose pictures corresponding to this context, consequently, the child can pick rapidly what he needs. The architecture of the system is based on four modules: event sensing, location sensing, behavior sensing, and adaptive content presentation. In addition, a module for sending messages was developed on children's tablets. The system has four categories and 400 pictures.

Usually, children with autism communicate with motions and gestures; parents and caregivers can understand their gestures but it is difficult for other people to understand the meaning of children's gestures (Siddiqui et al., 2021). Hence, to promote communication among those children, the study conducted by Siddiqui et al. (2021) proposed a sensing-based IoT platform that classifies gestures. The architecture of this project relies on a wearable sensor (the sensor contains an accelerometer and gyroscope) that collects and sends data to a classification server via Bluetooth. Several machine learning classifiers were used to process data: K-nearest neighbor, DT, random forest, and back-propagation-based neural networks. The authors used a data set composed of 24 gestures from 10 children with ASD. Despite the few amount of data, the accuracy of the system reaches 91% using the single-layer neural network. Another approach was introduced in Saini et al. (2019) for monitoring the interaction between two ASD individuals by adopting the bidirectional long short-term memory neural network (BLSTM-NN). The system was based on a Kinect sensor to collect data. During the communication, each individual's activities were tracked by 3D skeletal. A unique skeletal ID was attributed to each person. BLSTM-NN was used to identify those activities. A lexicon approach was applied to enhance the performance of system. 10 volunteers have participated in the validation stage. The system's accuracy reached f 58.51% without a lexicon and improved to 70.72% with a lexicon.

The next section describes the results of SLR to answer the research questions.

6.5 Results

6.5.1 RQ1: What are the results acquired by the use of the proposed IoT approaches?

Using comfortable and efficient wearable devices can provide parents and caregivers the accurate information about the health conditions children with. Therefore, they can understand better their behaviors and situations. In addition, IoT allows real-time access to data, parents, and caregivers can receive real-time alerts and notifications to react correctly. Selected papers belonging to the "Monitoring vital signs" category, reported the use of IoT to track several vital signs, in particular, heart rate, blood pressure, body temperature, motions, EEG signals, etc.

Parents and caregivers reported that social safety is a major issue when children with autism are outside a secured environment or home. For example, NT children can ask for help, ASD children may have communication problems and can't express what they need. Dealing with similar situations was the purpose of more than 10 researches of selected papers. In many cases, the authors proposed using a wearable device that includes GPS to track continuously the location of the child. Rather than that, some studies proposed defining secured areas, so parents and caregivers receive alerts when the child is outside this zone.

More than six papers considered the importance of detecting stereotypical movements as they can be dangerous and need early intervention from parents and caregivers. Most papers proposed using accelerometers to detect gestures, a machine learning model to recognize the motion, and a module for sending messages to parents and caregivers. Some proposed devices trigger music, images of audios to calm the child when detecting SMM.

In the selected papers, the deficit of expressing emotions among children with autism was revealed. Some research suggested using body movement, facial expressions, and other physiological signs to recognize the child's emotions and make him aware of his emotions.

Depending on the intellectual development of children with autism, they may have communication problems or not. In the presence of language and communication deficits, they can't reveal their needs and sometimes they can't understand what others say. To address this issue, more than six papers of our selection suggested the implementation of IoT to assist children when asking for a need and helping parents and caregivers recognize what children ask for. Analyzing gestures, developing a PECS-based IoT system, monitoring social interaction, and other techniques were adopted to improve the communication skills of children with autism and make their parents and caregivers able to know what they express.

6.5.2 RQ2: What IoT approaches have been used in assisting parents of children with autism?

We identify four areas where IoT can be used to monitor children and assist their parents and caregivers: monitoring vital signs, social safety monitoring, stereotypical movement monitoring, emotion recognition, and communication.

6.5.3 RQ3: What types of sensors have been utilized?

The development of a wearable sensor that tracks data for an IoT-based system is difficult. Children are supposed to wear wearable devices continuously. Even if the device is designed to be comfortable, well placed, Strong, and efficient, the possibility that the child can throw it away is apparent.

Most approaches that propose the monitoring of motions, gestures, and physiological signs suggested a wearable device placed on the wrist (smartwatch for example). The accelerometer was the main used sensor to track motions and gestures. The heart rate sensor, skin temperature sensor, and other sensors were used to monitor vital signs. Usually, cameras and audio sensors were used to monitor activities and behaviors. In all studies that use location tracking, a GPS sensor was required.

6.5.4 RQ4: What techniques (e.g., algorithms) have been used to analyze data for early intervention?

Techniques based on machine learning models (SVM, CNN, etc.) were applied to process data collected by sensors. The limited data sets can't prove the efficiency of the results. Still, these techniques were widely used for feature extraction, classification, decision-making, etc. Meters such as specificity, accuracy, precision, and sensitivity were calculated in the majority of selected papers (at least two) to demonstrate the proposed model efficiency.

6.5.5 RQ5: What metrics have been used for evaluation?

The validation step of most of the mentioned approaches was conducted by the participation of ASD and NT people. The number of participants in all selected research is few. However, the authors demonstrated the efficiency and the performance of the approach. Sometimes, they compare their prototype with existing solutions and show the impact of implementing their approach. For the validation, accuracy, sensitivity, latency and specificity are the most used measures.

6.6 Conclusion

People with autism, especially children, face many challenges. But their parents and caregivers are impacted as well. In this review, we noticed that IoT is a promising technology with a significant role in assisting parents and caregivers. We conducted our research on the following questions: (1) What are the results acquired by the use of the proposed IoT approaches? (2) What IoT approaches have been used in assisting parents of children with autism? (3) What types of sensors have been utilized? (4) What techniques (e.g., algorithms) have been used to analyze data for early intervention? and (5) What metrics have been used for evaluation?

From this review, it appeared the huge potential of IoT in the discussed field. However, several limitations exist in the considered papers and further work needs to be done.

6.6.1 Limitations and further work

This work has some limitations, we reviewed only papers that present IoT approaches for helping also parents and caregivers, and we selected papers based on specific keywords which can make us miss some relevant papers that explore IoT in monitoring children with autism. In addition, we reviewed only English; we think that other relevant papers may be written in other languages. Further work could explore useful IoT systems that could be used by the affected people with autism without the intervention of parents and caregivers.

References

Abdullah, N. M., & Al-Allaf, A. F. (2021). A support system for autistic children using Internet of Things technology. In *2021 international conference on advanced computer applications, ACA 2021* (pp. 51–56). Institute of Electrical and Electronics Engineers Inc. https://doi.org/10.1109/ACA52198.2021.9626825

Ahmed, I. U., Hassan, N., & Rashid, H. (2017). Solar powered smart wearable health monitoring and tracking device based on GPS and GSM technology for children with autism. In *4th international conference on advances in electrical engineering, ICAEE 2017* (Vol 2018, pp. 111–116). Institute of Electrical and Electronics Engineers Inc. https://doi.org/10.1109/ICAEE.2017.8255337

Al Banna, M. H., Ghosh, T., Taher, K. A., Kaiser, M. S., & Mahmud, M. (2020). *A monitoring system for patients of autism spectrum disorder using artificial intelligence* (Vol 12241, pp. 251–262). Springer Science and Business Media LLC. https://doi.org/10.1007/978-3-030-59277-6_23

Alwakeel, S. S., Alhalabi, B., Aggoune, H., & Alwakeel, M. (2016). A machine learning based WSN system for autism activity recognition. In *Proceedings – 2015 IEEE 14th international conference on machine learning and applications, ICMLA 2015* (pp. 771–776). Institute of Electrical and Electronics Engineers Inc. https://doi.org/10.1109/ICMLA.2015.46

Amiri, A., Peltier, N., Goldberg, C., Sun, Y., Nathan, A., Hiremath, S., & Mankodiya, K. (2017). WearSense: Detecting autism stereotypic behaviors through smartwatches. *Healthcare, 5*(1), 11. https://doi.org/10.3390/healthcare5010011

Bansode, S., Shinde, T., Garapati, S., & Abdel-Qader, I. (2019). Stereotypic repetitive hand flapping movement detector for children with autism. In *Proceedings of 2019 3rd IEEE international conference on electrical, computer and communication technologies, ICECCT 2019*. Institute of Electrical and Electronics Engineers Inc. https://doi.org/10.1109/ICECCT.2019.8869018

Benssassi, E. M., Gomez, J. C., Boyd, L. E., Hayes, G. R., & Ye, J. (2018). Wearable assistive technologies for autism: Opportunities and challenges. *IEEE Pervasive Computing, 17*(2), 11−21. https://doi.org/10.1109/MPRV.2018.022511239

Bergstrom, R., Najdowski, A. C., & Tarbox, J. (2012). Teaching children with Autism to seek help when lost in public. *Journal of Applied Behavior Analysis, 45*(1), 191−195. https://doi.org/10.1901/jaba.2012.45-191

Beukelman, D. R., & Light, J. C. (n.d.). Augmentative & alternative communication supporting children and adults with complex communication needs.

Bondy, A. S., & Frost, L. A. (1994). The picture exchange communication system. *Focus on Autistic Behavior, 9*(3), 1−19. https://doi.org/10.1177/108835769400900301

Bouras, C. J., Gkamas, A., Katsampiris Salgado, S. A., & Papachristos, N. (2021). *Search and Rescue system based on NB-IoT wearable device* (pp. 195−222). IGI Global. https://doi.org/10.4018/978-1-7998-4775-5.ch009

Cabibihan, J. J., Javed, H., Aldosari, M., Frazier, T. W., & Elbashir, H. (2017). Sensing technologies for autism spectrum disorder screening and intervention. *Sensors (Switzerland), 17*(1). https://doi.org/10.3390/s17010046

Clees, T. J., & Gast, D. L. (1994). *Social safety skills instruction for individuals with disabilities: A sequential model. Education and treatment of children* (Vol 17, pp. 163−185).

Coronato, A., De Pietro, G., & Paragliola, G. (2014). A situation-aware system for the detection of motion disorders of patients with Autism Spectrum Disorders. *Expert Systems with Applications, 41*(17), 7868−7877. https://doi.org/10.1016/j.eswa.2014.05.011

El Arbaoui, F. E. Z., El Hari, K., & Saidi, R. (2022). A survey on the application of the Internet of things in the diagnosis of autism spectrum disorder. In *Lecture notes on data engineering and communications technologies* (Vol 110, pp. 29−41). Springer Science and Business Media Deutschland GmbH. https://doi.org/10.1007/978-3-030-94188-8_4

Fadhil, T. Z., & Mandeel, A. R. (2018). Live monitoring system for recognizing varied emotions of autistic children. In *ICOASE 2018 - international conference on advanced science and engineering* (pp. 151−155). Institute of Electrical and Electronics Engineers Inc. https://doi.org/10.1109/ICOASE.2018.8548931

Faras, H., Al Ateeqi, N., & Tidmarsh, L. (2010). Autism spectrum disorders. *Annals of Saudi Medicine, 30*(4), 295−300. https://doi.org/10.4103/0256-4947.65261

Fazana, F., Alsadoon, A., Prasad, P. W. C., Costadopoulos, N., Elchouemi, A., & Sreedharan, S. (2017). Integration of assistive and wearable technology to improve communication, social interaction and health monitoring for children with autism spectrum disorder (ASD). In *TENSYMP 2017 - IEEE international symposium on technologies for smart cities*. Institute of Electrical and Electronics Engineers Inc. https://doi.org/10.1109/TENCONSpring.2017.8070018

Francese, R., & Yang, X. (2021). Supporting autism spectrum disorder screening and intervention with machine learning and wearables: A systematic literature review. *Complex & Intelligent Systems*, 1−16. https://doi.org/10.1007/s40747-021-00447-1

Goel, I., & Kumar, D. (2015). Design and implementation of android based wearable smart locator band for people with autism, dementia, and Alzheimer. *Advances in Electronics, 1–8.* https://doi.org/10.1155/2015/140762

Helmy, J., & Helmy, A. (2016). The alzimio app for dementia, autism & Alzheimer's: Using novel activity recognition algorithms and geofencing. In *2016 IEEE international conference on smart computing, SMARTCOMP 2016*. Institute of Electrical and Electronics Engineers Inc. https://doi.org/10.1109/SMARTCOMP.2016.7501720

Kashanian, H., Ajami, N. B., & Deghati, M. (2017). Communication with autistic people through wearable sensors and cloud technology. In *5th Iranian joint congress on fuzzy and intelligent systems - 16th conference on fuzzy systems and 14th conference on intelligent systems, CFIS 2017* (pp. 139–143). Institute of Electrical and Electronics Engineers Inc. https://doi.org/10.1109/CFIS.2017.8003672

Keele, S. (2007). *Guidelines for performing systematic literature reviews in software engineering*.

Khullar, V., Singh, H. P., & Bala, M. (2019). IoT based assistive companion for hypersensitive individuals (ACHI) with autism spectrum disorder. *Asian Journal of Psychiatry, 46*, 92–102. https://doi.org/10.1016/j.ajp.2019.09.030

Kitchenham, B., Brereton, O. P., Budgen, D., Turner, M., Bailey, J., & Linkman, S. (n.d.). Systematic literature reviews in software engineering – a systematic literature review. *Information and Software Technology, 51*.

Krishna, C. S., & Sampath, N. (2017). Healthcare monitoring system based on IoT. In *2nd international conference on computational systems and information technology for sustainable solution (CSITSS)*. https://doi.org/10.1109/CSITSS.2017.8447861

Lavanya, K. (2019). Emotion recognition of autistic children using IoT. *International Journal of Applied Engineering Research, 14*.

Lebedev, G., Klimenko, H., Fartushniy, E., Shaderkin, I., Kozhin, P., & Galitskaya, D. (2019). *Building a telemedicine system for monitoring the health status and supporting the social adaptation of children with autism spectrum disorders* (Vol 143, pp. 287–294). Springer Science and Business Media LLC. https://doi.org/10.1007/978-981-13-8303-8_26

Li, T. Y., & Lo, J. L. (2016). The predictors of uncertainty in mothers of children with autism spectrum disorder. *Children's Health Care, 45*(2), 147–164. https://doi.org/10.1080/02739615.2014.979924

Madhuri, M., Gill, A. Q., & Khan, H. U. (2020). IoT-enabled smart child safety digital system architecture. In *Proceedings - 14th IEEE international conference on semantic computing, ICSC 2020* (pp. 166–169). Institute of Electrical and Electronics Engineers Inc. https://doi.org/10.1109/ICSC.2020.00033

Mamun, M. I., Rahman, A., Khaleque, M. A., Hamid, M. A., & Mridha, M. F. (2019). Autilife: A healthcare monitoring system for autism center in 5G cellular network using machine learning approach. In *IEEE international conference on industrial informatics (INDIN), 2019* pp. 1501–1506). Institute of Electrical and Electronics Engineers Inc. https://doi.org/10.1109/INDIN41052.2019.8972179

Manocha, A., & Bhatia, M. (n.d.). IoT-inspired monitoring framework for real-time stereotypic movement analysis. *IEEE Systems Journal*.

Min, C. H., & Tewfik, A. H. (2010). Automatic characterization and detection of behavioral patterns using linear predictive coding of accelerometer sensor data. In *2010 annual international conference of the IEEE engineering in medicine and biology society, EMBC'10* (pp. 220–223). https://doi.org/10.1109/IEMBS.2010.5627850

Ortolan-Soto, A., Castro-García, J. A., Molina-Cantero, A. J., Merino-Monge, M., & Gómez-González, I. M. (2021). Smart bracelet for emotional enhancement in children with autism spectrum disorder. *Engineering Proceedings, 7*(1), 7. https://doi.org/10.3390/engproc2021007007

Papadopoulos, D. (2021). Mothers' experiences and challenges raising a child with autism spectrum disorder: A qualitative study. *Brain Sciences, 11*(3). https://doi.org/10.3390/brainsci11030309

Rad, M., Nastaran, B., Kia, S., Mostafa, J., Venuti, P., & Furlanello, C. (2015). *Convolutional neural network for stereotypical motor movement detection in autism.*

Rahman, M. A., & Bhuiyan, M. (2015). IOT enabled sensor in multimodal intelligent applications for children with special needs. In *2015 Internet technologies and applications, ITA 2015 - proceedings of the 6th international conference* (pp. 352–357). Institute of Electrical and Electronics Engineers Inc. https://doi.org/10.1109/ITechA.2015.7317425

Saini, R., Kumar, P., Kaur, B., Roy, P. P., Dogra, D. P., & Santosh, K. C. (2019). Kinect sensor-based interaction monitoring system using the BLSTM neural network in healthcare. *International Journal of Machine Learning and Cybernetics, 10*(9), 2529–2540. https://doi.org/10.1007/s13042-018-0887-5

Shattnawi, K. K., Bani Saeed, W. M., Al-Natour, A., Al-Hammouri, M. M., Al-Azzam, M., & Joseph, R. A. (2021). Parenting a child with autism spectrum disorder: Perspective of Jordanian mothers. *Journal of Transcultural Nursing, 32*(5), 474–483. https://doi.org/10.1177/1043659620970634

Shimmer sensor kit. (n.d.). http://www.shimmersensing.com/.

Siddiqui, U. A., Ullah, F., Iqbal, A., Khan, A., Ullah, R., Paracha, S., Shahzad, H., & Kwak, K. S. (2021). Wearable-sensors-based platform for gesture recognition of autism spectrum disorder children using machine learning algorithms. *Sensors, 21*(10). https://doi.org/10.3390/s21103319

Solingen, R., Basili, V., Caldiera, G., & Rombach, H. D. (2002). *Goal question metric (GQM) approach. Encyclopedia of software engineering.*

Srinivasa, K. G., Gayatri, K. S., Adeeb, M. S., & Nikhil, N. (2016). An Internet of things based software framework to handle medical emergencies. In *12th international conference distributed computing and internet technology.*

Sundhara Kumar, K. B., & Bairavi, K. (2016). IoT based health monitoring system for autistic patients. In *Smart innovation, systems and technologies* (Vol 49, pp. 371–376). Springer Science and Business Media Deutschland GmbH. https://doi.org/10.1007/978-3-319-30348-2_32

Tang, T. Y. (2016). Helping neuro-typical individuals to "read" the emotion of children with Autism Spectrum disorder: An internet-of-things approach. In *Proceedings of IDC 2016 - the 15th international conference on interaction design and children* (pp. 666–671). Association for Computing Machinery, Inc. https://doi.org/10.1145/2930674.2936009

Tang, T. Y., & Winoto, P. (2018). Poster: An interactive picture exchange communication system (PECS) embedded with augmented AIDS enabled by IoT and sensing technologies for Chinese individuals with autism. In *UbiComp/ISWC 2018 - adjunct proceedings of the 2018 ACM international joint conference on pervasive and ubiquitous computing and proceedings of the 2018 ACM international symposium on wearable computers* (pp. 299–302). Association for Computing Machinery, Inc. https://doi.org/10.1145/3267305.3267629

Zwaigenbaum, L., & Penner, M. (2018). Autism spectrum disorder: Advances in diagnosis and evaluation. *BMJ (Online)*, 361. https://doi.org/10.1136/bmj.k1674

CHAPTER

Regression analysis of the most frequent medical diagnoses in a Mediterranean country

7

Dominik Bezić, Marina Bagić Babac

University of Zagreb, Faculty of Electrical Engineering and Computing, Zagreb, Croatia

7.1 Introduction

During the pandemic of the SARS-CoV-2 virus in the nation, people tend to forget about "every day" diseases. While acute diseases generally develop rapidly and last a short time, often only a few days or weeks (Yew & Cheng, 2009), they can be a real nuisance to people, especially to ones with a weak immune system, and deal with them frequently. On the other hand, chronic conditions develop slowly and last a long time but have much more severe symptoms (Bernell & Howard, 2016).

Because of the character of acute diseases, it is reasonable not to worry about their occurrence, as there is no way to prepare for them (Yi et al., 2020). They are often caused by a virus or an infection and are accompanied by distinct symptoms that require urgent or short-term attention, which get better once treated (Lorenzl et al., 2012). Differently, chronic conditions cannot be cured but studies show that by making healthy choices, one can reduce the likelihood of getting a chronic disease and improve the quality of life (Martin, 2007).

An acute or chronic diagnosis is not necessarily fixed (Damhorst et al., 2019). An acute condition can sometimes become chronic, while a chronic condition may suddenly present with acute symptoms (Hennessy et al., 2004). Certain infections, for example, will progress from an acute phase (in which symptoms appear and resolve after the initial exposure) to a chronic phase (in which the infection persists, but progresses less aggressively; Mehdipoor et al., 2017).

Globally, chronic diseases have affected the health and quality of life of many citizens (Raghupathi & Raghupathi, 2018). According to the World Health Organization, the causes of chronic diseases are well established and well known; a small set of common risk factors are responsible for most of the main chronic diseases. These risk factors are modifiable and the same in men and women: unhealthy diet, physical inactivity, tobacco use. Aging is an important marker of the accumulation of modifiable risks for chronic disease as the impact of risk factors increases over the life course. The underlying determinants of chronic diseases reflect the major forces driving social, economic, and cultural change—globalization,

Computational Intelligence for Medical Internet of Things (MIoT) Applications
https://doi.org/10.1016/B978-0-323-99421-7.00002-7

urbanization, population aging, and the general policy environment (Hayes et al., 2017, pp. 339–353).

In addition, chronic diseases and poverty are interconnected in a vicious circle. At the same time, poverty and the worsening of already existing poverty are caused by chronic diseases. The poor are more vulnerable for several reasons, including greater exposure to risks and decreased access to health services. Psychosocial stress also plays a role (WHO, 2005).

The main objective of this paper is to show an in-depth overview of the most frequent chronic and acute diagnoses based on age and gender, which allows for the identification of future trends. Despite the limitation of this study that it relies on data acquired before the onset of the COVID-19 in the world as well as in Croatia, the predictive regression models are proposed to anticipate future trends in the state of the health of the nation.

7.2 Related work

Acute conditions occur suddenly, have immediate or rapidly developing symptoms, and are limited in their duration (e.g., the flu). Chronic conditions, on the other hand, are long-lasting. They develop and potentially worsen over time (e.g., Crohn's disease). Most, but not all, chronic diseases will lead to an acute event if left untreated (Linden et al., 2022). For example, atherosclerosis can lead to a heart attack or stroke if steps aren't taken to reduce arterial plaque build-up or reduce blood pressure. With early diagnosis and treatment, some chronic disorders may remain subclinical (without readily observed symptoms) and never manifest acutely (Providence et al., 2012).

The causes of chronic diseases are expressed through the intermediate risk factors of raised blood pressure, raised glucose levels, abnormal blood lipids, overweight, and obesity. The major modifiable risk factors, in conjunction with the nonmodifiable risk factors of age and heredity, explain most new events of heart disease, stroke, chronic respiratory diseases, and some important cancers. The relationship between the major modifiable risk factors and the main chronic diseases is similar in all regions of the world (WHO, 2005).

Despite increasing awareness of the range of positive health effects that physical activity provides us, about 60% of adults are irregularly active or completely inactive (Currie et al., 2012). Moreover, obesity is increasing globally and has been linked to major causes of death, such as diabetes and heart disease (Cnesin, 2019). In Croatia, it is worrying that children are increasingly physically inactive and that 35% of children aged 8 to 9 are overweight or obese (Rito et al., 2019). According to statistics (Starc et al., 2019), Croatia is among the top five European countries with this problem. Recent research has also shown differences among children in all three regions in Croatia (Adriatic, Continental, and the City of Zagreb); the smallest number of children with overweight and obesity was found in the City of Zagreb with 18.8% overweight and 11% obese children, while most concerning is the data showing that in the Continental region, almost every fourth child, 22.4%, is overweight and every sixth child, 15.6%, is obese (Music̀ Milanović, 2020).

It is not surprising that we can find plenty of studies on different factors that contribute to the occurrences of diseases (like obesity). Poor diet and its consequences like obesity is a common problem in urban societies (Farhud, 2015). The highest risk factors for some diseases are ones related to the process of urbanization (Lenzi, 2019). As we live in a modern age, the consequences of urbanization affect us all (Vlahov & Galea, 2002). More than half of the world's population lives in urban areas, e.g., in 2017, 4.1 billion people were living in urban areas (Sanyaolu & Sanyaolu, 2018). The UN estimated that by 2050, 70% of people will be living in an urban environment (UN, 2018). Although city life has many advantages, including better health and mental care, there is increasing awareness of the disadvantages that influence the health of the population.

One of the disadvantages is air pollution, and it is getting worse in the developing world (Ghorani-Azam et al., 2016). While it is getting better in some developed nations, the knowledge of how it damages our bodies and minds is growing even faster. Toxic air is now the biggest environmental risk of early death, responsible for one in nine of all fatalities (Zhang et al., 2019). The diseases caused by it kill seven million people a year, far more than HIV, tuberculosis, and malaria combined (Manisalidis et al., 2020). Exposure to high levels of air pollution increases the risk of respiratory infections, heart disease, and lung cancer (WHO, 2012), which is the most common cancer worldwide—causing more deaths than breast and prostate cancer put together. Certainly, cigarette smoking is also a major cause, but air pollution contributes to the risk greatly (LCE, 2020).

Furthermore, living in rural areas and being in touch with different plants and animals in early childhood is linked to a lower risk of allergies in adulthood and stronger lung function in women (Naleway, 2004). Given that allergies are one of the triggers of chronic bronchitis and asthma, urbanization has an impact on the creation of serious respiratory disorders that can last a lifetime (Smit et al., 2014).

7.3 Exploratory analysis

This study provides an analysis of an anonymized data set of acute and chronic diagnoses based on issued prescriptions in Croatia during 2017–19. Data is classified by the *International Statistical Classification of Diseases and Related Health Problems* (ICD – 10, 2020). It is important to note that our data set is based on the Croatian citizens who have health insurance, which is almost everyone in Croatia (CBS, 2019), thus making it possible to draw general conclusions for the nation based on this sample. Data is grouped for more specific analysis based on a variety of attributes in order to discover patterns, or check assumptions. Since the data do not contain all acute/chronic diseases, this study does not give a representation of all diseases in the entire nation, but the aim is rather to explore the most common and widely spread diseases.

Age groups are divided into 9 different age groups, namely 0–9, 10–19, ...,70–79, 80+.

It is important to note that the number of people who had a specific disease differs from the number of issued prescriptions recorded by these data for the same disease. That difference is present because a lot of people do not go to the doctor for prescribed medicine, but rather handle the disease by themselves, especially acute diseases. Other reasons could be that the person does not need medication, or is even unaware that they have a disease, etc.

Looking at the average number of cases in a year (for the years 2017–19) for each diagnosis based on issued prescriptions shown in Fig. 7.1, data need to be interpreted with caution—for example, when comparing the average number of cases for heart attack (I21) and common cold (J00), it might be falsely concluded that heart attack is more frequent than the common cold. Such a statement does not make sense, that is, the issue is that this data shows only prescription-based diagnoses, so a person with a common cold might not be prescribed medication, or even does not need medical attention. Second, this data set shows that most prescriptions occur within diseases of the respiratory system, followed by diseases of the skin and subcutaneous tissue.

From Fig. 7.1, it is easily distinguished the top three diagnoses from this dataset:

- J30: Vasomotor and allergic rhinitis: 648,633 average no. diagnoses yearly
- H10: Conjunctivitis (pink eye): 447,833 average no. diagnoses yearly
- N30: Cystitis (urinary tract infection): 355,491 average no. diagnoses yearly

The changes over time for these three diagnoses are shown in Fig. 7.2. Time of the year in the case of vasomotor and allergic rhinitis considerably affects the number of diagnoses (Varshney & Varshney, 2015.). The cause of this fluctuation in the number of diagnoses is a result of "seasonal allergies" (Emeryk et al., 2019). Most people are affected by pollen and mold, that is why there are two spikes for each year in the graph (Smit et al., 2014). At the beginning of spring trees, grasses, and weeds release pollen grains into the air to fertilize other plants (Hoyte & Nelson, 2018). Because of global warming, signs of pollination are present even in February and last until July, as depicted on the graph (first spike). The second spike on the graph is because August is a prime month for people with summer allergies due to mold spores, which peak during hot, humid weather (Larsen et al., 2016). Contrarily, conjunctivitis and cystitis are not greatly influenced by the time of the year.

7.4 Analysis of acute diseases

As shown in Fig. 7.2, seasons have been a factor in the number of diagnoses for vasomotor and allergic rhinitis. Furthermore, this study aims to explore different factors for which these kinds of anomalies could be recognized. Thus, we provide an insight into the relationship between the number of issued prescriptions (as a dependent

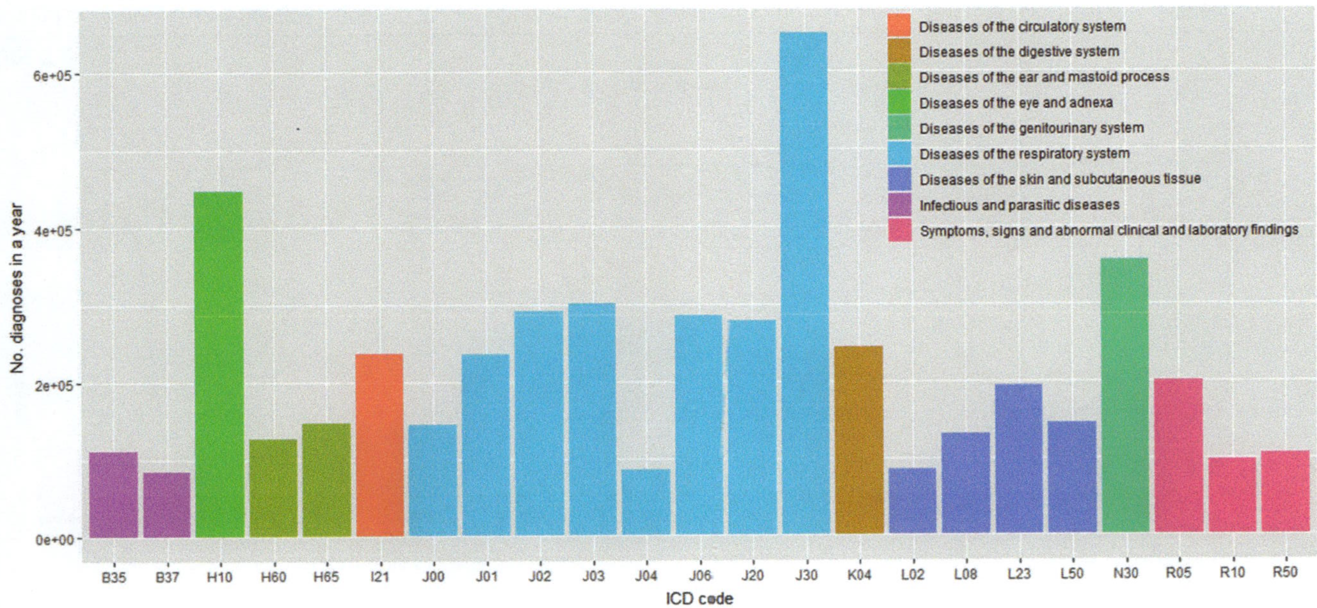

FIGURE 7.1

The average number of diagnoses in a year for a specific disease is based on issued prescriptions.

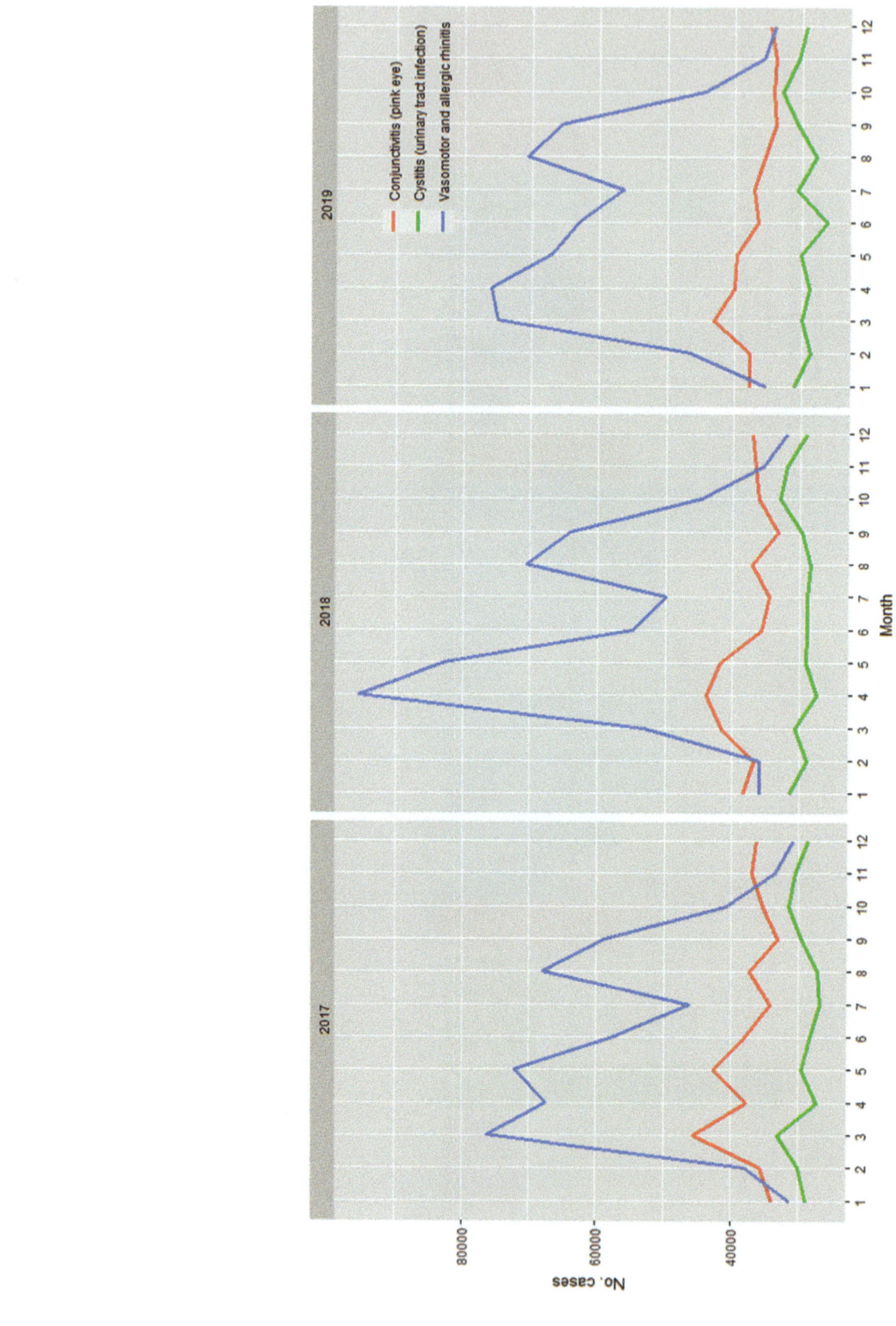

FIGURE 7.2

The number of diagnoses from 2017 until 2020 per month of the top three most common acute diseases based on this data set.

variable), and a set of independent (predictor) variables, namely age, gender, and location using linear regression as a predictive model.

7.4.1 Age as a factor

It is well known that age plays a substantial part in the occurrence of diseases (Castelo-Branco & Soveral, 2013). This can be observed from the regression model focusing on the number of diagnoses in a month per different age group, for which a summary of results is shown in Table 7.1.

From Table 7.1, it is safe to conclude that age has a high impact on the variation of the ratio when looking at the R^2 value of 79.56%. The base intercept is 18.5259, and it is based on the age group 0–9 which are the most susceptible to acute diseases. The slope for each of the remaining age groups is negative, which concludes that the occurrence of acute diseases drops significantly in other age groups. Furthermore, this variation in different age groups is better seen in Fig. 7.3.

Other factors influence the weakening of a person's immune system as well, but until some point in adulthood, our immune system develops more antibodies to the diseases we have overcome in the past (Chaplin, 2010). Because of this phenomenon, adults tend to get fewer diseases than children (Nicholson, 2016) as shown in Fig. 7.3. Data show that from all children aged 0–9, on average, 18.5% of them are diagnosed with some of the given acute diseases in a month. Compared to young adults (ages 20–29) who have an average of 6.6%, that percentage is almost tripled. The major reason for this is that children have had limited exposure to diseases and therefore have not built the immune system required to defend themselves from certain diseases (Simon et al., 2015). Children also do not always practice good hygiene and that makes them susceptible to diseases (Bloomfield et al., 2006).

Table 7.1 Regression results for the ratio of issued prescriptions based on age group (for acute diseases).

Coefficient	Estimate	Std. error	t value	Pr (>|t|)
(Intercept)	18.5259	0.3046	60.83	<2e − 16***
Age group 10–19	−9.1796	0.4307	−21.31	<2e − 16***
Age group 20–29	−11.8734	0.4307	−27.57	<2e − 16***
Age group 30–39	−11.6045	0.4307	−26.94	<2e − 16***
Age group 40–49	−10.6311	0.4307	−24.68	<2e − 16***
Age group 50–59	−9.1272	0.4307	−21.19	<2e − 16***
Age group 60–69	−7.6584	0.4307	−17.78	<2e − 16***
Age group 70–79	−6.2581	0.4307	−14.53	<2e − 16***
Age group 80+	−4.9928	0.4307	−11.59	<2e − 16***

Note: $R^2 = 0.7956$; *adjusted* $R^2 = 0.7904$; *F-statistic: 153.3 on 8 and 315 DF,* P-value: < 2.2e − 16.
Significance codes: ***P < .001, **P < .01, *P < .05, ° P < .01.

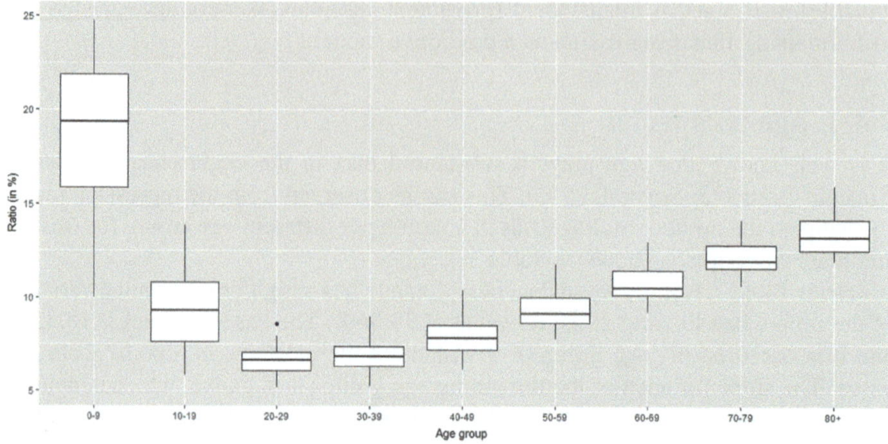

FIGURE 7.3

Side-by-side boxplot of the ratio of diagnosed people to the number of people in a month split by age groups.

Another noticeable thing from Fig. 7.3 is that children and teenagers are more susceptible to different random factors (e.g., environment, seasons), which is depicted from the thickness of the interquartile range (IQR) of the boxplot. As people get older, the chance of getting a disease does not vary based on such random factors, but rather on the persons' immune system (Montecino-Rodriguez et al., 2013). Because aging affects a person's immune system is why from ages 20–29 and forward there is a gradual slope in the average ratio of people in that age group with some diagnosed disease (Castelo-Branco & Soveral, 2013).

The total number of prescriptions issued in each month, with age groups as a coloring factor is depicted in Fig. 7.4. It can be observed that on average, the largest number of diagnoses in a month is for ages 0–9, and the lowest for ages 20–29 and 30–39, which confirms the conclusions made from Fig. 7.3.

The ratio of individual age groups in the total amount per month constantly changes according to the total amount which makes sense, but younger age groups tend to fluctuate much more from month to month. As an example, two age groups: 10–19 and 60–69 in the year 2018 are shown in Fig. 7.5.

There are slight fluctuations from month to month for ages 40–49 which could be because of the large number of allergy diagnoses and that diagnoses are drastically influenced by time. Focusing on ages 10–19, more extreme changes in the number of diagnoses for different months can be observed.

Grouping of the diagnoses from 2017 until 2019 to show the difference age has in the type of diseases a person is diagnosed with, is shown in Fig. 7.6. It can be noticed that the children and young adults do not have diagnoses for diseases of the cardiovascular system (in this dataset specifically heart attack) because increasing age is an independent risk factor for developing cardiovascular disease (Dhingra & Vasan,

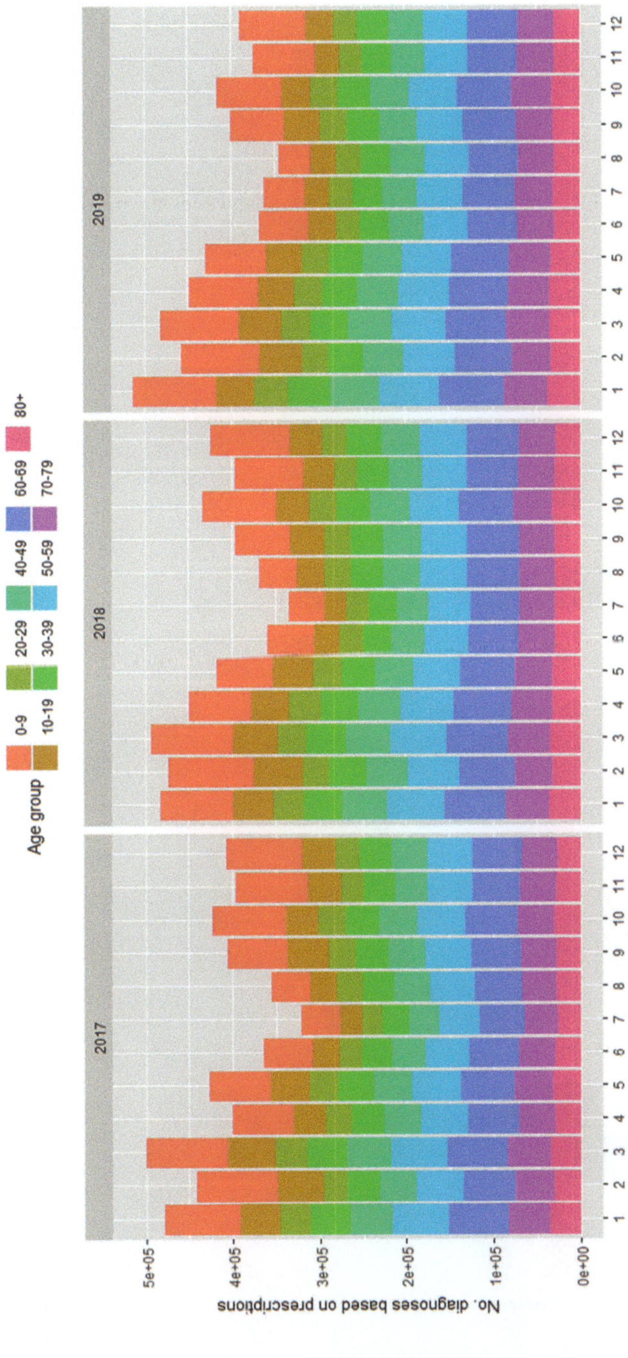

FIGURE 7.4

The total number of diagnoses based on prescriptions made per month in different years (with age group).

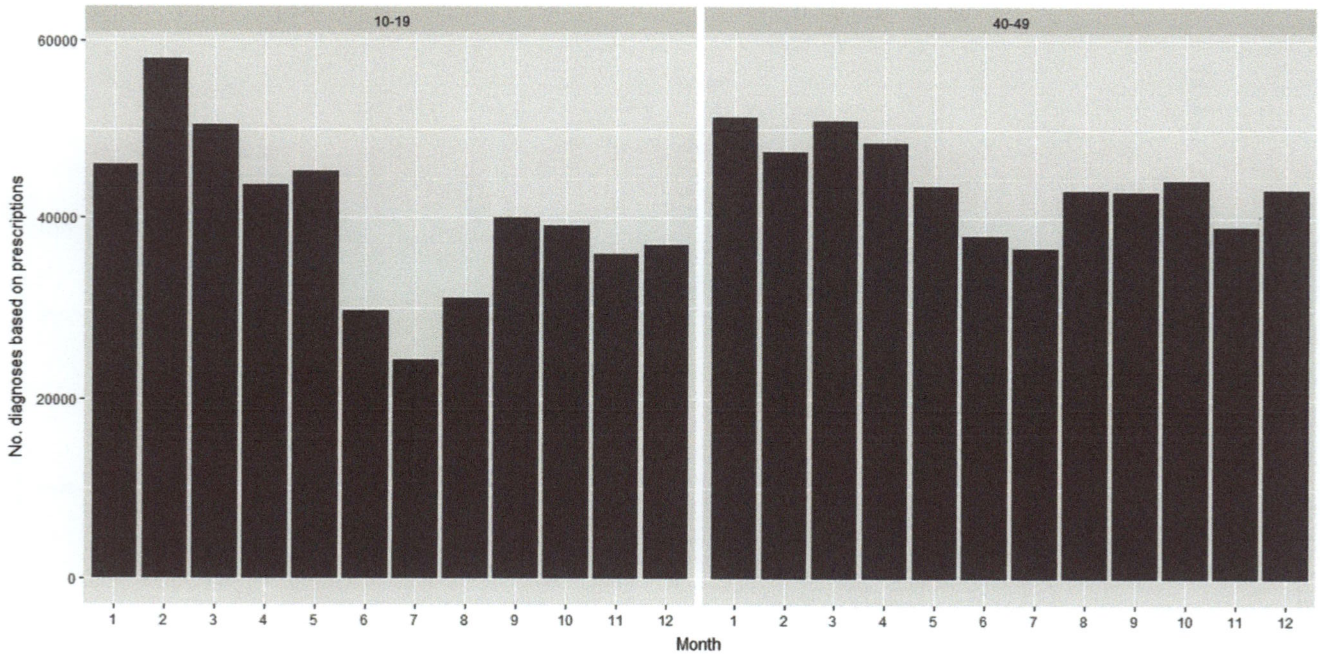

FIGURE 7.5

Difference between fluctuations of two age groups.

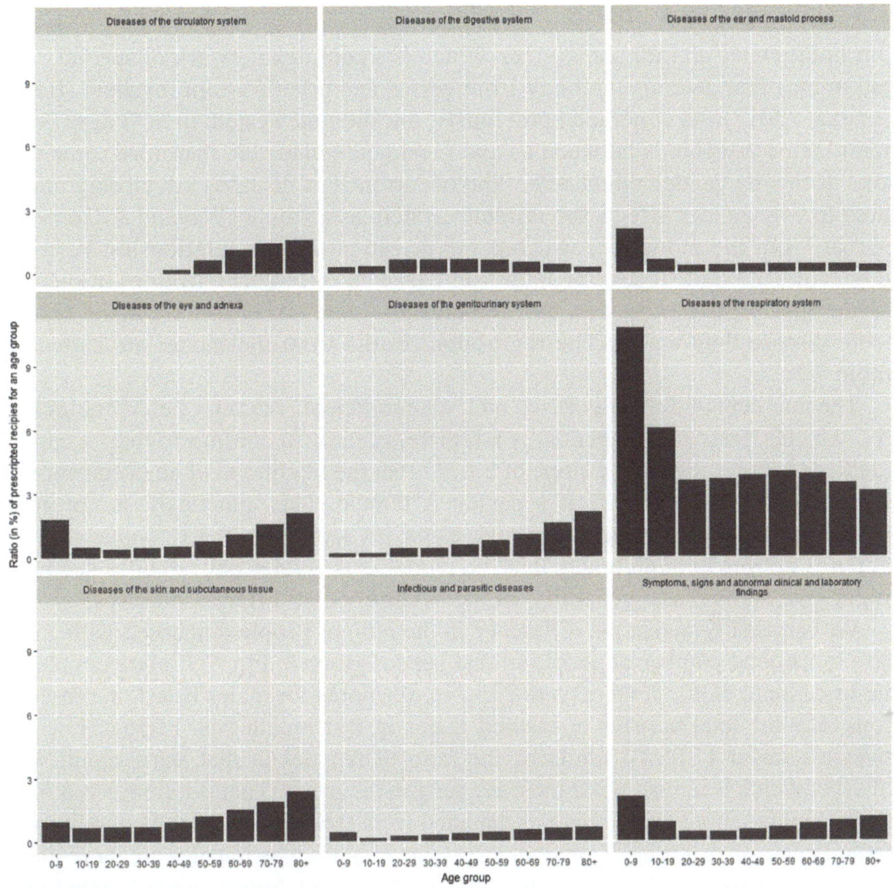

FIGURE 7.6

The ratio of prescriptions for an age group based on groups of diagnoses per month.

2012), which is depicted as a gradual increase in the ratio of people diagnosed with a heart attack. Also, it can be noted an exponential increase in diseases of the genitourinary system (UTI) because urinary tract infection is common in older adults (Rowe & Juthani-Mehta, 2013).

For children aged 0–9, a large ratio of them have been diagnosed with some sort of disease of the respiratory system or diseases of the ear and mastoid process. The reason for this is that the most common diseases for children are respiratory ones (common cold, bronchitis) and ones involving ear problems (acute otitis media) (Goodman et al., 2013). Also, it is obvious from Fig. 7.6 that a large ratio of them has been diagnosed with diseases of the eye and adnexa (from this dataset only conjunctivitis is in that group). Conjunctivitis is common for young children, who may rub their eyes and transmit infections to other children (Azari & Barney, 2013).

7.4.2 Gender as a factor

Our bodies have an immune system, which is a complex network of special cells and organs that defends the body from germs and other foreign invaders (Bagatini et al., 2017). As concluded previously, our immune system in later ages is the main factor that stands between us and most acute diseases, therefore some reasons as to why gender might affect the occurrence of diseases are closely correlated to why gender affects the immune system as a whole (Weyand & Goronzy, 2016). From the model constructed for investigating the relationship between gender and the ratio of several diagnoses based on issued prescriptions in specific gender groups, it can be seen that females are more likely to have some sort of acute disease than males. The regression results from the model are shown in Table 7.2.

The intercept of 8.8757 is based on if all coefficients are zero, i.e., if coefficient "F," which represents if a person is a female, is zero. According to that, it can be concluded from the positive slope of 2.6737 that the likelihood of an occurrence of disease increases by 2.6737 if a person is female. This, obviously, is not good enough to make that an accurate conclusion (as seen from the R^2 value of 55% which is not big enough to say that the model is accurate) but rather to see what might give an increase, generally, in the occurrence of different diseases.

We can clearly notice the difference in the ratio of people diagnosed with a disease to the total number of people in that gender group in Fig. 7.7. For example, in the first month of 2019, there were 215,746 diagnoses for males based on prescriptions, and the total number of insured males in that month was 1,956,451 which gives a ratio of 11.02%. Similarly, the ratio of females in that same month was 13.96%, which is almost a 3% increase per gender group. That difference is almost the same throughout each month as depicted from the gap between the two lines. A natural question that arises from looking at this graph is why females are more likely to have some sort of disease. A study by the American Autoimmune Related Diseases Association (AARDA) showed that females are much more likely to suffer from some sort of autoimmune disease and reported that 75% of the people diagnosed with an autoimmune illness are women (Regitz-Zagrosek, 2012). That reason, for example, might be why the immune system of females is much weaker than for a male, thus making them more prone to acute diseases.

Table 7.2 Regression results for the ratio of issued prescriptions based on gender (for acute diseases).

Coefficient	Estimate	Std. error	t value	Pr (>|t|)
(Intercept)	8.8757	0.2035	43.607	<2e − 16***
F	2.6737	0.2878	9.289	7.84e − 14***

Note: *$R^2 = 0.5521$; adjusted $R^2 = 0.5457$; F-statistic: 86.28 on 1 and 70 DF,* P-value = *7.836e−14.*
Significance codes: ***P < .001, **P < .01, *P < .05, ° P < .01.

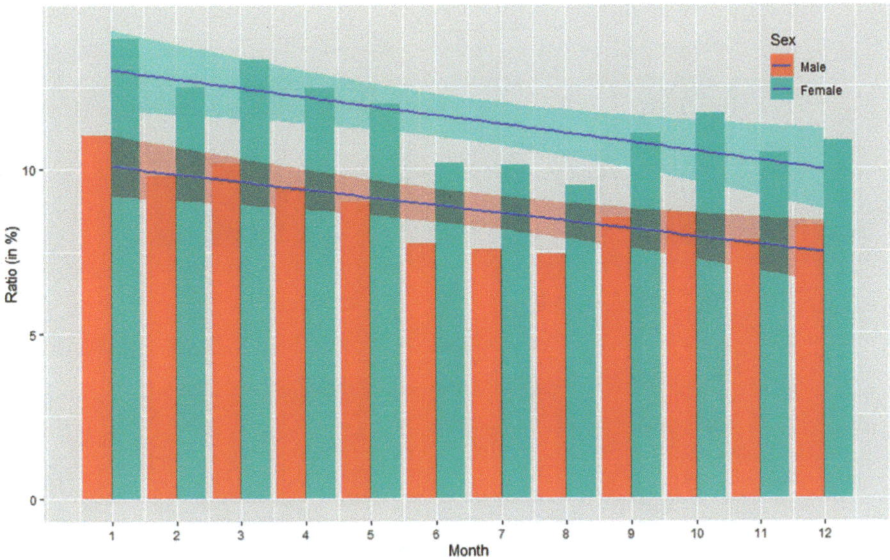

FIGURE 7.7

The ratio of the number of diagnoses based on issued prescriptions in specific gender groups. The data is shown for the year 2019 and throughout each month.

Generally speaking, it can be noticed that females are more likely overall to develop some acute disease, as to reasons why is that is still unclear, but looking at different groups of acute diseases might give an inside on what is really going on.

The graph in Fig. 7.8 suggests that still, women are affected more by different disease groups than men. The large difference in the ratios might be explained by the large percentage of women with problems with the genitourinary system. This data set from the genitourinary system diseases only covers cystitis (urinary tract infection, or UTI) which is known to affect more females than males. Some studies suggest that overall UTIs are 14 times more frequent in females than males (Matuszkiewicz-Rowińska et al., 2015).

The only group of diseases where males have a higher occurrence of the diseases is for diseases of the circulatory system. This observation is limited by the number of diseases in each group, so for the group of circulatory diseases, there is only a record for acute myocardial infarction (heart attack). Heart attack is known from different studies to be twice as common in males than females, as seen in this graph (Maas & Appelman, 2010).

Another noticeable difference is infectious and parasitic diseases. Two diseases recorded for that group are dermatophytosis (ringworm) and candidiasis. Some studies found that there is no statistical difference between male and female subjects with dermatophytosis (Rashidian et al., 2015). The difference-maker in the group of infectious and parasitic diseases is candidiasis. Candidiasis is an infection caused by a yeast (fungus) called Candida (de Oliveira Santos et al., 2018). Candida normally

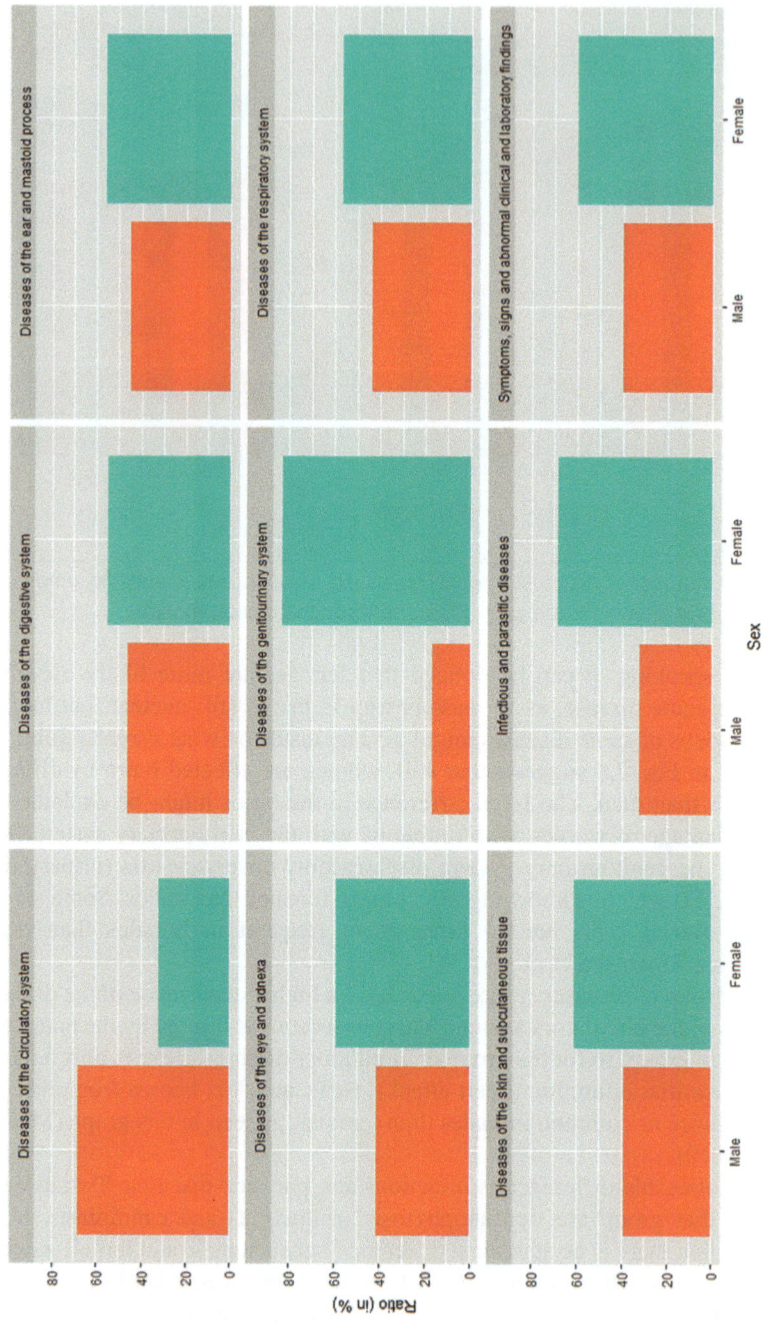

FIGURE 7.8

The average ratio of males and females diagnosed with a disease is divided into groups of diseases.

lives inside the body (in places such as the mouth, throat, gut, and vagina) and on the skin without causing any problems. The real problem starts when it multiplies and causes an infection (Spampinato & Leonardi, 2013). The most common of those infections are vaginal yeast infection, and as the name suggests, it affects only females. Vaginal yeast infection is so common that it affects up to 3 out of four women at some point in their lifetimes, many of them experience at least two episodes (Barousse et al., 2004).

Other specific diseases that affect females more than males in a noticeable amount (around 65%–70%) gathered from this data set are the following ranked by the difference: abdominal and pelvic pain (stomachache), urticaria (hives), and allergic contact dermatitis as shown in Fig. 7.9.

7.5 Analysis of chronic diseases

Humans historically died of acute diseases, like infections and trauma. Similarly, the experience of the 2020 COVID-19 pandemic (Yi et al., 2020) resurrects that paradigm because there are more than 700,000 deaths worldwide at the time of writing this study (Dong et al., 2020). As people turn their focus toward the new acute disease because it is unknown, chronic diseases seem to be forgotten but are the bigger killers society needs to worry about. Of all deaths globally, 60% of them are due to chronic diseases (Willett et al., 2006). The projected total of deaths from all causes in 2005 was 58 million, it was then estimated that chronic diseases would account for 35 million, which is double the number of deaths from all infectious diseases (including HIV/AIDS, tuberculosis, and malaria), maternal and perinatal conditions, and nutritional deficiencies combined (Taubenberger & Morens, 2006). Numbers from the study of mortality done in the United States in 2018 (Xu et al., 2020) point that the top two causes of death in the United States are heart disease and cancer.

Unlike acute diseases which are highly time-dependent, as new cases of the disease come and go, chronic diseases do not go away. The definition of "chronic disease" by the National Cancer Institute states (NCI, 2020) says "A disease or condition that usually lasts for 3 months or longer and may get worse over time. Chronic diseases tend to occur in older adults and can usually be controlled but not cured." Because of that, when looking at the total number of diagnoses based on prescriptions of a disease per month in Fig. 7.10, we can see that there is almost no fluctuation from month to month as depicted from the straight lines for each diagnosis, i.e., the number of sick people in the nation stays the same.

Because the total number of diagnoses stays the same from month to month, it does not make sense to look at a larger scale of data, for example, the average number of diagnoses of a disease per year. If we would do that, it would require us to sum up all the diagnoses from each month and the result would give a false sense of the scale of occurrences of a disease in a year because the conditions are long-term. We were able to do that in the case of acute diseases because one cannot be a lifetime patient of, for example, conjunctivitis.

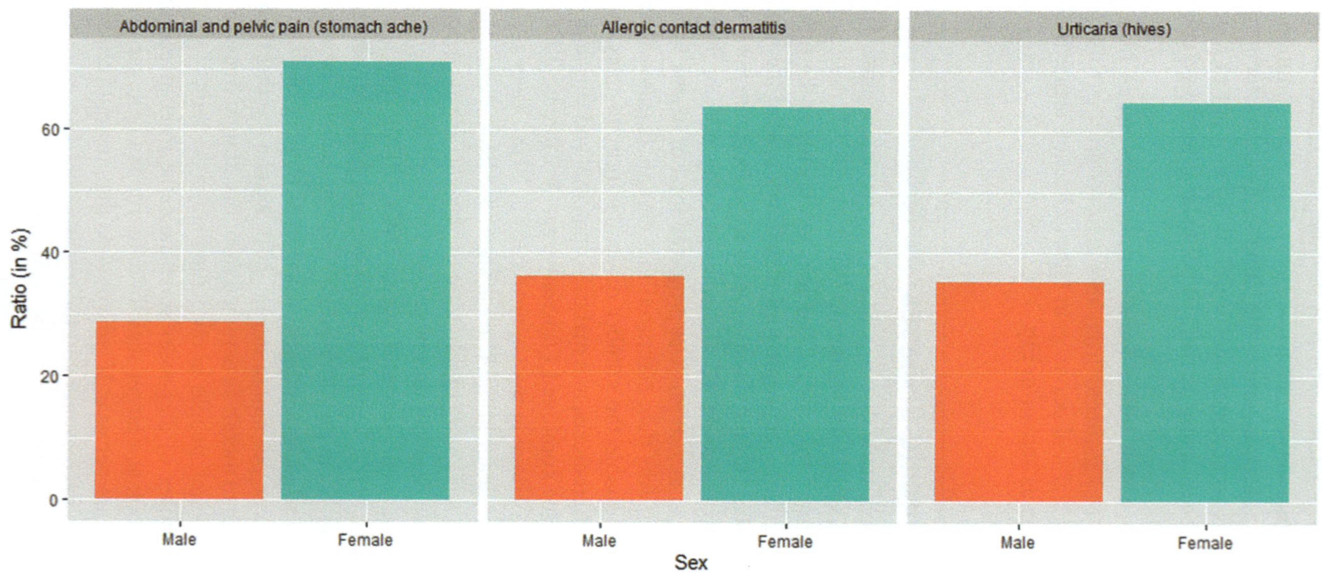

FIGURE 7.9

The average ratio of males and females diagnosed with a disease for three specific diseases: abdominal and pelvic pain (stomach-ache), urticaria (hives), and allergic contact dermatitis.

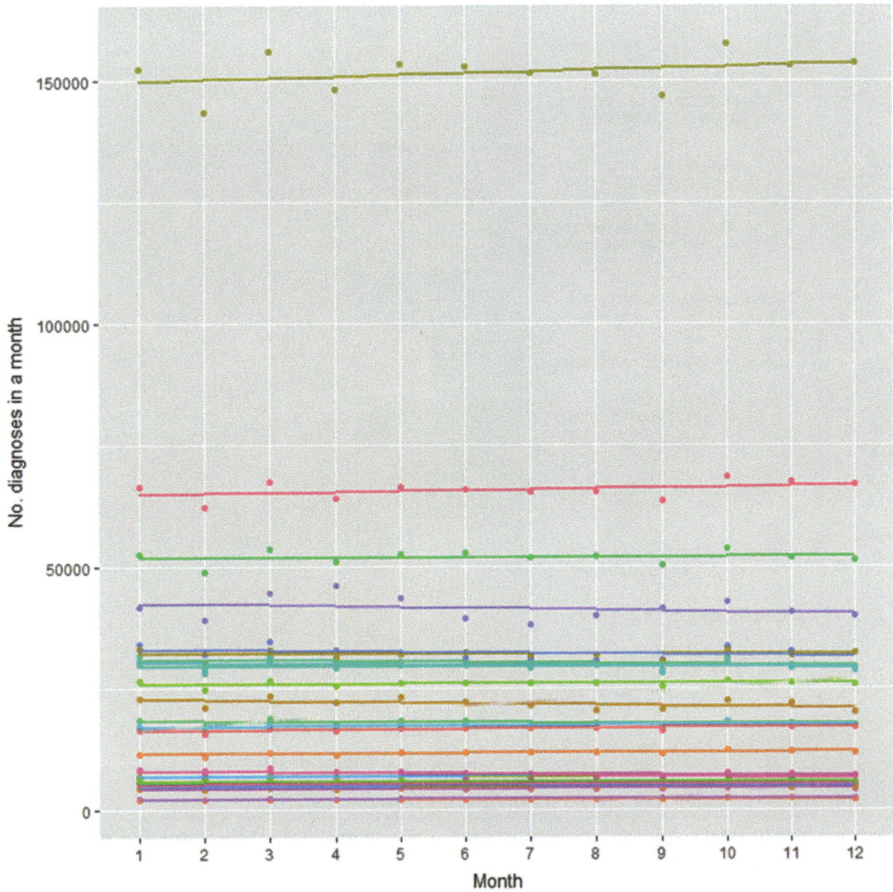

FIGURE 7.10

A number of total diagnoses based on prescriptions of different diseases (different color) per month in 2018. A number of total diagnoses based on prescriptions of different diseases (different color) per month in 2018. The *dots* represent the number of people in a month diagnosed with a specific disease, and the line represents the correlation between the month and number of diagnoses in a month – the flatter the line is the more the correlation of the variables approaches zero.

Keeping that in mind, looking at the graph in Fig. 7.11, it can be noticed what are, on average, the most common chronic diseases in a month (for the year 2018). The highest number of diagnoses in a month are for the group colored purple—endocrine, nutritional, and metabolic diseases.

Fig. 7.12 presents the number of total diagnoses based on prescriptions of different diseases (different colors) per month in 2018.

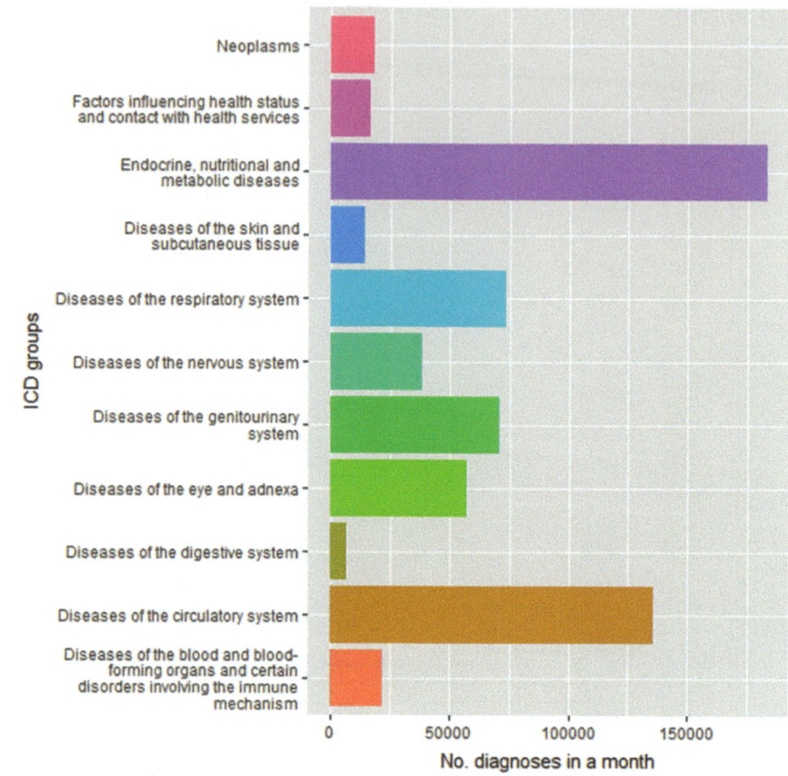

FIGURE 7.11

The number of total diagnoses based on prescriptions of different diseases (different colors) per month in 2018.

That group consists of two types of diabetes: type 1 and type 2 (the more common of the two). Diabetes (especially type 2 diabetes), being one of the most common chronic diseases in the world, has a risk factor that is a huge problem in Croatia—obesity. Globally, Croatia is part of the group of "fat nations" (Musić Milanović, 2009). It ranks fifth overall in Europe, ahead of only Malta, Greece, Turkey, and England. According to estimates by the World Health Organization in 2005, Croats are ranked sixth in the world (67.7%) by people overweight, and Croatian women are in 22nd place (58.2%) (Starc et al., 2019).

Another group of diseases that emerges from the left graph is diseases of the cardiovascular system. As the study of the National Council on Aging from the United States show, in the top five most common chronic conditions in adults over the age of 65, three of them are conditions of the cardiovascular system (Atella et al., 2019). That ratio alone might explain why this is the second most common group of diseases. Other diseases that stand out are N40—hyperplasia of the prostate and H40—glaucoma.

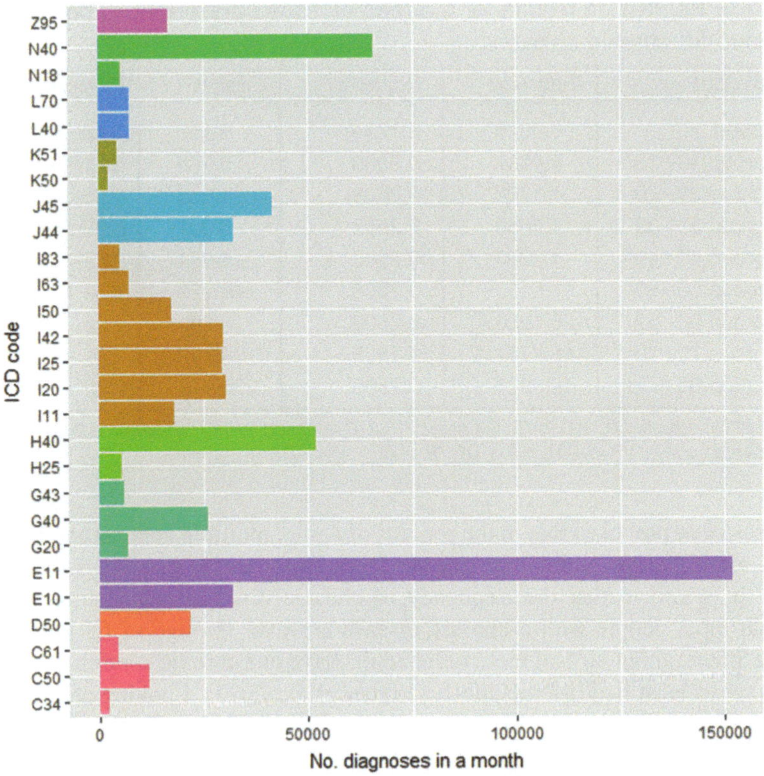

FIGURE 7.12

The number of total diagnoses based on prescriptions of different diseases (different colors) per month in 2018.

7.5.1 Age as a factor

As shown before, age plays a huge part in the occurrence of diseases, the weakening of a person's immune system throughout the years alone plays a big part, but for chronic diseases, the difference is much more profound. This can be seen when looking at the summary statistic of a model that depicts the relationship with the ratio of prescriptions in a specific age group for chronic diseases shown in Table 7.3.

It can be noticed that this linear model can predict approximately 99% of the variation in the ratio of issued prescriptions in a month using age as a factor. The intercept is based on the age group 0–9 and is 1.4376. For the older age groups, the slope increases drastically from ages 50 and older. For example, if a person is in the age group 60–69, the chances of a chronic disease increase by 28.1656 (from the base of 1.4376). Age was an important factor in the analysis of acute diseases, but not as important as for chronic diseases.

Table 7.3 Regression results for the ratio of issued prescriptions based on age group for chronic diseases.

Coefficient	Estimate	Std. error	t value	Pr (>|t|)
(Intercept)	1.4376	0.1774	8.105	1.18e − 14***
Age group 10–19	1.4987	0.2508	5.975	6.21e − 09***
Age group 20–29	1.1702	0.2508	4.665	4.56e − 06***
Age group 30–39	1.5053	0.2508	6.001	5.38e − 09***
Age group 40–49	4.2293	0.2508	16.861	<2e − 16***
Age group 50–59	11.5180	0.2508	45.920	<2e − 16***
Age group 60–69	28.1656	0.2508	112.291	<2e − 16***
Age group 70–79	48.7731	0.2508	194.449	<2e − 16***
Age group 80+	59.1227	0.2508	235.711	<2e − 16***

$R^2 = 0.9976$; adjusted $R^2 = 0.9975$; F-statistic: 16,370 on 8 and 315 DF, P-value: *< 2.2e − 16.*
*Significance codes: ***P < .001, **P < .01, *P < .05, ° P < .01.*

It has been proposed that in the process of aging, multiple cellular and molecular events malfunctions, ultimately leading to various chronic diseases (Atella et al., 2019). It is known that the frequency of chronic disease rises sharply with age and that most people with a chronic disease are over the age of 65 years. In the United States, about 80% of these older adults have one chronic condition, and about 68% have at least two (Montecino-Rodriguez et al., 2013). Looking at the graph in Fig. 7.13 we can see exactly how sharp the frequency of chronic diseases rises with

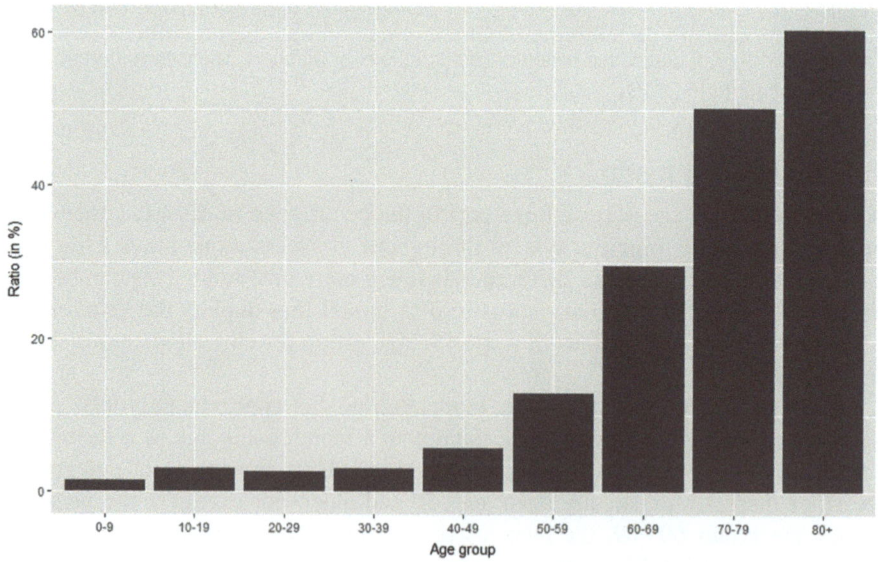

FIGURE 7.13

Average ratios of number of diagnoses to number of people in a specific age group.

age. This graph shows the average ratio of diagnoses based on prescriptions to the number of people with health insurance in specific age groups. There is an exponential increase in the ratio, which confirms the assumptions explored previously.

Comparing the monthly changes to the number of diagnoses made, we can recognize, unlike acute diseases, the number of diagnoses fluctuates slightly around 60,000, as depicted in. Also, it is noticeable that the most diagnoses based on prescriptions are for the age group 70—79, followed by age group 60—69.

Average ratios of diagnoses for a specific month in different age groups (grouped by different disease groups) to the average number of people with insurance for that age group.

We have already concluded that, generally, with age comes the greater chance of getting a chronic disease, let us see for which of the given groups of diagnosis from this data set age makes a significant factor. Observing the average ratio of diagnoses for a specific month in different age groups (grouped by different disease groups) to the average number of people with insurance for specific age groups, shown in Fig. 7.14, we can see that, indeed, for different groups of diseases age makes a difference.

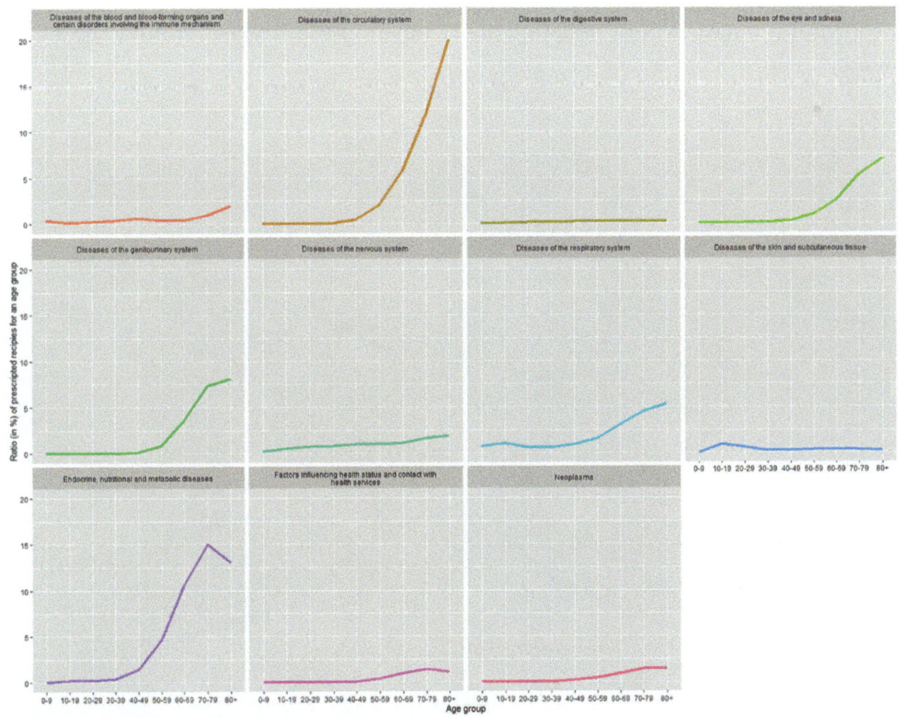

FIGURE 7.14

Average ratios of diagnoses for a specific month in different age groups (grouped by different disease groups) to the average number of people with insurance for that age group.

For most of the disease groups, we can see that the ratio increases the older the age group gets. Unlike most, diseases of the skin and subcutaneous tissue are more common among younger age groups - especially teenagers. The real reason is that in that group there are diseases that mostly develop during puberty - acne, and psoriasis. Acne commonly starts during puberty between the ages of 10 and 13 and psoriasis often develops between the ages of 15 and 35, but it can develop at any age (Dogan Gunaydin & Atakan, 2013; Tan et al., 2017). Teenage acne usually lasts for five to 10 years, normally going away during the early 20s, which explains the graph. That group is the only one depicted where the ratio drops with age, others, like diseases of the circulatory system, genitourinary system, and diseases of the eye and adnexa have exponential growth with age and are very common among older people.

Some, like the diseases of the nervous system, have linear growth. The reason being is that in that group there are the following diseases: Parkinson's, epilepsy, and migraine. Looking at the graphs for each of them in Fig. 7.15, we can see that epilepsy (G40) and migraine (G43) are differently affected by age. Migraine peaks during the ages 40–49. Rates of new cases of epilepsy are the most common in children, especially in the group 0–9, then the ratio gradually falls, and again, from 50 to 59, it rises (Dito & Ikrar, 2014). Parkinson's follows the exponential curve, where people usually develop the disease around age 60 or older.

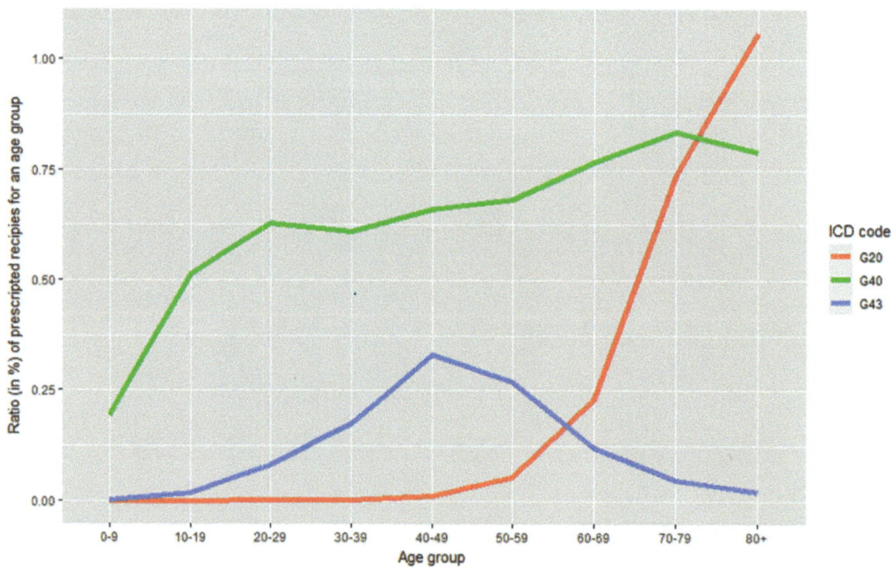

FIGURE 7.15

Average ratios for epilepsy (green), migraine (blue), and Parkinson's (red).

7.5.2 Gender as a factor

We have concluded from the analysis of acute diseases that there are many differences in the occurrences of acute diseases according to gender. In the model constructed for correlation between gender and ratio, we can see that males are more likely to have some sort of chronic disease than females. The results from the model are shown in Table 7.4. In contrast to acute diseases, men are more likely to develop some chronic disease (seen in the negative slope for "F" which represents if a person is a female). The two lines that represent the model approximation can also be seen in Fig. 7.16.

Generally, females were shown to be more prone to diseases (ones explored from this data set), but looking at the graph in Fig. 7.16. We can see a difference in chronic diseases.

Table 7.4 Regression results for the ratio of prescriptions based on gender for chronic diseases.

Coefficient	Estimate	Std. error	t value	Pr (>|t|)
(Intercept)	17.4944	0.1322	132.30	<2e − 16***
F	−3.1266	0.1870	−16.72	5.43e − 14***

$R^2 = 0.927$; adjusted $R^2 = 0.9237$; F-statistic: 279.5 on 1 and 22 DF, P-value = *5.429e−14.*
*Significance codes: ***P < .001, **P < .01, *P < .05, ° P < .01.*

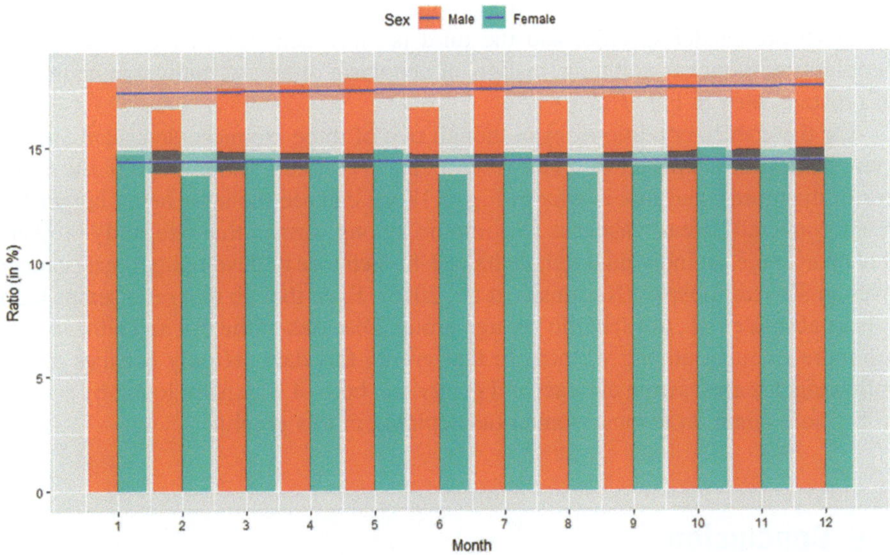

FIGURE 7.16

The ratio of the number of diagnoses based on issued prescriptions in specific gender groups. The data is shown for the year 2019 and throughout each month.

For example, in January of 2019, there are 349,402 cases of different chronic diagnoses for males, and a total of 1,956,451 males insured which results in a ratio of 17.85%. For females, that ratio is 14,71%, and the difference is around 3% and is constant as it was the case for acute diseases. One study confirms this proposition that males had a higher incidence of chronic disease than women—2.09 versus 1.90 per 100 person-years, respectively (Turabian, 2018).

Looking at the average ratio of men and women per month for specific groups of diseases in Fig. 7.17. We can see why the difference from Fig. 7.18 is so noticeable.

The most noticeable ratio is for diseases of the genitourinary system, the reason being that in that group there are only two diseases—chronic renal failure and hyperplasia of the prostate. Hyperplasia of the prostate, obviously, only affects men and is very common. About one-third of men experience moderate to severe symptoms by age 60, and about half do so by age 80.

Looking at the other groups where men are more dominant we can spot that for factors influencing health status and contact with health services, more specifically as there is only one condition in that group, presence of cardiac and vascular implants and grafts there are about 70% males and only 30% females.

As for the groups where females are more affected than males, we can see that, for example, group of diseases of the blood and blood-forming organs and certain disorders involving the immune mechanism, which only includes iron-deficiency anemia, number of diagnoses include about 72% females. A woman loses with their period from 10 to 250 mL of blood (4–100 mg of iron; Rushton & Barth, 2009). These iron losses in women double their need to absorb iron in comparison to males, which explains the graph above. In the neoplasms group, we have three diseases, two of which are gender-specific, and the third is more common in men—malignant neoplasm of bronchus and lung, malignant neoplasm of breast, malignant neoplasm of prostate, seen in Fig. 7.17.

For these three conditions, even though two of three are more dominant among men, malignant neoplasm of breast (breast cancer) outnumbers the two in the number of diagnoses, and that is why in Fig. 7.18 we can see the ratio being bigger for females overall. Breast cancer is so common among women that one study projects that on average, an individual female has a 1-in-8 chance of developing breast cancer over an 80-year lifespan (Kamińska et al., 2015). Even though that ratio seems high it is an absolute risk, not specific per age group. Diseases of the eye and adnexa also are more frequent among women. In that group, this data set only consists of the following diseases: senile cataract and glaucoma, both of which are found by studies to be more common among women (as depicted in this graph).

7.6 Conclusion

This paper is an attempt to paint a general picture of the occurrence of different diseases within Croatia, a Mediterranean country situated at the heart of Europe. It is well known that diseases vary by geographic region and population, and they change

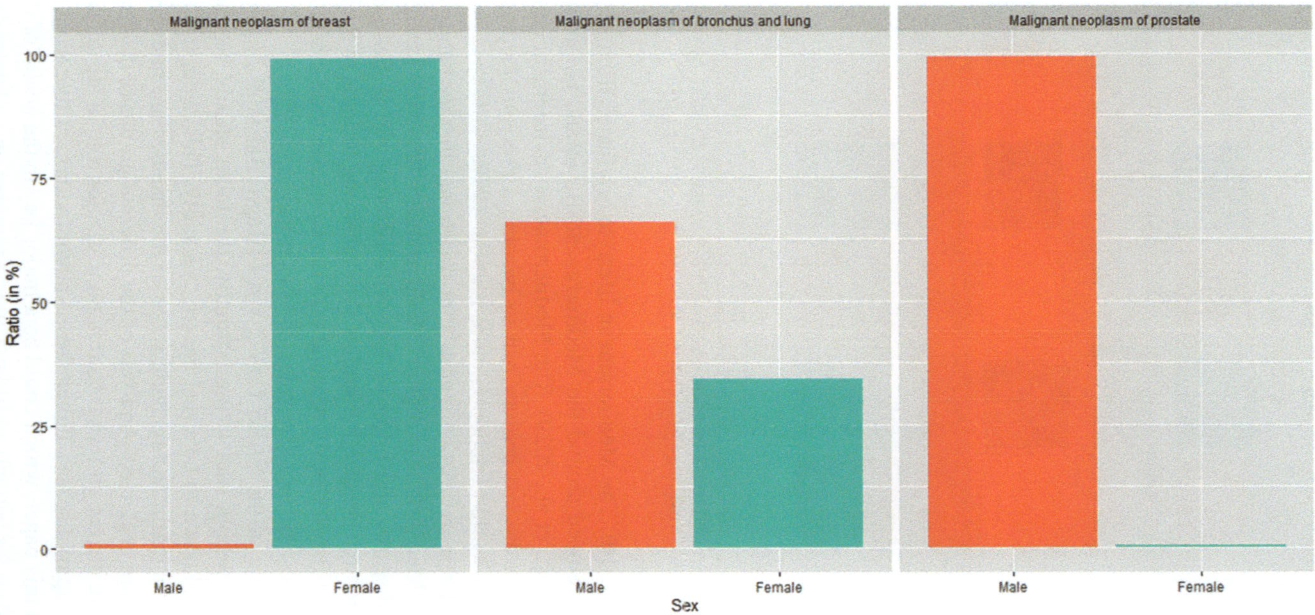

FIGURE 7.17

The average ratio of males and females diagnosed with a disease for three specific diseases—malignant neoplasm of bronchus and lung, malignant neoplasm of breast, and malignant neoplasm of the prostate.

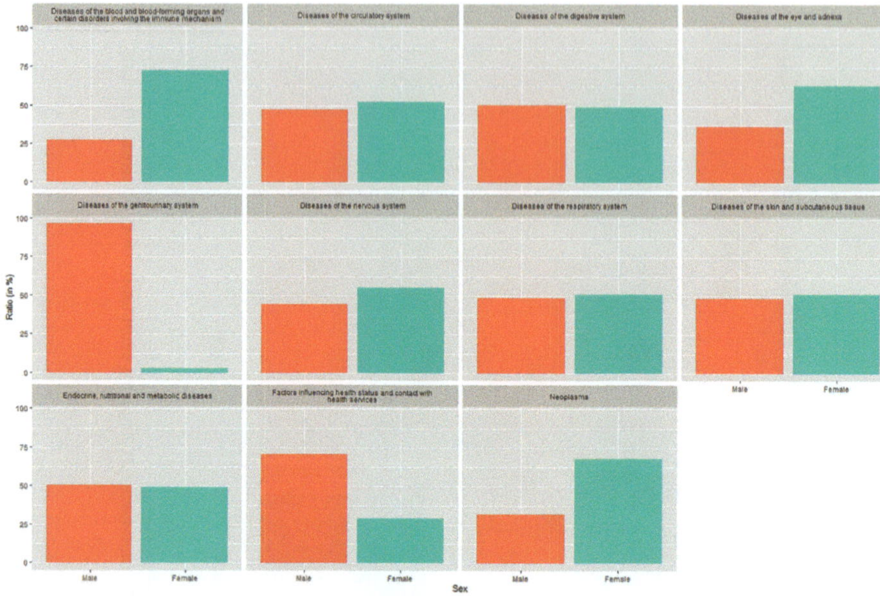

FIGURE 7.18

The average ratio of males and females diagnosed with a disease is divided into groups of diseases.

over time (Wilson, 2010). The Mediterranean lifestyle originates from ancient civilizations which developed around the Mediterranean Basin and is famous for its food cultures (Lăcătuşu et al., 2019). The Mediterranean environment came to acquire new valences in the last century and to become a precious medical tool in the contemporaneous world (Trichopoulou & Lagiou, 1997).

A large body of research data suggests that traditional dietary habits and lifestyles unique to the Mediterranean region (Mediterranean diet, MD) lower the incidence of chronic diseases and improve longevity (Romagnolo & Selmin, 2017). Recent reports from large perspective studies showed strong benefits of the Mediterranean diet to reduce the risk of myocardial infarction, stroke, total mortality, heart failure, and disability (Martinez-Gonzalez & Martin-Calvo, 2016).

After the pandemic of the SARS-CoV-2 virus (Bagić Babac & Mornar, 2020) gets diminished and people start living normally, the focus should be returned to the diseases that are known to be a real hazard to society. This paper tried to bring attention to how meaningful and realistic some of the diseases are in everyday life and how often they are neglected. Analysis of the different groups of diseases (acute and chronic) gave an insight into what factors play a major role in the occurrence of each disease or group of diseases. Given these known factors, further work could be done to expand on this paper, which could be a major key in the health of the nation and the world. Caring for patients in today's world requires an understanding of the basic factors that underlie the geography of human diseases and events that cause shifts in the distribution and burden of specific diseases (Wilson, 2010).

References

Atella, V., Piano Mortari, A., Kopinska, J., Belotti, F., Lapi, F., Cricelli, C., & Fontana, L. (2019). Trends in age-related disease burden and healthcare utilization. *Aging Cell, 18*(1), e12861.

Azari, A. A., & Barney, N. P. (2013). Conjunctivitis: A systematic review of diagnosis and treatment. *Journal of the American Medical Association, 310*(16), 1721–1729.

Bagatini, M. D., Cardoso, A. M., Dos Santos, A. A., & Carvalho, F. B. (2017). Immune system and chronic diseases. *Journal of Immunology Research*, 4284327.

Bagić Babac, M., & Mornar, V. (2020). Resetting the initial conditions for calculating epidemic spread: COVID-19 outbreak in Italy. *IEEE Access, 8*, 148021–148030. https://doi.org/10.1109/ACCESS.2020.3015923

Barousse, M. M., Van Der Pol, B. J., Fortenberry, D., Orr, D., & Fidel, P. L., Jr. (2004). Vaginal yeast colonisation, prevalence of vaginitis, and associated local immunity in adolescents. *Sexually Transmitted Infections, 80*(1), 48–53.

Bernell, S., & Howard, S. W. (2016). Use your words carefully: What is a chronic disease? *Frontiers in Public Health, 4*, 159.

Bloomfield, S. F., Stanwell-Smith, R., Crevel, R. W., & Pickup, J. (2006). Too clean, or not too clean: The hygiene hypothesis and home hygiene. *Clinical and Experimental Allergy: Journal of the British Society for Allergy and Clinical Immunology, 36*(4), 402–425.

Castelo-Branco, C., & Soveral, I. (2013). The immune system and aging: A review. *Gynecological Endocrinology: The Official Journal of the International Society of Gynecological Endocrinology, 30'*.

Censin, J. C., Peters, S., Bovijn, J., Ferreira, T., Pulit, S. L., Mägi, R., Mahajan, A., Holmes, M. V., & Lindgren, C. M. (2019). Causal relationships between obesity and the leading causes of death in women and men. *PLoS Genetics, 15*(10), e1008405. https://doi.org/10.1371/journal.pgen.1008405

Chaplin, D. D. (2010). Overview of the immune response. *The Journal of Allergy and Clinical Immunology, 125*(2 Suppl. 2), S3–S23.

Currie, I., Zanotti, C., Morgan, A., Currie, D., de Looze, M., Roberts, C., & Barnekow, V. (2012). *'Social determinants of health and well-being among young people. Health behaviour in school-aged children (HBSC) study', international report from the 2009/2010 survey (Health Policy for Children and Adolescents, No. 6)*. Copenhagen: WHO Regional Office for Europe.

Damhorst, G. L., Tyburski, E. A., Brand, O., Martin, G. S., & Lam, W. A. (2019). Diagnosis of acute serious illness: The role of point-of-care technologies. *Current Opinion in Biomedical Engineering, 11*, 22–34. https://doi.org/10.1016/j.cobme.2019.08.012

Dhingra, R., & Vasan, R. S. (2012). Age as a risk factor. *The Medical Clinics of North America, 96*(1), 87–91.

Dito, D., & Ikrar, T. (2014). Treatment of epilepsy: Background and future directions. *Progress and Communication in Sciences, 1*(27).

Dogan Gunaydin, S., & Atakan, N. (2013). *Psoriasis - types, causes and medication, chapter 5 psoriasis: A disease of systemic inflammation with comorbidities*.

Dong, E., Du, H., & Gardner, L. (2020). An interactive web-based dashboard to track COVID-19 in real time. *Lancet Infectious Diseases*.

Emeryk, A., Emeryk-Maksymiuk, J., & Janeczek, K. (2019). New guidelines for the treatment of seasonal allergic rhinitis. *Postepy Dermatologii I Alergologii, 36*(3), 255–260.

Farhud, D. D. (2015). Impact of lifestyle on health. *Iranian Journal of Public Health, 44*(11), 1442–1444.

Ghorani-Azam, A., Riahi-Zanjani, B., & Balali-Mood, M. (2016). Effects of air pollution on human health and practical measures for prevention in Iran. *Journal of Research in Medical Sciences: The Official Journal of Isfahan University of Medical Sciences, 21*, 65.

Goodman, D. M., Lynm, C., & Livingston, E. H. (2013). Ear problems in children. *Journal of the American Medical Association, 309*(21), 2284. https://doi.org/10.1001/jama.2013.4428

Hayes, C., West, C., & Egger, G. (2017). *Chapter 22—Rethinking chronic pain in a lifestyle medicine context*. Cambridge, MA, USA: Academic Press.

Hennessy, T. W., Marcus, R., Deneen, V., Reddy, S., Vugia, D., Townes, J., Bardsley, M., Swerdlow, D., & Angulo, F. J. (April 15, 2004). Emerging infections Program FoodNet working group. Survey of physician diagnostic practices for patients with acute diarrhea: Clinical and public health implications. *Clinical Infectious Diseases, 38*(Suppl. 3), S203–S211. https://doi.org/10.1086/381588. PMID: 15095191.

Hoyte, F., & Nelson, H. S. (2018). Recent advances in allergic rhinitis. *F1000Research, 7*, F1000. Faculty Rev-1333.

ICD – 10. (2020). https://en.wikipedia.org/wiki/ICD-10 (Last Accessed 9 June 2020).

Kamińska, M., Ciszewski, T., Łopacka-Szatan, K., Miotła, P., & Starosławska, E. (2015). Breast cancer risk factors. *Menopausal Review, 3*, 196–202.

Lăcătuşu, C. M., Grigorescu, E. D., Floria, M., Onofriescu, A., & Mihai, B. M. (2019). The Mediterranean diet: From an environment-driven food culture to an emerging medical prescription. *International Journal of Environmental Research and Public Health, 16*(6), 942.

Larsen, J. N., Broge, L., & Jacobi, H. (2016). Allergy immunotherapy: The future of allergy treatment. *Drug Discovery Today, 21*(1), 26–37.

LCE (Lung Cancer Europe), 'Lung Cancer' https://www.lungcancereurope.eu/lung-cancer/ (Last Accessed 9 June 2020).

Lenzi, A. (2019). Why urbanisation and health? *Acta Bio-Medica: Atenei Parmensis, 90*(2), 181–183.

Linden, M., Linden, U., Goretzko, D., & Gensichen, J. (2022). Prevalence and pattern of acute and chronic multimorbidity across all body systems and age groups in primary health care. *Science Reports, 12*, 272. https://doi.org/10.1038/s41598-021-04256-x

Lorenzl, S., Füsgen, I., & Noachtar, S. (2012). Acute confusional States in the elderly–diagnosis and treatment. *Deutsches Arzteblatt International, 109*(21), 391–400.

Maas, A. H., & Appelman, Y. E. (2010). Gender differences in coronary heart disease. *Netherlands Heart Journal: Monthly Journal of the Netherlands Society of Cardiology and the Netherlands Heart Foundation, 18*(12), 598–602.

Manisalidis, I., Stavropoulou, E., Stavropoulos, A., & Bezirtzoglou, E. (2020). Environmental and health impacts of air pollution: A review. *Frontiers in Public Health, 8*, 14.

Martin, C. M. (2007). Chronic disease and illness care: Adding principles of family medicine to address ongoing health system redesign. *Canadian family physician Medecin de famille canadien, 53*(12), 2086–2091.

Martinez-Gonzalez, M. A., & Martin-Calvo, N. (2016). Mediterranean diet and life expectancy; beyond olive oil, fruits, and vegetables. *Current Opinion in Clinical Nutrition and Metabolic Care, 19*(6), 401–407.

Matuszkiewicz-Rowińska, J., Małyszko, J., & Wieliczko, M. (2015). Urinary tract infections in pregnancy: Old and new unresolved diagnostic and therapeutic problems. *Archives of Medical Science: AMS, 11*(1), 67–77.

Mehdipoor, G., Salmani, F., & Shabestari, A. A. (August 18, 2017). Survey of practitioners' competency for diagnosis of acute diseases manifest on chest X-ray. *BMC Med Imaging, 17*(1), 49. https://doi.org/10.1186/s12880-017-0222-8. PMID: 28821227; PMCID: PMC5563017.

Montecino-Rodriguez, E., Berent-Maoz, B., & Dorshkind, K. (2013). Causes, consequences, and reversal of immune system aging. *The Journal of Clinical Investigation, 123*(3), 958–965.

Music Milanović, S., Morović, M. L., Križan, H., Pezer, M., Seferović, J., & Missoni, S. (2020). Exploring the effect of socioeconomic development on child growth in post-transitional Croatia: A cross-sectional study. *International Journal of Public Health*, 1–9.

Music Milanović, S., Uhernik, A. I., & Fišter, K. (2009). Health behavior factors associated with obesity in the adult population in Croatia. *Collegium Antropologicum, 33*.

Naleway, A. L. (2004). Asthma and atopy in rural children: Is farming protective? *Clinical Medicine & Research, 2*(1), 5–12.

NCI (National Cancer Institute), 'NCI dictionary of cancer terms', www.cancer.gov/publications/dictionaries/cancer-terms (Last Accessed 9 June 2020).

Nicholson, L. B. (2016). The immune system. *Essays in Biochemistry, 60*(3), 275–301.

de Oliveira Santos, G. C., Vasconcelos, C. C., Lopes, A., de Sousa Cartágenes, M., Filho, A., do Nascimento, F., Ramos, R. M., Pires, E., de Andrade, M. S., Rocha, F., & de Andrade Monteiro, C. (2018). Candida infections and therapeutic strategies: Mechanisms of action for traditional and alternative agents. *Frontiers in Microbiology, 9*, 1351.

Providence, C., Gommans, J., & Burns, A. (January 2012). Managing acute medical admissions: A survey of acute medical services and medical assessment and planning units in New Zealand. *Intern Med J, 42*(1), 51–56. https://doi.org/10.1111/j.1445-5994.2010.02331.x. Epub 2010 Jul 30. PMID: 20681959.

Raghupathi, W., & Raghupathi, V. (2018). An empirical study of chronic diseases in the United States: A visual analytics approach. *International Journal of Environmental Research and Public Health, 15*(3), 431. https://doi.org/10.3390/ijerph15030431

Rashidian, S., Falahati, M:, Kordbacheh, P., Mahmoudi, M., Safara, M., Sadeghi Tafti, H., Mahmoudi, S., & Zaini, F. (2015). A study on etiologic agents and clinical manifestations of dermatophytosis in Yazd, Iran. *Current Medical Mycology, 1*(4), 20–25. https://doi.org/10.18869/acadpub.cmm.1.4.20.28681000.

Regitz-Zagrosek, V. (2012). Sex and gender differences in health', Science & Society Series on Sex and Science. *EMBO Reports, 13*(7), 596–603.

Rito, A. I., Buoncristiano, M., Spinelli, A., Salanave, B., Kunešová, H., Hejgaard, T., García Solano, M:, Fijałkowska, A., Sturua, L., Hyska, J., Kelleher, C., Duleva, V., Music Milanović, S., Farrugia Sant'Angelo, V., Abdrakhmanova, S., Kujundzic, E., Peterkova, V., Gualtieri, A., Pudule, I., & Breda, J. (2019). Association between characteristics at birth, breastfeeding and obesity in 22 countries: The WHO European childhood obesity surveillance initiative–COSI 2015/2017. *Obesity Facts, 12*(2), 226–243. https://doi.org/10.1159/000500425.31030194.

Romagnolo, D. F., & Selmin, O. I. (2017). Mediterranean diet and prevention of chronic diseases. *Nutrition Today, 52*(5), 208–222.

Rowe, T. A., & Juthani-Mehta, M. (2013). Urinary tract infection in older adults. *Aging Health, 9*(5).

Rushton, D., & Barth, J. (2009). What is the evidence for gender differences in ferritin and hemoglobin? *Critical Reviews in Oncology/hematology, 73*, 1–9.

Sanyaolu, P., & Sanyaolu, C. (2018). *Urbanization 1*. https://doi.org/10.13140/RG.2.2.23495.96161

Simon, A. K., Hollander, G. A., & McMichael, A. (2015). Evolution of the immune system in humans from infancy to old age. *Proceedings: Biological Sciences, 282*(1821), 20143085.

Smit, L. A., Hooiveld, M., van der Sman-de Beer, F., Opstal-van Winden, A. W., Beekhuizen, J., Wouters, I. M., Yzermans, C. J., & Heederik, D. (2014). Air pollution from livestock farms, and asthma, allergic rhinitis and COPD among neighbouring residents. *Occupational and Environmental Medicine, 71*(2), 134–140. https://doi.org/10.1136/oemed-2013-101485

Spampinato, C., & Leonardi, D. (2013). Candida infections, causes, targets, and resistance mechanisms: Traditional and alternative antifungal agents. *BioMed Research International, 2013*, 204237.

Starc, G., Popović, S., Đordić, V., Ostojić, S., Musić Milanović, S., & Kujundžić, E. (2019). Differences in body height between the contemporary Western Balkan children and the WHO growth references core sample. *Anthropological Notebooks, 25*(3).

Tan, A. U., Schlosser, B. J., & Paller, A. S. (2017). A review of diagnosis and treatment of acne in adult female patients. *International Journal of Women's Dermatology, 4*(2), 56–71.

Taubenberger, J. K., & Morens, D. M. (2006). 1918 influenza: The mother of all pandemics. *Emerging Infectious Diseases, 12*(1), 15–22.

Trichopoulou, A., & Lagiou, P. (1997). Healthy traditional Mediterranean diet: An expression of culture, history, and lifestyle. *Nutrition Reviews, 55*, 383–389.

Turabian, J. (2018). Gender differences in prevalence of chronic diseases: Facts and hypothesis. *Melody and Harmony*, 1–3.

Varshney, J., & Varshney, H. (2015). Allergic rhinitis: An overview. *Indian Journal of Otolaryngology and Head and Neck Surgery: Official Publication of the Association of Otolaryngologists of India, 67*(2), 143–149.

UN. (2018). *68% of the world population projected to live in urban areas by 2050, says UN*. https://www.un.org/development/desa/en/news/population/2018-revision-of-world-urbanization-prospects.html.

Vlahov, D., & Galea, S. (2002). Urbanization, urbanicity, and health. *Journal of Urban Health: Bulletin of the New York Academy of Medicine, 79*(4 Suppl. 1), S1–S12.

Weyand, C. M., & Goronzy, J. J. (2016). Aging of the immune system. Mechanisms and therapeutic targets. *Annals of the American Thoracic Society, 13*(Suppl. 5), S422–S428.

WHO (World Health Organization). (2005). *Chronic diseases are the major cause of death and disability worldwide*. https://www.who.int/chp/chronic_disease_report/media/Factsheet1.pdf.

WHO (World Health Organization). (2012). *Effects of urbanization on the incidence of non-communicable diseases*. https://applications.emro.who.int/dsaf/EMPUB_2012_864.pdf (Last Accessed 9 June 2020).

Willett, W. C., Koplan, J. P., Nugent, R., Dusenbury, C., Puska, P., & Gaziano, T. A. (2006). Chapter 44: Prevention of chronic disease by means of diet and lifestyle changes. In D. T. Jamison, J. G. Breman, A. R. Measham, et al. (Eds.), *Disease control priorities in developing countries* (2nd ed.). Oxford University Press.

Wilson, M. E. (2010). Geography of infectious diseases. *Infectious Diseases*, 1055–1064.

Xu, J., Sherry, L., Murphy, S. L., Kenneth, D., Kochanek, M. A., & Arias, E. (2020). *Mortality in the United States, 2018*. https://www.cdc.gov/nchs/products/databriefs/db355.htm (Last Accessed 9 June 2020).

Yew, K. S., & Cheng, E. (2009). Acute stroke diagnosis. *American Family Physician, 80*(1), 33–40.

Yi, Y., Lagniton, P., Ye, S., Li, E., & Xu, R. H. (2020). COVID-19: What has been learned and to be learned about the novel coronavirus disease. *International Journal of Biological Sciences, 16*(10), 1753–1766.

Zhang, J. J., Adcock, I. M., Bai, Z., Chung, K. F., Duan, X., Fang, Z., Gong, J., Li, F., Miller, R. K., Qiu, X., Rich, D. Q., Wang, B., Wei, Y., Xu, D., Xue, T., Zhang, Y., Zheng, M., & Zhu, T. (2019). Health effects of air pollution: What we need to know and to do in the next decade. *Journal of Thoracic Disease, 11*(4), 1727–1730.

Further reading

Carinanos, P. (2013). 'Urban green zones and related pollen allergy: A review', some guidelines for designing urban green areas of low allergy impact. *Landscape and Urban Planning*.

Casale, M., Moffa, A., Cassano, M., Carinci, F., Lopez, M. A., Trecca, E., Torretta, S., Rinaldi, V., & Pignataro, L. (2018). Saline nasal irrigations for chronic rhinosinusitis: From everyday practice to evidence-based medicine. An update. *International Journal of Immunopathology and Pharmacology, 32*, 2058738418802676.

CBS (Croatian Bureau of Statistics). (2019). *Population estimate of Republic of Croatia, 2018*. www.dzs.hr/Hrv_Eng/publication/2019/07-01-03_01_2019.htm (Last Accessed 9 June 2020).

Murphy, S., Xu, J., Kochanek, K., & Arias, E. (2018). *Mortality in the United States, 2017 key findings data from the national vital statistics system, NCHS data brief.*

Petruccelli, B. P. (2012). Infectious disease: A geographic guide and Atlas of human infectious diseases. *Emerging Infectious Diseases, 18*(7), 1216–1217.

Platts-Mills, T. A. (2015). The allergy epidemics: 1870-2010. *The Journal of Allergy and Clinical Immunology, 136*(1), 3–13.

CHAPTER

A conceptual framework for Artificial Intelligence of Medical Things (AIoMT) 8

Hamed Nozari[1], Reza Tavakkoli-Moghaddam[1], Javid Ghahremani-Nahr[2], Esmaeil Najafi[3]

[1]*School of Industrial Engineering, College of Engineering, University of Tehran, Tehran, Iran;*
[2]*Faculty Member of Academic Center for Education, Culture and Research (ACECR), Tabriz, Iran;*
[3]*Department of Industrial Engineering, Science and Research Branch, Islamic Azad University, Tehran, Iran*

8.1 Introduction

The Internet of Things (IoT) devices, which can report in a real-time without human intervention, has provided a new level of efficiency, convenience, and automation in medicine and telemedicine. For example, healthcare is one of the front lines of the IoT business. The growth of the IoT in various fields has brought astonishing results in the achievements and progress of mankind in the 21st century (Nozari, Fallah, Kazemipoor et al., 2021). Although the concept of the IoT is often seen alongside the construction, warehousing, and smart factories of the future, IoT applications in healthcare are another lesser-known area among interconnected object enthusiasts. Using the IoT can benefit physicians, patients, and the general public because the accuracy of measurement and speed of operation of intelligent systems and computers is thousands of times higher than humans. Applying technology to medicine can significantly help reduce treatment costs and mortality rates (Nozari et al., 2021). The Internet of Medical Things (IoMT) is a collection of medical devices that connect to the internal network of internal health systems and physicians via the International Internet of Things. Through IoMT, a person's health data is stored in a database on the internet and made available to the relevant organization or individuals, such as physicians, nurses, or the World Health Organization (Jain et al., 2021).

On the other hand, artificial intelligence (AI) is used in different layers of the IoT. It can be seen at varying levels of this technology; however, one of the main functions of AI in the IoT is on information collected from IoT equipment. Large volumes with the concept of big data require precise processing to obtain acceptable results, for which AI is used and helps in processing (Alhayani et al., 2021). An AI system can analyze data and make decisions when needed. Therefore, objects that connect to the internet must also have artificial intelligence. Thus, the combination of this technology can play a significant role in increasing the efficiency and effectiveness of services and activities of healthcare systems. In this chapter, a

Computational Intelligence for Medical Internet of Things (MIoT) Applications
https://doi.org/10.1016/B978-0-323-99421-7.00007-6

concept called Artificial Intelligence of Medical Things (AIoMT) is defined and introduced to show the capabilities and functions of this technology in health systems (Sun et al., 2020). The data collected by millions of IoT devices in medical procedures is so large that it is difficult to separate and extract useful information. To organize the unstructured data into a meaningful data set, artificial intelligence-based algorithms are used to remove useless data and maximize the use of the data in therapeutic processes (Nozari, Fallah, Szmelter-Jarosz, & Krzemiński, 2021).

This research has attempted to provide a conceptual framework for an AI-based health system that combines a powerful AI computing system with powerful IoT technology as one of the most important sources of big data generation. For this purpose, using literature review, the most important components and effective parts in a health system were extracted. Then using the opinions of experts in the field of treatment and IT professionals familiar with the concepts of artificial intelligence and IoT causal relationship, the defects of these components were identified with technologies. Finally, the framework's validity was confirmed using the opinion of experts active in these fields. Using this framework, we can identify the essential elements in implementing a health system, emphasizing big data and the use of transformative computing technologies, and taking steps to create an intelligent treatment structure.

8.2 IoT in healthcare

The concept of the IoT requires the use of electronic tools to record information to connect to the Internet, Bluetooth, or other networks, the ability to perform specific tasks (e.g., sending to the server and processing) to the system. The use of many industrial products and equipment can change if the internet can be used because there are a lot of changes in the field of healthcare every year. New technologies improve patient care methods and make physicians' treatments more efficient. The field of medicine has great potential for using IoT. The integration of IoT with other medical devices has played an essential role in the development of the medical field of countries. In general, the IoT has significantly reduced treatment costs and improved treatment outcomes by providing tools for integrating treatment and medical systems and increasing their accuracy and efficiency. Patients and healthcare providers can also benefit from the use of the IoT in health. Some IoT applications can be found in mobile health software or devices that record personal health information. Many hospitals also use this technology in medical equipment, staff, and patients (Maksimović et al., 2015). The main reason for using this technology is to reduce the human role and avoid human errors that lead to the provision of services in health. This technology can provide medical services to patients by remote access and control and facilities to record patient information and transfer them for review. The IoT can be used in various medical fields, including emergency alert systems, remote patient care systems, chronic illnesses, fitness programs, and geriatric care. These include heart rate monitoring systems, health monitoring systems, blood pressure monitoring systems, hearing aids, and artificial pacemakers. In more advanced cases, the devices monitor the course of treatment and medications and their amount. Also, there are programs on the IoT that allow physicians to monitor their patients after they are discharged from the hospital (Yuehong et al., 2016). One of the most important uses of the IoT in the health sector is to monitor vital signs and specific parameters of people with chronic and common diseases. Common diseases include heart disease, respiratory diseases, and diabetes. To reduce costs and increase patient care, the use of smart health devices is increasing day by day (Yehia et al., 2015). Fig. 8.1 shows how the Internet of Things affects the healthcare industry.

IoT-enabled smart and connected solutions such as smart sensors, wearables, and smart health monitoring systems are being used to unleash the potential growth of the healthcare industry. They will do this by improving treatment using effective health tracking. The growing popularity of the Internet of Things in the field of healthcare and medicine has been enhanced by modern techniques such as IoMT. IoMT is an ecosystem of smart devices that can communicate in a real-time environment and formulate results. This greatly reduces human error and eliminates many decision delays (Baker et al., 2017).

Digital healthcare systems use IoT and big data to bring seamless digital communication with the patient. These systems are also increasingly connecting to the

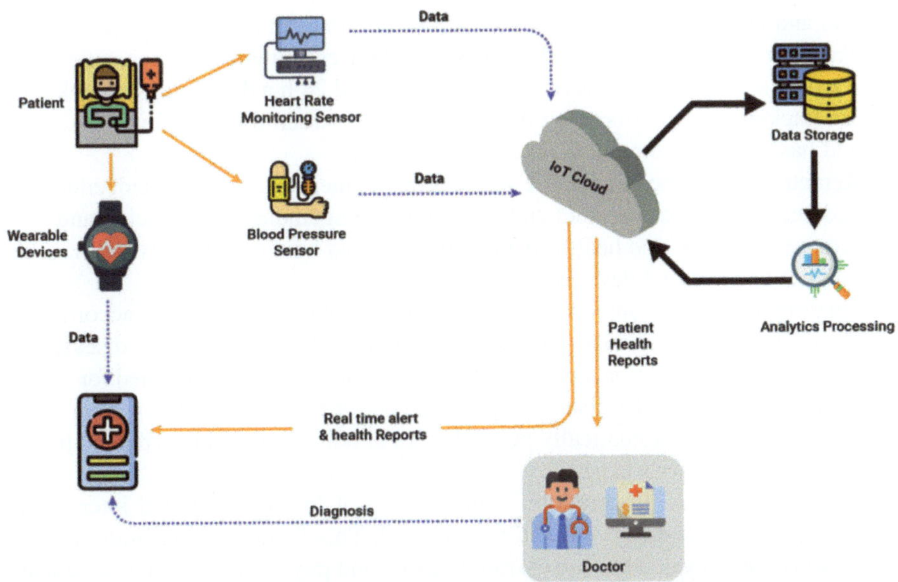

FIGURE 8.1

How IoT is Transforming the Healthcare Industry (Shrimali, 2020).

internet through various wearable medical technologies to assist us in real-time patient information.

The desire of people to live daily life without worries and assurance of supervision, as well as the unwillingness to spend long days in the hospital and even the willingness of some patients to live in small towns or villages without advanced medical facilities are also factors in using smart health tools (Shrimali, 2020). Typically, the IoT solution in health systems includes the following functions:

- Collecting vital signs continuously: Vital signs, including heart rate, blood pressure, body temperature, and respiration are collected and stored all day and night using intelligent tools equipped with a communication system.
- Collect vital signs periodically: Vital signs, including heart rate, blood pressure, body temperature, and respiration, are collected and regularly stored at adjustable times at all hours of the day and night using intelligent tools equipped with a communication system.
- Collect specific parameters related to chronic and common diseases continuously: Specific parameters about chronic and common conditions such as blood sugar, blood lipids, body water percentage, stress level, and seizure probability using intelligent tools equipped with a continuous communication system collected and stored at all hours of the day.
- Collection of specific parameters related to chronic and common diseases periodically: Specific parameters related to chronic and common conditions such as blood sugar, blood lipids, body water percentage, stress level, and seizure probability using intelligent tools equipped with periodic communication system and are collected and stored at adjustable times at all hours of the day.
- Tracking and monitoring: All objects and their communication capacities with wireless sensor network devices can be measured 24 h a day, 7 days a week and are tracked and monitored by the identification screen that exists in all places and has a high communication capacity.
- Remote services: health and life services (e.g., emergency and first aid, education and health of residence, diet and medicine management, telemedicine and remote diagnosis, and health social networks) can be remotely provided via the internet and optimal devices.
- Sending intelligent content to the user: The system has the ability to according to the vital signs and specific parameters related to chronic. Common diseases collected by each person, and according to the threshold levels defined for them, if the symptoms of the disease appear, the user page modifies the person accordingly and automatically posts articles or educational videos related to the disease on the user's page.
- Interorganizational integration: With the help of IoT an integrated interorganizational information system can be achieved. This feature allows authorized persons (i.e., physicians, nurses, radiologists, and physiotherapists) to access all patients' medical information in different locations (i.e., hospitals and doctors' offices).

Fig. 8.2 shows how this revolution in medicine manifests itself in practice in ordinary IoT hospitals. The patient will have an ID card that, when scanned, will be connected to a secure cloud that stores essential e-health information, laboratory results, medical history, and prescription.

The IoT in most healthcare systems is designed to enter, store, receive, and exchange health information. The system increases the number of devices and increases the mobility of data to support health professionals in their consultations. In addition to the benefits of using the IoT in hospitals, reliability, several challenges related to availability, scalability of management, mobility, performance, security, interoperability, and privacy should be taking into consideration during its application.

The IoT helps monitor equipment status in hospital wards and track patients' health with special sensors. Such devices can monitor patients' health status from the moment they enter the hospital, collecting and updating information about them without a nurse (thus saving time and money). One of the essential features of IoT medical solutions is the remote provision of some medical services and health monitoring. This concept means replacing the medical staff with intelligent programs in different devices. For example, special flexible devices are used to rehabilitate strokes. They are attached to the neck to track swallowing and speech disorders. Clinics with intelligent systems can provide more straightforward and faster solutions to the care process (Nozari, Szmelter-Jarosz, & Ghahremani-Nahr, 2021).

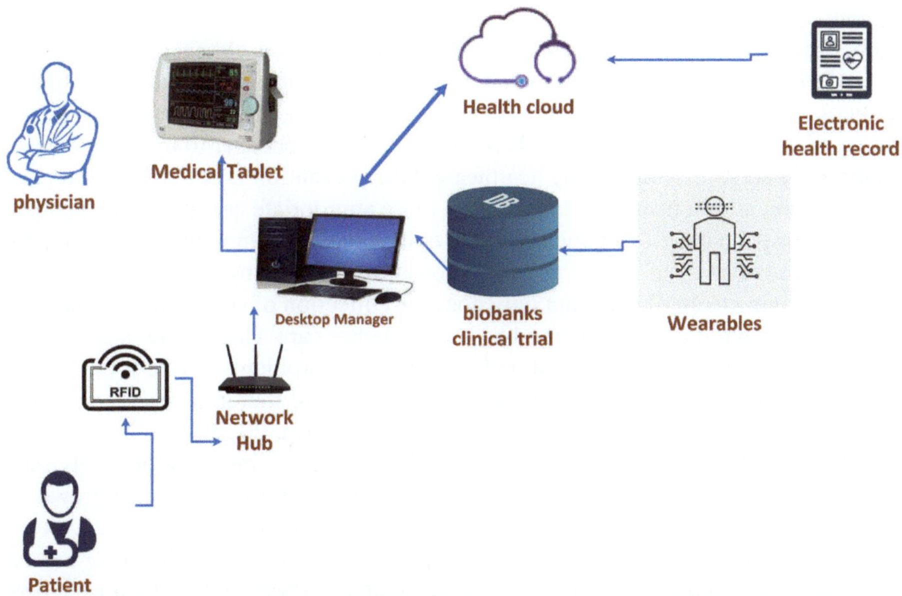

FIGURE 8.2

Hospital IoT scenario (Dauwed & Meri, 2019).

IoT devices in medicine reduce doctors' errors in diagnosis and help monitor the work of a medical center. Such tools can analyze the information obtained and provide solutions that also contribute to employee efficiency. With the advent of the medical IoT, healthcare is now finding completely new ways to monitor and treat health. The world can now use smart drugs with sensors inside: they allow doctors to learn more about a patient's health.

According to forecasts and analyzes, healthcare is the most important part of the Internet of Things. Intelligent devices and systems are not created to replace doctors and nurses, but to help improve their work. The main driver of the growth of the IoT is the need for tools and programs to maintain health.

8.3 Big data in healthcare

As mentioned in the previous section, the IoT is one of the most important sources of big data production. Through this big data and calculations on this data, we can use these revolutionary technologies to serve patients. win. For this reason, in this section we will describe some of the most important effects of big data on treatment systems.

The use of big data analysis in healthcare has positive results and life-saving. Big data refers to the vast amounts of information generated by the digitization of everything that is synthesized and analyzed by specific technologies. Here, big data uses health services to use specific population health data (or a specific individual) and potentially help prevent disease pandemics, treat diseases, reduce costs, and more. Now, treatment models have changed, and many of these changes are driven by data. Doctors want to know as much as possible about a patient and his life as soon as possible so that they can recognize the warning signs of a serious illness when it occurs (Nahr et al., 2021). It is much easier and cheaper to treat any disease in the early stages. By analyzing healthcare data, prevention is better than cure, and management allows insurance to provide a more appropriate cost package to paint a comprehensive picture of a patient. In fact, collecting large amounts of data for medical purposes has been costly and time-consuming for many years. With today's ever-improving technologies, not only does the collection of such data become relevant insights, but it can also be used to provide better care. Healthcare data analysis aims to use data-driven findings to predict and solve problems before it is too late. This speeds up the evaluation of treatment methods and therefore leads to a better follow-up of individual health (Mokliakova & Srivastava, 2022).

Physicians' decisions are increasingly evidence-based, meaning they rely on a wealth of research and clinical data. Like many other industries, as data grows, so does data management, and experts need help. This new therapeutic approach means that there is more demand for big data analysis in medical centers than ever before.

Using big data in healthcare allows strategic plans to better understand what people think. Care managers can analyze the survey results among different population groups and consider the determining factors to prevent the use of treatment. In the field of health, big data covers a wide range of information, including physiological, behavioral, molecular, clinical, medical imaging, disease management, medication history, nutrition, or exercise parameters.

Data sources can be categorized as follows:

1. Traditional medical records: including electronic medical records (EMRs), electronic health records (EHRs), medical history, and laboratory reports that help better understand disease outcomes and optimize healthcare delivery.
2. Genomic, microbiomic, proteomic, and metabolic data used to understand disease mechanisms and accelerate the personalization of medical therapies.
3. Social media data, biometric data (wearable systems and sensors) that provide information about people's behavior and lifestyle (Kashani et al., 2021).

Although health data provide potential value for optimizing care, they are still considered a by-product of healthcare. Since this electronic information is not widely used and wasted, it is essential that raw data be converted into meaningful and practical information.

Despite the many potential benefits of big data analytics, the health industry is in the early stages of using this technology. Despite the large amount of data available, lack of knowledge, lack of infrastructure, and the need for massive initial investment make using big data more difficult. The challenge of storing large amounts of data can be tackled using cloud computing. This feature solves cost and data storage problems, especially for small hospitals and care organizations. Another problem is the weakness of data governance, which imposes huge costs on IT investment for healthcare organizations. With proper data management and monitoring, the entire company's data sources can create business value. By developing a culture of information sharing and data aggregation, it is possible to create interoperability and effectively use big data analysis and forecasting capabilities. Fig. 8.3 shows the relationship between big data analysis as well as the Internet of Things.

8.4 Artificial intelligence in healthcare

Artificial intelligence is used in many industries, but its impact is certainly critical in medical science, where many deaths occur based on human error. This transformative technology has revolutionized medicine. With this technology, while receiving positive treatment results, it is possible to see a reduction in costs. Artificial intelligence can be considered a relatively new technology that is in its infancy in the medical industry. As AI tools and machine learning become more sophisticated, artificial intelligence in medicine is becoming more widespread. Of course, as we said, we are still the first way and different companies are trying to find a specific strategy for it. Due to the complexity of medical decisions, information systems to support these decisions have increased. In the meantime, the role of intelligent systems in assisting physicians is prominent. AI is used for a variety of therapeutic and research purposes, including diagnosis, management of chronic diseases, medical services,

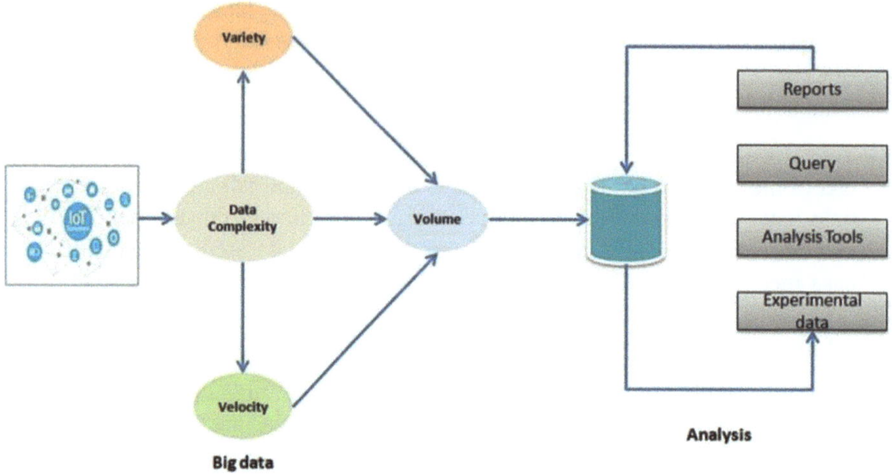

FIGURE 8.3

IoT big data processing.

and drug discovery. AI technology has better patient-care potential, administrative processes of pharmaceutical organizations, and the ability to diagnose disease than humans (Jiang et al., 2017). AI health programs provide the conditions for people to assess their symptoms and take care of themselves if possible. AI systems enhance the quality of life of individuals. Hospitals look for AI solutions to increase cost savings, improve patient satisfaction, and meet staffing and workforce needs. As the digital world continues to grow in the field of healthcare, more and more data are being generated and stored in this space every day (Reddy et al., 2019). The amount of data available is growing at a staggering rate, and the volume of this data is multiplying almost every two years. In other words, the amount of information that we have today in healthcare is considerable, and AI can quickly classify and organize this huge mass of data (Schönberger, 2019).

Existing AI solutions are divided into six main areas in which AI directly impacts the patient and three areas of the healthcare value chain that they can benefit from. Fig. 8.4 shows these key areas.

The potential of AI for the use in the field of medicine is extremely high. Thus, AI can help simplify drug production processes to quickly provide appropriate treatments for new and old diseases. This system can even help identify previously unknown diseases. AI can increasingly be used in the following cases:

- It helps doctors act faster to treat serious illnesses, thus reducing mortality in hospitals worldwide.
- Provides a quick and accurate diagnosis that is virtually impossible using human intelligence alone.
- Mistakes made as a result will limit human fatigue.

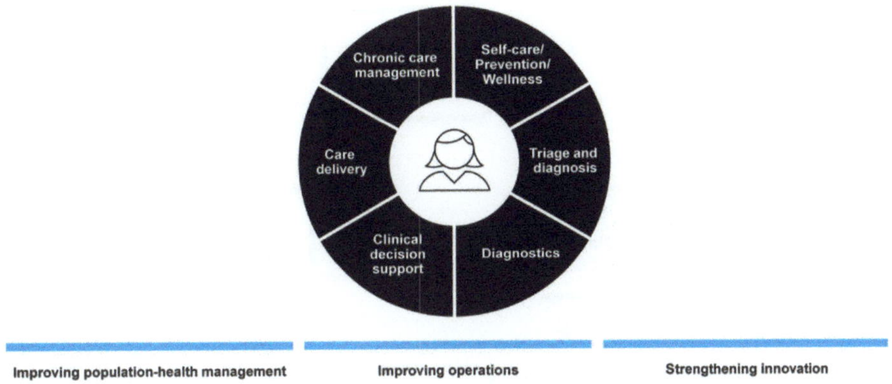

FIGURE 8.4

Six key areas of artificial intelligence solutions in health systems.

However, the important thing is that AI has not been offered to replace doctors in healthcare. Instead, AI is practically provided to enhance the capabilities of medical professionals and can bridge the gap in their abilities. Also, although AI technology can have many benefits for the healthcare industry, finding a way to implement this new technology in the current healthcare system and finding training solutions for medical professionals can always be a significant challenge (Bohr & Memarzadeh, 2020).

Given the above, it can be seen that AI is used for all three classic medical tasks: diagnosis, prognosis, and treatment, but more in the field of medical diagnosis. In general, the medical diagnosis cycle includes observing and examining the patient, collecting the patient data, interpreting the data using the physician's knowledge and experience, and then formulating the diagnosis and treatment plan by the physician. The diagnostic treatment cycle is shown in Fig. 8.5.

All AI systems used in medical engineering and medicine use deep learning algorithms to diagnose the disease. Data from healthcare centers are used to train these systems. Then, these AI systems employ specific techniques to achieve the diagnosis. There is a challenge and problem in deep learning techniques is transparency. The inputs and outputs given to the system are transparent; however, it is not clear how AI can diagnose the disease. Another point in this regard is that the quality of the AI system in detection depends directly on the quality of the data (Szolovits et al., 1988).

Artificial intelligence applications have helped to increase the speed and accuracy of medical diagnosis. Artificial intelligence is used in the research and development of new medical products. It also helps automate repetitive tasks of medical staff such as routine office work, scheduling and scheduling to improve efficiency and reduce costs. Artificial intelligence has also helped physicians analyze historical data to identify insights for better treatment (Li et al., 2020).

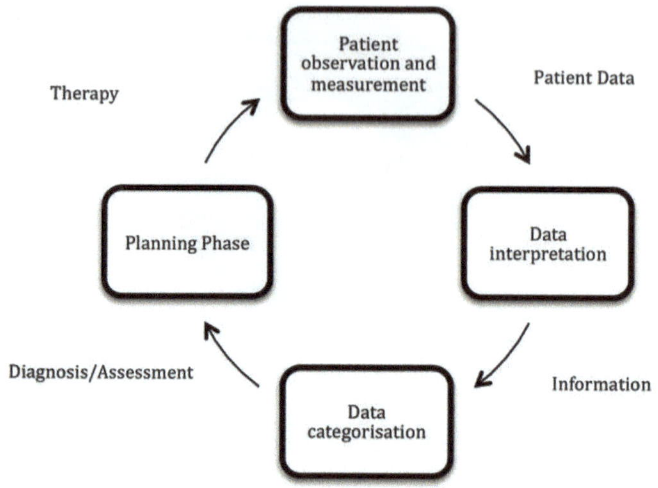

FIGURE 8.5

Diagnostic-therapeutic cycle of medicine (Mokliakova & Srivastava, 2022).

Machine learning, and more specifically deep learning algorithms, have recently made great strides in medicine. These algorithms automatically detect diseases and make the process cheaper and more accessible. However, how do machines learn to diagnose disease? Machine learning algorithms can learn to see disease patterns like doctors. The main difference is that these algorithms require thousands of interconnected examples to learn. And these examples need to be cleaned and digitized; machines do not know how to read from the lines of books! Therefore, machine learning is particularly useful in cases where physician test information is stored in a database. This data is processed in such a way that it can be used as a result, which is the input of another type of system that provides the proposed differential. It provides input, diagnosis, and conclusion based on a set of rules. A tree-like hierarchy is provided using data that these systems can help with. These systems are based on the "expert systems" rule. Systems experts consider this experience to make the final decision. Most of these systems are able to answer the questions with "what" instead of "how" and at the same time explain the reasoning behind them (Fallah et al., 2021).

The increasing availability of electronic data in the field of healthcare has provided an important opportunity to discover and apply various methods in improving healthcare. While artificial intelligence can and often is well used, it can also detect and exploit vulnerabilities. Machine learning has the power to be used for both good and, unfortunately bad purposes. As more connected medical devices are built on artificial intelligence, the risks of cybersecurity increase, and it is even more important for manufacturers to use advanced security protections in the design phase to ensure the safety of healthcare organizations, providers, and patients.

8.5 Artificial Intelligence of Medical Things (AIoMT)

There have been powerful combinations throughout history, each with unique characteristics, but miracles happened when they were put together. Similarly, the complete combination of the IoT with AI, known as AIoT, allows companies to take advantage of both (Nozari & Sadeghi, 2021). AIoT means using the IoT to perform intelligent tasks with the help of AI integration. AIoT helps connect IoT devices to sensors with AI capabilities, which is done without human intervention. AIoT has the following features (Kishor & Chakraborty, 2021):

- AIoT is the brain that controls the nervous system to make better business decisions.
- AIoT that provides intelligent decisions requires software code written by programmers to carried out various tasks.
- AIoT is the next generation of the IoT, and its primary design goal is independent operation without human support using predictive maintenance and AI algorithms.
- In AIoT, IoT self-correction devices are created by analyzing data for better decision-making.

With excellent personalization experience, active intervention, and intelligent automation, AIoT offers countless benefits to companies and consumers. The benefits of AIoT are shown in Fig. 8.6.

Maintaining health is a difficult challenge and takes time. In today's world, with all kinds of challenges, everyone is very cautious about their health, and technologies (e.g., IoT and AI) use the entire healthcare sector. Frequent visits to doctors for regular checkups are difficult for a large population. This problem is solved with

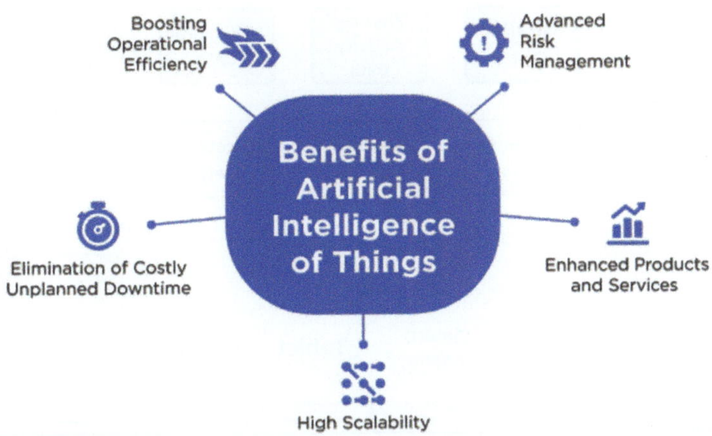

FIGURE 8.6

Benefits of AI of things (AIoT).

wearable devices (e.g., smartwatches, fitness trackers, panic buttons to track blood sugar levels, and cholesterol levels). The healthcare industry has to deal with vast data, and the IoT is adding significant volume to wearable devices. AI provides meaningful insights into data and helps with real-time responses, inventory management, human resource management, and affiliate pharmaceutical services. AIoT applications help to collect data to provide preventive measures for the individual, early diagnosis, and medication administration (Reddy, 2018). Fig. 8.7 provides a framework for giving relationships between the parameters affecting AIoT on the healthcare system, called Artificial Intelligence of Medical Things (AIoMT).

In order to create a conceptual framework for expressing the connections between transformational tools such as the Internet of Things and artificial intelligence

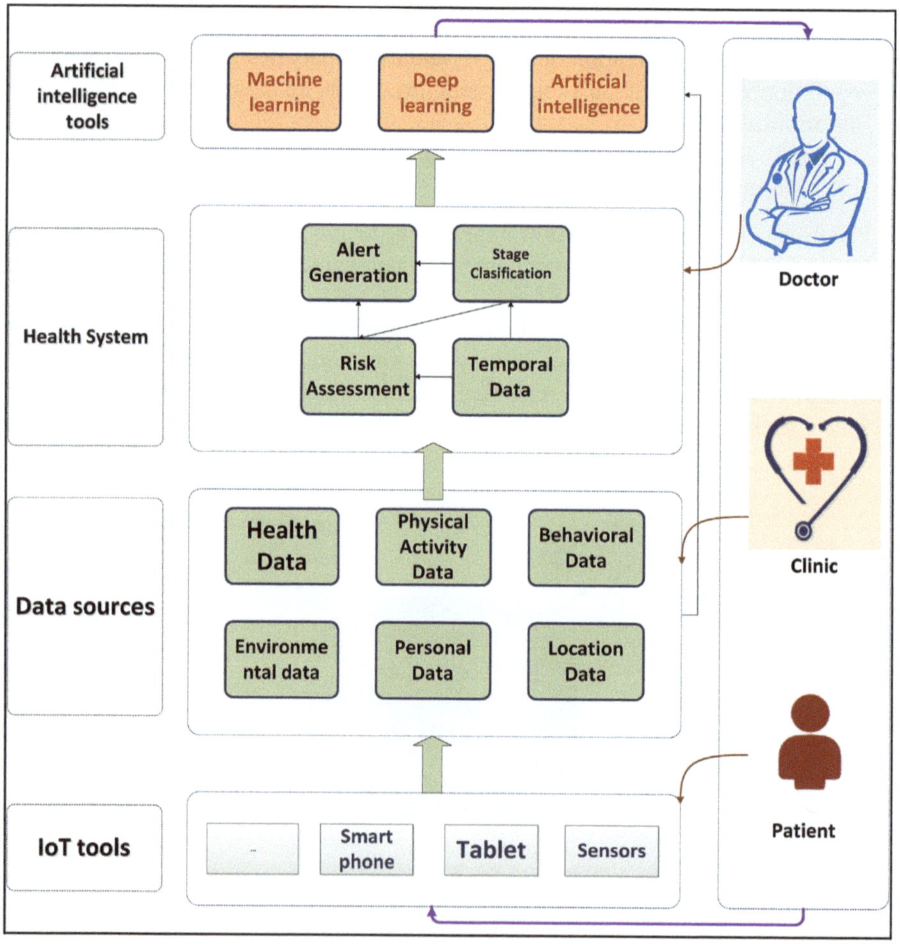

FIGURE 8.7

Framework of the proposed system (AIoMT).

and the big impact of big data from IoT technology on the industry, all the basic parts of the field were separated using the opinions of experts. Then, by reviewing the literature, the key elements in each section were extracted and confirmed by experts active in Jose Medical Services and familiar with information technology and transformational technologies. Then the causal relationship between the elements was identified and put together in a conceptual framework. Active experts in related fields also approved this framework.

This framework shows the clear relationships between the effective parameters in the treatment systems based on AI of objects. Using this framework, significant points can be identified in specific situations and increasing efficiency can be an optimal effort, which is one of the main tasks of IoT-based systems.

8.6 Conclusion

There are many changes in the field of healthcare every year. New technologies improve patient care methods and make physicians' treatments more efficient. The field of medicine has great potential for using IoT. The integration of the IoT with other medical devices has been able to play an essential role in the development of the medical field of countries. On the other hand, AI has various applications in treatment and medicine. The meaning of these users is that everyone is among the users of AI in the medical field, from recognizing the connection between genetic codes to using AI robots for complicated surgeries. With all these applications, AI has created a modern course in health services and taken it to another level. When these technologies are combined, they reduce costs and activate the next level of automation and productivity. As consumers, businesses, and governments begin to use the IoT in various environments, our world will change dramatically, allowing all of us to make better choices. This process is rapidly changing everything in the healthcare chain, and the IoT with AI capability can also transform the healthcare industry with smart solutions. This combination creates a concept called Artificial intelligence of Things or AIoT. Due to the very high efficiency of this concept, this chapter provides a framework for implementing an AIoT-based treatment system or AIoMT. Using this framework, we can understand the factors affecting creating an intelligent structure of the medical system, emphasizing AI and the IoT.

References

Alhayani, B., Mohammed, H. J., Chaloob, I. Z., & Ahmed, J. S. (2021). Effectiveness of artificial intelligence techniques against cyber security risks apply of IT industry. *Materials Today: Proceedings*. https://www.sciencedirect.com/science/article/pii/S2214785321016722. Available online 10 March 2021.

Baker, S. B., Xiang, W., & Atkinson, I. (2017). Internet of things for smart healthcare: Technologies, challenges, and opportunities. *IEEE Access, 5*, 26521–26544.

Bohr, A., & Memarzadeh, K. (2020). The rise of artificial intelligence in healthcare applications. In *Artificial intelligence in healthcare* (pp. 25–60). Academic Press.

Dauwed, M., & Meri, A. (2019). IOT service utilisation in healthcare. In *Internet of things (IoT) for automated and smart applications* (p. 41).

Fallah, M., Sadeghi, M. E., & Nozari, H. (2021). Quantitative analysis of the applied parts of internet of things technology in Iran: An opportunity for economic leapfrogging through technological development. *Science and Technology Policy Letters, 11*(4).

Jain, S., Nehra, M., Kumar, R., Dilbaghi, N., Hu, T. Y., Kumar, S., & Li, C. Z. (2021). Internet of medical things (IoMT)-integrated biosensors for point-of-care testing of infectious diseases. *Biosensors and Bioelectronics*, 113074.

Jiang, F., Jiang, Y., Zhi, H., Dong, Y., Li, H., Ma, S., & Wang, Y. (2017). Artificial intelligence in healthcare: Past, present and future. *Stroke and Vascular Neurology, 2*(4), 230–243.

Kashani, M. H., Madanipour, M., Nikravan, M., Asghari, P., & Mahdipour, E. (2021). A systematic review of IoT in healthcare: Applications, techniques, and trends. *Journal of Network and Computer Applications, 192*, 103164.

Kishor, A., & Chakraborty, C. (2021). Artificial intelligence and internet of things based healthcare 4.0 monitoring system. *Wireless Personal Communications*, 1–17.

Li, R. C., Asch, S. M., & Shah, N. H. (2020). Developing a delivery science for artificial intelligence in healthcare. *NPJ Digital Medicine, 3*(1), 1–3.

Maksimović, M., Vujović, V., & Perišić, B. (June 2015). A custom Internet of Things healthcare system. In *Proceedings of the 2015 10th Iberian Conference on information systems and technologies (CISTI)* (pp. 1–6). IEEE.

Mokliakova, K., & Srivastava, G. (2022). Privacy issues in smart IoT for healthcare and industry. In *Intelligent internet of things for healthcare and industry* (pp. 307–326). Cham: Springer.

Nahr, J. G., Nozari, H., & Sadeghi, M. E. (2021). Green supply chain based on artificial intelligence of things (AIoT). *International Journal of Innovation in Management, Economics and Social Sciences, 1*(2), 56–63.

Nozari, H., Fallah, M., Kazemipoor, H., & Najafi, S. E. (2021). Big data analysis of IoT-based supply chain management considering FMCG industries. *Business Informatics, 15*(1), 78–96.

Nozari, H., Fallah, M., & Szmelter-Jarosz, A. (2021). A conceptual framework of green smart IoT-based supply chain management. *International Journal of Research in Industrial Engineering, 10*(1), 22–34.

Nozari, H., Fallah, M., Szmelter-Jarosz, A., & Krzemiński, M. (2021). Analysis of security criteria for IoT-based supply chain: A case study of FMCG industries. *Central European Management Journal, 29*(4).

Nozari, H., & Sadeghi, M. E. (2021). Artificial intelligence and machine learning for real-world problems (a survey). *International Journal of Innovation in Engineering, 1*(3), 38–47.

Nozari, H., Szmelter-Jarosz, A., & Ghahremani-Nahr, J. (2021). The ideas of sustainable and green marketing based on the internet of everything—the case of the dairy industry. *Future Internet, 13*(10), 266.

Reddy, S. (2018). Use of artificial intelligence in healthcare delivery. In *eHealth-making health care smarter*. IntechOpen.

Reddy, S., Fox, J., & Purohit, M. P. (2019). Artificial intelligence-enabled healthcare delivery. *Journal of the Royal Society of Medicine, 112*(1), 22–28.

Schönberger, D. (2019). Artificial intelligence in healthcare: A critical analysis of the legal and ethical implications. *International Journal of Law and Information Technology, 27*(2), 171–203.

Shrimali, R. (June 30, 2020). How IoT is transforming the healthcare industry. *Embedded Computing*. Retrieved from: https://www.embeddedcomputing.com/application/healthcare/telehealth-healthcare-iot/how-iot-is-transforming-the-healthcare-industry.

Sun, L., Jiang, X., Ren, H., & Guo, Y. (2020). Edge-cloud computing and artificial intelligence in internet of medical things: Architecture, technology and application. *IEEE Access, 8*, 101079–101092.

Szolovits, P., Patil, R. S., & Schwartz, W. B. (1988). Artificial intelligence in medical diagnosis. *Annals of Internal Medicine, 108*(1), 80–87.

Yehia, L., Khedr, A., & Darwish, A. (2015). Hybrid security techniques for Internet of Things healthcare applications. *Advances in Internet of Things, 5*(3), 21–25.

Yuehong, Y. I. N., Zeng, Y., Chen, X., & Fan, Y. (2016). The internet of things in healthcare: An overview. *Journal of Industrial Information Integration, 1*, 3–13.

CHAPTER

Framework for integrating healthcare big data using IoMT technology

9

Youness Khourdifi[1], Alae Elalami[2], Mohamed Bahaj[2], Mounia Zaydi[2], Omar Er-Remyly[2]

[1]*Polydisciplinary Faculty of Khouribga, Sultan Moulay Slimane University, Beni Mellal, Morocco;* [2]*Faculty of Sciences and Techniques, Hassan 1st University, Settat, Morocco*

9.1 Introduction

Big data in healthcare is derived from enormous collections of electronic health records. The challenge is to manage these data sets using standard software and hardware. Existing data management methods and technologies don't really provide for the most effective use of all of this data.

Big data in healthcare is a challenging and important topic Fig. 9.1, not only because of the large volume of data, but also because of its heterogeneity and the speed with which it must be managed (Katal et al., 2013).

The difficulty of "big data" in the health industry is the collection of patient data and their well-being. In healthcare, big data analytics has become a big and critical topic. By proposing new issues in data knowledge representation, data integration,

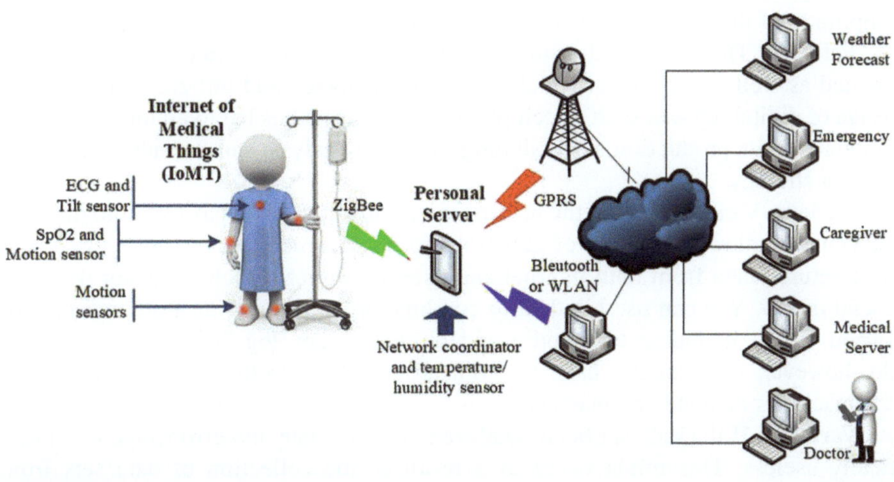

FIGURE 9.1

Internet of Medical Things for e-health.

Computational Intelligence for Medical Internet of Things (MIoT) Applications
https://doi.org/10.1016/B978-0-323-99421-7.00012-X

database architecture, data querying, and clinical decision-making, e-health contributes to the advancement of big data analytics technology (Auffray et al., 2016).

Big data has sparked a lot of attention and debate in recent years as a way to change the world, and the easiest way to grasp it is to look at how important data is used in the healthcare industry (Dash et al., 2019). In this industry, critical data is used to save costs, control diseases, increase revenues, anticipate epidemics, and improve the quality of life by preventing mortality.

Big data analysis is used by scientific research laboratories, hospitals, and other medical organizations to reduce healthcare expenses by changing treatment patterns. The adventure of big data in healthcare begins here, with a focus on the most extensively utilized uses of big data in the healthcare industry (Liu & Park, 2013).

Big data has recently emerged as a hot topic in the worlds of technology and information. Almost every facility or tool is now connected to the network and the cloud. Success can be attributed to recent technological advancements. "Big data" is a notion that allows for a new way of capturing and analyzing data.

Every day, everyone creates more than one piece of data on their cell phones, computers, or other devices, and the amount of data produced will continue to grow. Because data will rise at a breakneck pace, we'll need to figure out how to process it so that we can utilize it for something beneficial, such as an e-health service.

The concept of "big data" was originally associated with the 3V (volume, velocity, and variety), which are the three dimensions of big data.

Considered to be a new technology concept that satisfies the 7V requirement, which stands for (Katal et al., 2013) variety, velocity, veracity, value, variability, visualization, and volume of data.

Volume: Big data is offered in another format: since many companies produce a high volume of data internally or assemble other vast volumes of data on the external side, they are now infused with data, and large is the most well-known attribute. The amplitude of the data is referred to as volume.

Velocity: This is typically time-sensitive, referring to the rate at which data is created as well as the rate at which it must be analyzed and utilized. The growing usage of digital devices such as cell phones and sensors has led to an unprecedented amount of data production, necessitating real-time analysis and a results-based data mining strategy.

Variety: Variety refers to the heterogeneity of data formats, as technological advancements allow for the use of numerous forms of structured, semistructured, and unstructured data from both internal and external sources, such as sensor data and social media. You can use big data to combine organized and unstructured data of various types, including text, audio, video, clickstream, log files, and more. They do, however, occasionally have to work around the structural arrangements that the machines demand for analysis.

Veracity: If the data set being analyzed is inadequate and erroneous, it is practically useless. This might occur as a result of the collection of data sets from numerous sources in varied forms, as well as noise and mistakes. Cleaning up this noisy data, rather than analyzing it, might take a long time.

Value: Big data analytics has a lot of potential utility. Big data analytics has reduced costs in applications such as the US healthcare system by 12%–17%. Big data not only enables new and successful marketing tactics, but also new products to meet previously unmet market demands. Many sectors utilize big data to save money for their businesses and their clients.

Variability: The term "variability" refers to a data collection whose meaning and interpretation vary on a regular basis. Depending on the situation, these adjustments take place. This is especially true in the case of natural language processing. A single word can have a variety of meanings. New meanings may emerge in the future to replace the previous ones. Being able to interpret them is crucial in applications such as social media analytics. As a result, big data's inexhaustible variety provides a unique challenge for data scientists.

Visualization: The data collection should be given in a legible way once it has been processed. Many factors and variables may be included in a visualization that cannot be represented using standard graphical formats or spreadsheets. Even three-dimensional visualizations may not be of assistance. As a result, visualization has emerged as a new big data analytics issue. AT&T has unveiled a new visualization package dubbed nanocubes.

Fig. 9.2 depicts the 7Vs of big data.

Big data is a concept that defines the massive amounts of organized and unstructured data that a company is bombarded with on a regular basis. It isn't, however, about the volume of big data. What matters is what organizations and enterprises do with the data. It may be analyzed for insights that lead to improved business choices and strategic movements.

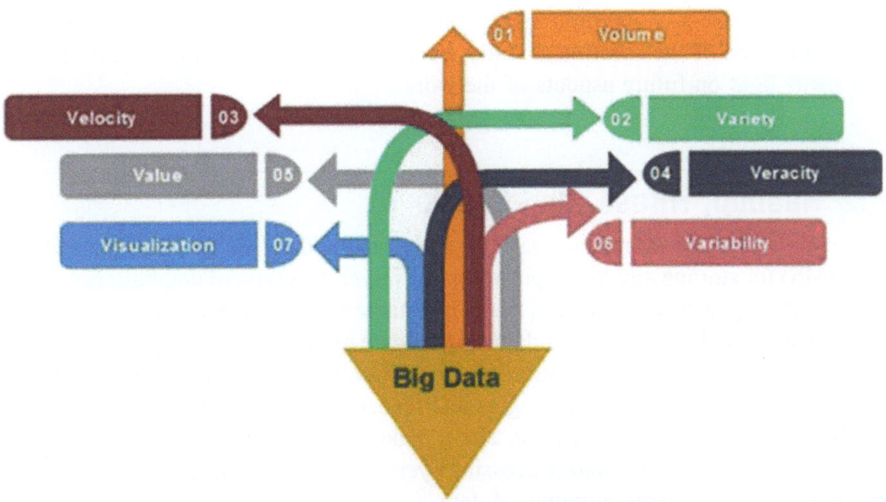

FIGURE 9.2

The 7V's of big data.

In this context, e-health or healthcare 4.0 (Aceto et al., 2020) is a complex field involving multiple markets and players, as well as multiple application areas, all of which are subject to regulations that are more or less adapted to today's reality, especially as new connected devices emerge, allowing patients to take real-time control of their own health. Modern information and communication technologies are at the heart of our healthcare system's progress, allowing information to flow freely between the many actors.

Big data and the IoMT open up new avenues for efficiency gains in research, prevention, illness knowledge, and medical efficacy. The analysis of the obtained data allows for contextualization, and cross-referencing aids in the construction of a more realistic image of the topic under consideration.

The progress of these new technologies, such as HBase as a column-oriented database management system and Spark in the Hadoop ecosystem, now allows for the processing of increasingly large volumes of data in real time with high speed through the use of in-memory and distributed parallel computing methods.

In this chapter, we present our complete E-Health Big Data Architecture (E-HBDA), which provides capabilities to collect, store, and analyze IoMT-generated data in relational or NoSQL format with HBase via a transformation framework. The latter stores this data in a Hadoop ecosystem while using the Spark Framework to analyze streaming IoMT sensor data.

This Section 9.4 is structured as follows: We briefly describe each pillar of our contribution, starting with the Hadoop framework, HBase, and finally Spark. In the second section, we present related work in the field of e-health with massive data. Section 9.2 proposes our E-HBDA model to load the raw data from e-health sensors into the Hadoop system using the HBase column-oriented database management system, then process the raw data with Spark so that it can be analyzed, and provides the details of its implementation. Section 9.8 discusses and interprets the implementation of the solution. Finally, Section 9.9 concludes the current research and sheds light on future aspects of the work.

9.2 Hadoop, HBase, and Spark

For many years, companies mainly stored their data in relational databases (RDBMS) for storage and query purposes. However, this type of database is not suitable for storing unstructured data, nor is it suitable for the large volumes of big data.

Actually, the digitalization and the appearance of many technologies such as IoT, IoMT, and smartphones have caused an explosion in the volume of raw data. Faced with this revolution, new technologies are needed for data storage and processing.

The Hadoop framework (Taylor, 2010) makes it possible to meet these new constraints. It is a file storage and processing system adapted to big data since it allows the management of large amounts of data.

Hadoop is an open-source framework based on Java. Hadoop supports the processing of large amounts of data in distributed computing environments. Hadoop is an integral part of the Apache project. It allows applications to be run on clustered systems with thousands of nodes, involving hundreds of terabytes of data.

Its distributed file system, HDFS (Borthakur, 2008), promotes a high rate of data transfer between nodes and allows uninterrupted operation of the system in the event of a node failure. This approach reduces the risk of a major failure, even when a large number of nodes become inoperative.

Hadoop is inspired by Google MapReduce, a software model that breaks an application into many small components. Each of these components (called a fragment or block) can run on any node in the cluster.

The Apache Hadoop ecosystem Fig. 9.3 consists of the Hadoop kernel, MapReduce, the Hadoop Distributed File System (HDFS), and a number of related projects, including Hbase, which is a nonrelational database (NoSQL), based on the concept and functionality of Google Big Table. The difference is that HBase is open source. This database generally runs on the HDFS. It provides real-time, random and consistent read and write access to tables containing billions of rows and millions of columns.

It also allows data sources based on different structures and schemas to be combined. It is therefore a very good choice for multi-structured data storage. It is also possible to perform queries for a specific time frame, which makes it possible to perform data retrieval queries. HBase is natively integrated with Hadoop and works with other data access engines through YARN. Its programming language is Java.

Apache HBase (George, 2011; Li, 2010; White, 2012) Fig. 9.4 includes all the features of Google Big Table. These include Bloom filters, in-memory operations, and compression. The tables in this database can be used as input for MapReduce tasks in the Hadoop ecosystem, and can also be used as output after processing the data with MapReduce or Spark.

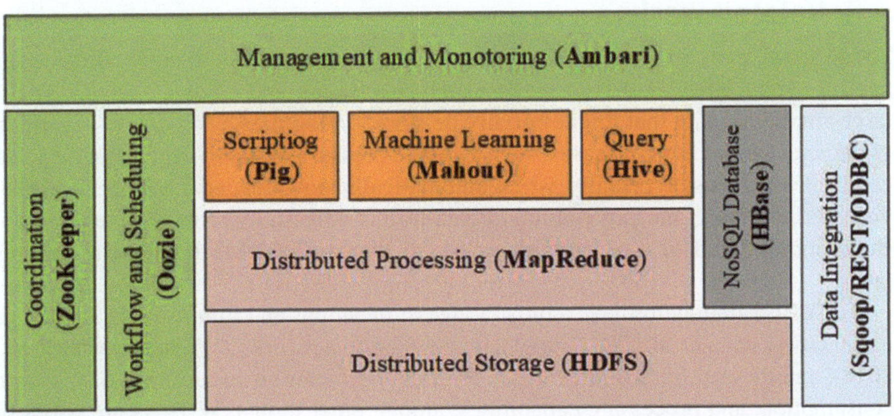

FIGURE 9.3

Hadoop ecosystem.

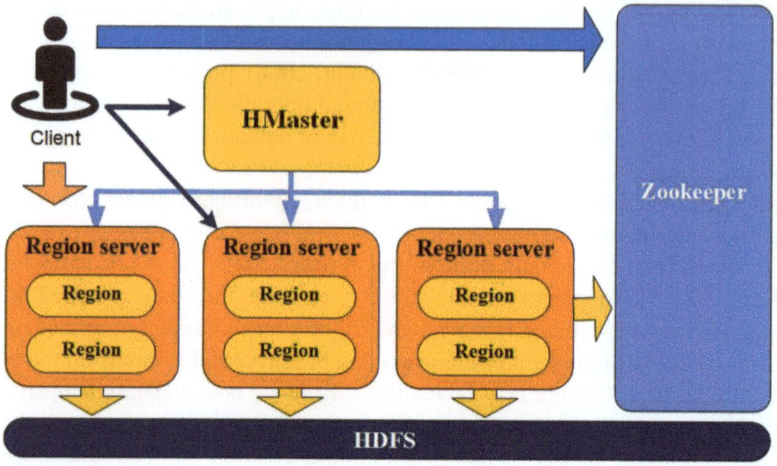

FIGURE 9.4

HBase architecture.

The last one is a unified and ultrafast analysis engine for large-scale data processing. It allows for large-scale analysis through cluster machines. It is mainly dedicated to big data. Spark is a framework (Gupta et al., 2003) Fig. 9.5 that allows working on data in a distributed way. It is one of the main processing solutions in the Hadoop ecosystem. By linking Spark to Hadoop, it becomes possible to distribute the data workload over multiple servers for storage and processing. This configuration is very popular for the analysis of large volumes of data.

9.3 Related works

Today, users, patients, and healthcare professionals upload data to applications such as PHRs and EMRs. There is a need to analyze, cleanse, and reconcile an extremely large amount of data that might initially be stored in log files. Medical observations of patients with chronic diseases, such as blood pressure or blood sugar, can be good candidates for this, especially when automatically downloaded from medical devices. Furthermore, the aggregation of data from a potentially large number of sources is more suited to a processing paradigm than to RDBMS-based data mining tasks.

IoT compatible items have a broad range of meanings and implications, including RFID (Ilie-Zudor et al., 2011) and wireless sensor networks (WSNs; Rawat et al., 2014), and they all have to meet a set of strict specifications in terms of size, power consumption, and processing capabilities, among other things. WBANs are wireless devices that are connected to or implanted in the human body (Cao et al., 2009; Chen et al., 2011). They are of special importance in healthcare.

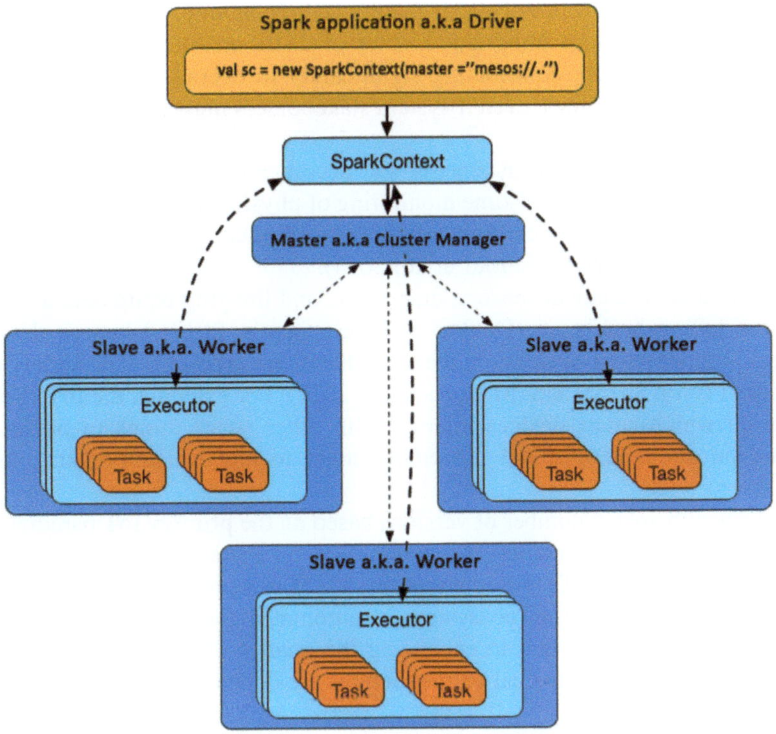

FIGURE 9.5

Spark architecture.

Because of this complicated and varied situation, IoT-related subjects are frequently addressed in terms of logical levels (Trappey et al., 2017), starting with the perception layer and progressing to the transmission layer, calculation layer, and ultimately the application layer. The transmission layer and related communication protocols have received the most attention in IoT research.

Despite the fact that designing and implementing a low-power, highly dependable, and internet-enabled communication stack is a widely acknowledged necessity, the concept of IoT is still a little hazy in some areas. For a more extensive discussion of standards, difficulties, and possibilities, see (Palattella et al., 2013; Sheng et al., 2013).

When applied to industry, the last vision of IoT essentially coincides with industry 4.0. This may be considered a step beyond IoT, either by including reference designs with logistics and manufacturing details (Weyrich & Ebert, 2016) or, on the other hand, by incorporating IoT technology into existing automated processes, resulting in a slew of new opportunities and difficulties (Shrouf et al., 2014).

One of the most appealing sectors for IoT use has been shown to be healthcare (Botta et al., 2016; Islam et al., 2015). The success of this paradigm is reshaping modern healthcare with promising technological, economic, and social prospects: IoT is arguably the most important enabler of distributed healthcare applications (Couturier et al., 2012), contributing significantly to overall cost reduction while improving health outcomes, even if system stakeholders must change their behavior (Osmani et al., 2008).

Wireless technology advancements and accompanying performance improvements considerably assist real-time monitoring of physiological indicators, allowing for continuous treatment of chronic diseases as well as early identification and management of medical crises (Shrouf et al., 2014).

In this context, medical sensors, diagnostic, and imaging equipment are critical for using IoT in healthcare (Doukas & Maglogiannis, 2012; Islam et al., 2015). General-purpose smart devices, on the other hand, are used in a wide variety of applications (Terry, 2016), and (Marques et al., 2017). For example, the IoT offers situations in which smart devices interact with other smart things to obtain fresh information about people and the environment to aid decision-making (Santos et al., 2016).

In the health area, a number of versions based on the primary IoT paradigm have been developed, each with its own unique set of characteristics. The Wearable Internet of Things (WIoT) (Hiremath et al., 2015) is a project that attempts to use telemedicine to establish an ecosystem of automated treatments. WIoT provides monitoring of data important to enhancing the quality of people's everyday lives and linking patients to medical infrastructures by depending on sensors worn on the body.

The Internet of Health Things (IoHT) makes use of professional-grade, always-on, context-aware sensor medical equipment, as well as mobile applications, wearables, and other connected devices (Terry, 2016). Alan Hong et al. (n.d.) describe an application of the Cloudera Distribution Hadoop (CDH)-based big data ecosystem, concentrating on the technical architecture of the CDH-based big data ecosystem and analyzing the system's hierarchical structure.

More research is being done on huge data analysis using Apache Hive (Konagala, 2022, pp. 979–992) in the Hadoop environment, as well as in the context of smart health and smart city applications (Renugadevi et al., 2021). We refer to Hu et al. (2014) for a full technological examination of the emergence of big data. Big data and related concepts are directly involved in a variety of ways in industry 4.0 in general and healthcare 4.0 applications in particular. To realize the full usefulness of big data as applied to healthcare 4.0, it is critical to be aware of the large diversity of data sources accessible.

Online social network data (Aggarwal, 2011, pp. 1–15) is the most conventional source of big data, and it has traditionally pushed big data applications and the development of the requisite technologies. Data from online social networks is the most conventional source of big data, which has traditionally pushed big data applications and the development of the requisite technologies. Originally meant for targeted advertising and market analysis, this data is now being utilized more directly in the context of industry 4.0 to automatically change the value chain.

In some ways, industry 4.0 may be viewed as an effort to encourage such fast feedback from data collected in the field during the design-production-delivery cycle. In terms of the health industry specifically, social networking is transforming the way health professionals evaluate medical records and distribute medical information. Social media and associated technologies are drastically transforming the practice of medicine (Waxer et al., 2013), thanks to increased access to digital sites that provide more relevant information.

Corporate data is another form of big data that is already existing and growing in relevance in industry 4.0. Companies already generate and handle significant amounts of data. In addition to internal accounting, personnel data, and internal communications, there are also regulatory data retention obligations.

This also applies to healthcare facilities, where this sort of data, even if it is not primarily and strictly tied to the healthcare profession, adds to the list of available sources, allowing research that is not simply focused on biological and medical elements to be carried out.

Due to the emphasis on comprehensive exploitation of the data stream, augmented by additional data sources and metadata on the process itself, this trend is projected to intensify in industry 4.0. External data from items sold, consumers, and suppliers/partners will be combined with this data, necessitating the use and advancement of big data technology (Santoso & Yulia, 2017).

The growth in data is attributed to technological advancements. Indeed, because of the quick and considerable market penetration of personal devices, developments in wireless sensors, and mobile communication technologies, workflow systems monitor the health status of individuals in real time, creating vast volumes of organized and unstructured data (Ullah et al., 2012).

Furthermore, clinical information on patients is collected through records that can take different forms and names as a result of medical tests, pictures, and physicians' descriptions (Simon et al., 2007; Smolij & Dun, 2006). Electronic health records, electronic medical records (Akanbi et al., 2012), and personal health records (Archer et al., 2011; Caligtan & Dykes, 2011) are the most common. While electronic health records are designed to track episodes of treatment across various care providers, electronic medical records are real-time patient health records with access to evidence-based decision support systems that can help physicians make better decisions.

Patients often handle personal health records, which are universally comprehensible instruments used throughout life to manage pertinent health information, encourage health maintenance, and aid in the treatment of chronic conditions. Furthermore, scientific literature continues to be an important source of biomedical information (Martin-Sanchez & Verspoor, 2014). It necessitates specific web-based text mining tools for indexing and cataloging, allowing users to search for and retrieve relevant articles rapidly and effectively.

Finally, as the cost of data capture and analysis reduces with technological advancements, enormous volumes of biological data in various formats are currently being created and gathered at an unprecedented speed and scale (Chen & Snyder, 2013). This data may be divided into four categories (Herland et al., 2014).

9.4 The proposed model

9.4.1 CRISP-DM methodology

We present our complete E-HBDA (Fig. 9.7), which allows us to gather, store, and analyze data generated by the medical Internet of Things in relational and NoSQL format using Hbase via a transformation framework.

This data is then stored in a Hadoop ecosystem, with IoMT sensor data being analyzed using the Spark Framework.

We used the CRISP-DM approach (Wirth & Hipp, 2000) to do this. It was created with the intention of serving the demands of industrial data mining operations. CRISP-DM is defined as a hierarchical process with four levels of abstraction: phase, generic task, specialized task, and process instance.

CRISP-DM quickly became the most extensively utilized method for developing data mining projects following its introduction. CRISP-DM (Oprean, 2010) stands for "CRoss-industry Standard for Data Mining" and is divided into six steps, as indicated in Fig. 9.6:

1. **Business understanding:** This first phase is all about figuring out what the project's goals and requirements are. The knowledge gathered will be used to outline the problem as well as a preliminary plan for achieving these goals.
2. **Data understanding:** This starts with data gathering and progresses to actions like as familiarizing oneself with the data, identifying data quality concerns, detecting subsets, and developing hypotheses about hidden information.
3. **Data preparation:** This phase includes all of the tasks required to construct the final database.
4. **Modeling**: Several approaches are chosen and applied to the data during this phase, and their parameters are calibrated with ideal values. Because there are so many different types of data creation, it's usually essential to go back one step.
5. **Evaluation (Assessment):** From this stage, the model(s) is/are examined, as well as the procedures used to develop the model, to verify that the project satisfies the business objectives set out at the outset.
6. **Deployment:** The model's construction does not signify the project's completion. Even if the project's primary purpose is to expand data understanding, the information gathered must be organized and presented in a way that the customer can understand.

Even if the project's primary purpose is to expand data understanding, the information gathered must be organized and presented in a way that the customer can understand.

Our proposal will focus on the four main phases of this methodology, as described in the implementation section. Fig. 9.6 shows the overall structure of the framework. The architecture consists of three main blocks, namely the medical Internet of Things data, storage, and analysis.

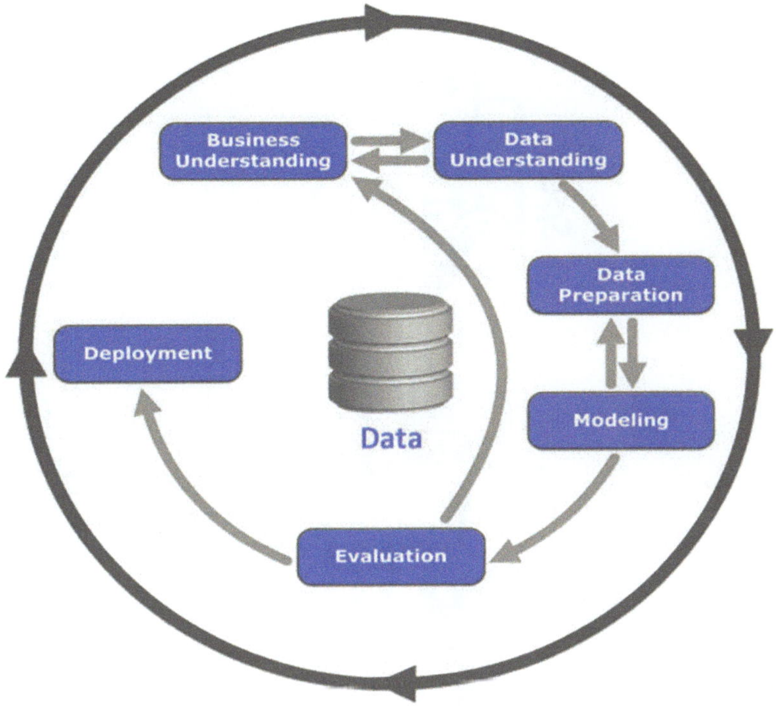

FIGURE 9.6

The CRISP-DM life cycle.

Spark is the big data processing method, and HBase is the storage method.

In our model Fig. 9.7, we will integrate the patient data collected by the IoMT into a relational database, and through our transformation framework (Khourdifi et al., 2018), we will migrate this data to the column-oriented database management system or a large table, which in our case is HBase. The HBase database based on Hadoop works with Spark in-memory to process the data collected from the sensors to produce a decision. The significant advantage of our model is the saving of insertion time and the processing of the data with Spark at high speed.

9.5 IoMT big data integration

This stage entails combining and translating the information into a format that may be used for further analysis. Big health data, on the other hand, is very huge, scattered, unstructured, and diverse, making integration and transformation in a relational database much more difficult. The database administrator faces a significant problem when it comes to integrating unstructured data (DBA) (El Alami & Bahaj, 2017).

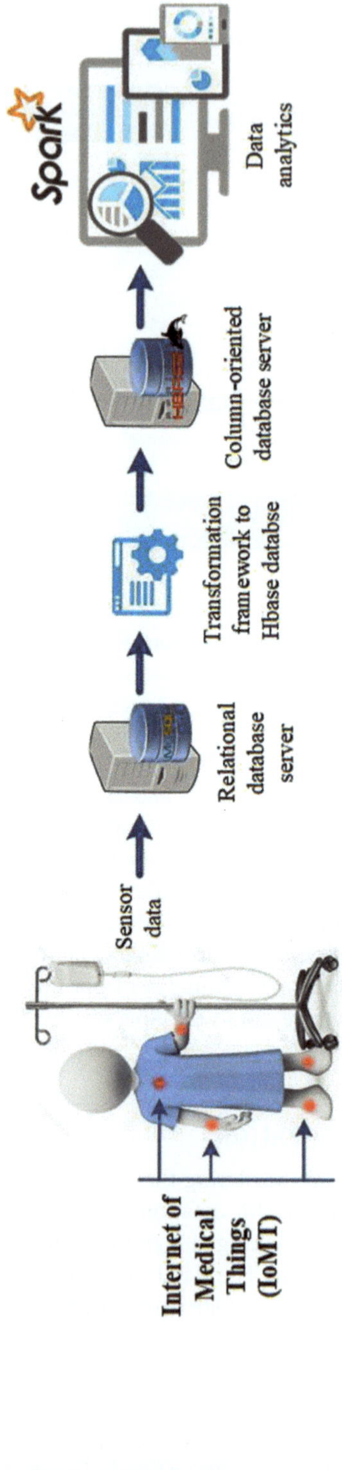

FIGURE 9.7

E-health big data architecture (E-HBDA).

In this part, we create an integration platform that can link and coordinate a range of applications in big companies with transactional integrity using web services, data transformation, and intelligent indexing. Adding additional apps or capabilities to the entire system is safer with data service integration.

In addition, each application's connection becomes more frictionless. Many researchers have utilized a relational database as an input database (El Alami & Bahaj, 2014), then loaded the data onto the Hadoop cluster using Sqoop (Ting & Cecho, 2013) or another tool (El Alami et al., 2018), or straight into HBase using integration scripts (Khourdifi & Bahaj, 2017).

In our model, we use an Internet Web Application Protocol called CoAP (Constrained Application Protocol) (Bormann et al., 2012) to integrate the data collected by the sensors into a relational database, and then we use our Transformation Framework to migrate the collected data into an HBase database via the Hadoop cluster.

9.6 IoMT big data storage

Big data storage is difficult to perform efficiently, and it has been a topic of debate in recent years. Given the properties of big data, such as volume, speed, variety, value, and complexity, a broad range of storage methods are available to accommodate it. The distributed file system is the most common and well-established approach.

In this work, we use HBase from HDFS to store IoMT big data (Vora, 2011). HBase is an open-source Apache project with a simplified and highly scalable column-based database without an HDFS database (Skeirik et al., 2013). Like the HDFS and MapReduce architectures, HBase also adopts the master-slave architecture. HBase consists of a master and a series of workers, commonly called local servers, and a zookeeper, used to create distributed applications. Zookeeper (Junqueira & Reed, 2013) is a high-performance configuration management service that supports distributed applications over the Internet. The master uses the node to give the available servers (Zhang et al., 2013). The HBase storage classes are initially assigned by the master to a region server. When the region exceeds its normal size, it is split into two parts, and the rows are distributed among the new region servers for additional data storage.

In the first step, we stored the data collected from the IoMTs in a relational database and then used our transformation framework Fig. 9.8 (Khourdifi et al., 2018) from a relational database to a column-oriented Hbase database.

9.7 Big data analysis in IoMT

Apache Spark is a distributed cluster computing tool (Salloum et al., 2016; Zaharia et al., 2016). Spark employs an in-memory computing engine instead of Hadoop's two-stage MapReduce computation engine. Spark usually has higher performance than Hadoop's disk-based storage since it is in-memory.

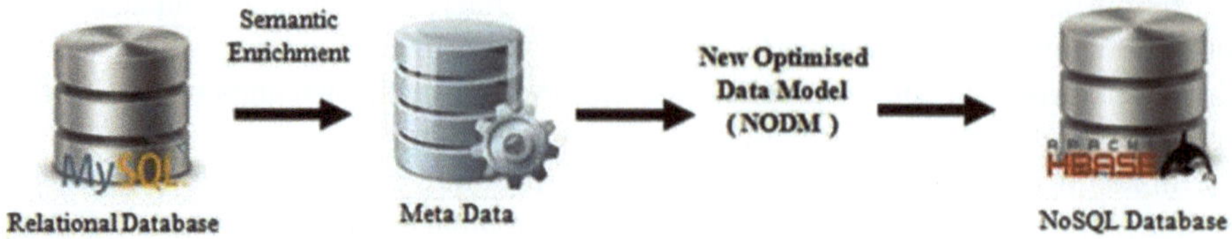

FIGURE 9.8

Framework for transformation processes.

The architecture of Spark is master-slave Fig. 9.5. The master or cluster manager is communicated with via a driver. The executors running on multiple worker/slave processes interact with the cluster management.

The architecture of Spark is seen in Fig. 9.5. The cluster manager and the driver application negotiate system resources. The executing agents on the worker nodes are then started by the cluster management. The executors are the widely scattered individuals who are in charge of completing assignments. In the form of resilient distributed data sets, data pieces are kept in memory by worker processes.

Actions and transformations are two types of operations supported by resilient distributed data sets in Spark. A directed acyclic graph is used to describe these operations, with each node representing a division of resilient distributed data sets. The two-stage paradigm of Hadoop MapReduce is eliminated when the sequence of operations is represented as a directed acyclic graph, resulting in increased performance over Hadoop.

9.8 Discussions

In the field of information and business technology, the management of vast and heterogeneous data in the IoMT is a fairly new issue, and the study findings need to be demystified.

Several parts of the IoMT have been investigated, as stated in the preceding section on research. Nonetheless, there are two major concerns concerning the IoMT that need to be investigated further (1). A typical IoMT system's interference consists of a few light and tiny sensors, each of which monitors one or more physiological or physical sensors.

When the IoMT is used in a crowded network setting like a school, hospital, or retail mall, when these are near each other, they can cause interference (Skeirik et al., 2013). The inference will reduce the system's performance, resulting in quick burnout. Furthermore, interference becomes more problematic when the IoMT runs in a congested network environment.

As a result, it's critical to address the interference issue in order to keep the IoMT running smoothly in the face of massive data issues (2). Although HDFS satisfies the need for IoMT large data, storage shortages still exist. According to a study on massive data storage, there are difficulties such as the tiny file problem and the load balancing method (Zhang & Xu, 2013), which take longer to fix. For our concept, we concentrated on utilizing modern database management technologies, notably NoSQL and, more precisely, Hadoop, which is a suite of tools dedicated to the storage and analysis of massive amounts of unstructured data.

Hadoop clusters' key benefit is their capacity to store enormous amounts of data. Big data is largely unstructured and dispersed. Because of the way the Hadoop framework works, which slices data into pieces and assigns each of these parts to a node for analysis, it's ideal for analyzing this sort of data.

The data does not have to be homogeneous since each piece of data is processed by a distinct process on a different node in the cluster. Hadoop clusters also have the benefit of scalability. One of the issues with big data analysis, like with any form of data, is that it is always growing. Furthermore, real-time analysis of big data is more beneficial.

Hadoop's parallel processing capabilities can speed up analysis, but as the amount of data to be analyzed grows, the cluster's processing capacity may become inadequate. Fortunately, the framework can scale with the addition of nodes. The expense of this form of architecture is a third benefit. This remark could surprise you: big data analysis is a type of corporate computing that has hitherto been prohibitively expensive.

Hadoop clusters, on the other hand, might be a cost-effective option. This is due to two factors. To begin with, the software necessary is free and open source. The Apache Hadoop software can even be downloaded for free.

Second, by using common hardware, a Hadoop project's expenses may be kept low. You don't need to spend a bunch on servers to develop a robust cluster. Another benefit of these clusters is their failure resilience.

When data is given to a node for analysis, it is replicated to other nodes as well, allowing the data to be copied and analyzed even if one node fails. Given the impossibility of obtaining a real database containing data generated by the IoT, we proceeded to build our own database by simulating the number of data points generated by the sensor network using the network simulator (NS2) tool (Issariyakul & Hossain, 2008, pp. 1—18), estimating the amount of data for a given period, inserting the generated data into a relational database, applying our HBase transformation framework using a bulk insert script, and finally analyzing the data with the Splunk tool.

9.9 Conclusion and future works

In this chapter, we first present the components of big data and then combine IoMT with big data to form the IoMT big data model. Then, taking into consideration the unique properties of the IoMT, we suggest a core processing architecture for handling massive data.

The E-HBDA is a comprehensive architecture that enables the IoMT to gather, store, and analyze data in relational and NoSQL formats using HBase and a transformation framework. The data is then stored in a Hadoop environment, and the Spark Framework is used to analyze streaming IoMT sensor data.

Spark and HBase are used to process and store large IoMT data sets, respectively. Spark's parallel structure achieves the objective of obtaining meaningful and valuable information from enormous amounts of data quickly.

The real-time data we obtain is useful for illness prediction and has a wide range of applications in health care. This massive data was used with machine learning or deep learning approaches to predict illness in the following research.

References

Aceto, G., Persico, V., & Pescapé, A. (2020). Industry 4.0 and health: Internet of Things, big data, and cloud computing for healthcare 4.0. *Journal of Industrial Information Integration, 18*, 100129. https://doi.org/10.1016/j.jii.2020.100129

Aggarwal, C. C. (2011). *An introduction to social network data analytics*. Springer Science and Business Media LLC. https://doi.org/10.1007/978-1-4419-8462-3_1

Akanbi, M. O., Ocheke, Amaka, N., Agaba, P. A., et al. (2012). Use of electronic health records in sub-Saharan Africa: Progress and challenges. *Journal of Medicine in the Tropics, 14*.

Archer, N., Fevrier-Thomas, U., Lokker, C., McKibbon, K. A., & Straus, S. E. (2011). Personal health records: A scoping review. *Journal of the American Medical Informatics Association, 18*(4), 515–522. https://doi.org/10.1136/amiajnl-2011-000105

Auffray, C., Balling, R., Barroso, I., Bencze, L., Benson, M., Bergeron, J., Bernal-Delgado, E., Blomberg, N., Bock, C., Conesa, A., Del Signore, S., Delogne, C., Devilee, P., Di Meglio, A., Eijkemans, M., Flicek, P., Graf, N., Grimm, V., Guchelaar, H. J., … Zanetti, G. (2016). Making sense of big data in health research: Towards an EU action plan. *Genome Medicine, 8*(1). https://doi.org/10.1186/s13073-016-0323-y

Bormann, C., Castellani, A. P., & Shelby, Z. (2012). CoAP: An application protocol for billions of tiny internet nodes. *IEEE Internet Computing, 16*(2), 62–67. https://doi.org/10.1109/MIC.2012.29

Borthakur, D. (2008). HDFS architecture guide. In *Hadoop Apache project* (Vol. 53).

Botta, A., De Donato, W., Persico, V., & Pescapé, A. (2016). Integration of cloud computing and Internet of Things: A survey. *Future Generation Computer Systems, 56*, 684–700. https://doi.org/10.1016/j.future.2015.09.021

Caligtan, C. A., & Dykes, P. C. (2011). Electronic health records and personal health records. *Seminars in Oncology Nursing, 27*(3), 218–228. https://doi.org/10.1016/j.soncn.2011.04.007

Cao, H., Leung, V., Chow, C., & Chan, H. (2009). Enabling technologies for wireless body area networks: A survey and outlook. *IEEE Communications Magazine, 47*(12), 84–93. https://doi.org/10.1109/MCOM.2009.5350373

Chen, M., Gonzalez, S., Vasilakos, A., Cao, H., & Leung, V. C. M. (2011). Body area networks: A survey. *Mobile Networks and Applications, 16*(2), 171–193. https://doi.org/10.1007/s11036-010-0260-8

Chen, R., & Snyder, M. (2013). Promise of personalized omics to precision medicine. *Wiley Interdisciplinary Reviews: Systems Biology and Medicine, 5*(1), 73–82. https://doi.org/10.1002/wsbm.1198

Couturier, J., Sola, D., Borioli, G., & Raiciu, C. (2012). How can the Internet of Things help to overcome current healthcare challenges. *Communications & Strategies*, 67–81.

Dash, S., Shakyawar, S. K., Sharma, M., & Kaushik, S. (2019). Big data in healthcare: Management, analysis and future prospects. *Journal of Big Data, 6*(1). https://doi.org/10.1186/s40537-019-0217-0

Doukas, C., & Maglogiannis, I. (2012). Bringing IoT and cloud computing towards pervasive healthcare. In *Proceedings – 6th international conference on innovative mobile and internet services in ubiquitous computing, IMIS 2012* (pp. 922–926). https://doi.org/10.1109/IMIS.2012.26

El Alami, A., & Bahaj, M. (2014). Migration of the relational data base (RDB) to the object relational data base (ORDB). *International Journal of Computer, Electrical, Automation, Control and In-Formation Engineering, 8*, 242–248.

El Alami, A., & Bahaj, M. (2017). Migration of a relational databases to NoSQL: The way forward. In *International conference on multimedia computing and systems –proceedings* (Vol. 0, pp. 18–23). IEEE Computer Society. https://doi.org/10.1109/ICMCS.2016.7905665

El Alami, A., Bahaj, M., & Khourdifi, Y. (2018). Supply of a key value database Redis in-memory by data from a relational database. In *19th IEEE mediterranean electrotechnical conference (MELECON)*. IEEE.

George, L. (2011). *HBase: The definitive guide: Random access to your planet-size data.*

Gupta, S., Dutt, N., Gupta, R., & Nicolau, A. (2003). Spark: A high-level synthesis framework for applying parallelizing compiler transformations. In *Proceedings of the IEEE international conference on VLSI design* (Vol. 2003, pp. 461–466). IEEE Computer Society. https://doi.org/10.1109/ICVD.2003.1183177

Herland, M., Khoshgoftaar, T. M., & Wald, R. (2014). A review of data mining using big data in health informatics. *Journal of Big Data, 1*(1). https://doi.org/10.1186/2196-1115-1-2

Hiremath, S., Yang, G., & Mankodiya, K. (2015). Wearable Internet of Things: Concept, architectural components and promises for person-centered healthcare. In *Proceedings of the 2014 4th international conference on wireless mobile communication and healthcare – \transforming healthcare through innovations in mobile and wireless technologies, MOBIHEALTH 2014* (pp. 304–307). Institute of Electrical and Electronics Engineers Inc. https://doi.org/10.1109/MOBIHEALTH.2014.7015971

Hong A. (n.d.). Big data analysis system based on Cloudera distribution hadoop. In: *2021 7th IEEE intl conference on big data security on cloud (BigDataSecurity), IEEE intl conference on high performance and smart computing, (HPSC) and IEEE intl conference on intelligent data and security* (pp. 169–173).

Hu, H., Wen, Y., Chua, T. S., & Li, X. (2014). Toward scalable systems for big data analytics: A technology tutorial. *IEEE Access, 2*, 652–687. https://doi.org/10.1109/ACCESS.2014.2332453

Ilie-Zudor, E., Kemény, Z., Van Blommestein, F., Monostori, L., & Van Der Meulen, A. (2011). A survey of applications and requirements of unique identification systems and RFID techniques. *Computers in Industry, 62*(3), 227–252. https://doi.org/10.1016/j.compind.2010.10.004

Islam, S. M. R., Kwak, D., Kabir, M. H., Hossain, M., & Kwak, K. S. (2015). The Internet of Things for health care: A comprehensive survey. *IEEE Access, 3*, 678–708. https://doi.org/10.1109/ACCESS.2015.2437951

Issariyakul, T., & Hossain, E. (2008). *Introduction to network simulator 2 (NS2)* (pp. 1–18). Springer Science and Business Media LLC. https://doi.org/10.1007/978-0-387-71760-9_2

Junqueira, F., & Reed, B. (2013). *ZooKeeper: Distributed process coordination.*

Katal, A., Wazid, M., & Goudar, R. H. (2013). Big data: Issues, challenges, tools and good practices. In *2013 6th international conference on contemporary computing, IC3 2013* (pp. 404–409). https://doi.org/10.1109/IC3.2013.6612229

Khourdifi, Y., & Bahaj, M. (2017). Hadoop and MapReduce technology as a solution for wireless body area networks in e-health. In *ACM international conference proceeding series.* Association for Computing Machinery. https://doi.org/10.1145/3167486.3167503

Khourdifi, Y., Bahaj, M., & Elalami, A. (2018). A new approach for migration of a relational database into column-oriented nosql database on hadoop. *Journal of Theoretical and Applied Information Technology, 96*(19), 6607. www.jatit.org/volumes/Vol96No19/27Vol96No19.pdf

Konagala, P. (2022). *Big data analytics using apache hive to analyze health data.* IGI Global. https://doi.org/10.4018/978-1-6684-3662-2.ch046

Li, C. (2010). Transforming relational database into HBase: A case study. In *Proceedings 2010 IEEE international conference on software engineering and service Sciences, ICSESS 2010* (pp. 683–687). https://doi.org/10.1109/ICSESS.2010.5552465

Liu, W., & Park, E. K. (2013). E-Healthcare cloud computing application solutions: Cloud-enabling characteristices, challenges and adaptations. In *2013 international conference on computing, networking and communications, ICNC 2013* (pp. 437–443). https://doi.org/10.1109/ICCNC.2013.6504124

Marques, R., Gregório, J., Da Silva, M. M., & Lapão, L. V. (2017). The promise of the Internet of Things in healthcare: How hard is it to keep?. In *Studies in health technology and informatics* (Vol. 228, pp. 665–669) IOS Press. https://doi.org/10.3233/978-1-61499-678-1-665

Martin-Sanchez, F., & Verspoor, K. (2014). Big data in medicine is driving big changes. *Yearbook of Medical Informatics, 9*, 14–20. https://doi.org/10.15265/IY-2014-0020

Oprean, C. (2010). *État de l'art sur les aspects méthodologiques et processus en Knowledge Discovery in Databases.*

Osmani, V., Balasubramaniam, S., & Botvich, D. (2008). Human activity recognition in pervasive health-care: Supporting efficient remote collaboration. *Journal of Network and Computer Applications, 31*(4), 628–655. https://doi.org/10.1016/j.jnca.2007.11.002

Palattella, M. R., Accettura, N., Vilajosana, X., Watteyne, T., Grieco, L. A., Boggia, G., & Dohler, M. (2013). Standardized protocol stack for the internet of (important) things. *IEEE Communications Surveys and Tutorials, 15*(3), 1389–1406. https://doi.org/10.1109/SURV.2012.111412.00158

Rawat, P., Singh, K. D., Chaouchi, H., & Bonnin, J. M. (2014). Wireless sensor networks: A survey on recent developments and potential synergies. *Journal of Supercomputing, 68*(1), 1–48. https://doi.org/10.1007/s11227-013-1021-9

Renugadevi, N., Saravanan, S., & Naga Sudha, C. M. (2021). Revolution of smart healthcare materials in big data analytics. *Materials Today: Proceedings.* https://doi.org/10.1016/j.matpr.2021.04.256

Salloum, S., Dautov, R., Chen, X., Peng, P. X., & Huang, J. Z. (2016). Big data analytics on Apache Spark. *International Journal of Data Science and Analytics, 1*(3–4), 145–164. https://doi.org/10.1007/s41060-016-0027-9

Santoso, L. W., & Yulia. (2017). Data warehouse with big data technology for higher education. *Procedia Computer Science, 124*, 93–99. https://doi.org/10.1016/j.procs.2017.12.134

Santos, J., Rodrigues, J. J. P. C., Silva, B. M. C., Casal, J., Saleem, K., & Denisov, V. (2016). An IoT-based mobile gateway for intelligent personal assistants on mobile health environments. *Journal of Network and Computer Applications, 71*, 194–204. https://doi.org/10.1016/j.jnca.2016.03.014

Sheng, Z., Yang, S., Yu, Y., Vasilakos, A., McCann, J., & Leung, K. (2013). A survey on the IETF protocol suite for the Internet of Things: Standards, challenges, and opportunities. *IEEE Wireless Communications, 20*(6), 91–98. https://doi.org/10.1109/MWC.2013.6704479

Shrouf, F., Ordieres, J., & Miragliotta, G. (2014). Smart factories in industry 4.0: A review of the concept and of energy management approached in production based on the Internet of Things paradigm. In *IEEE international conference on industrial engineering and engineering management* (Vol. 2015, pp. 697–701). IEEE Computer Society. https://doi.org/10.1109/IEEM.2014.7058728

Simon, S. R., Kaushal, R., Cleary, P. D., Jenter, C. A., Volk, L. A., Orav, E. J., Burdick, E., Poon, E. G., & Bates, D. W. (2007). Physicians and electronic health records: A statewide survey. *Archives of Internal Medicine, 167*(5), 507–512. https://doi.org/10.1001/archinte.167.5.507

Skeirik, S., Bobba, R. B., & Meseguer, J. (2013). Formal analysis of fault-tolerant group key management using ZooKeeper. In *Proceedings - 13th IEEE/ACM international symposium on cluster, cloud, and grid computing, CCGrid 2013* (pp. 636–641). https://doi.org/10.1109/CCGrid.2013.98

Smolij, K., & Dun, K. (2006). Patient health information management: Searching for the right model. *Perspectives in Health Information Management, 3*.

Taylor, R. C. (2010). An overview of the Hadoop/MapReduce/HBase framework and its current applications in bioinformatics. *BMC Bioinformatics, 11*(12). https://doi.org/10.1186/1471-2105-11-S12-S1

Terry, N. P. (2016). Will the Internet of Things transform healthcare. *Vanderbilt Journal of Entertainment and Technology Law, 19*.

Ting, K., & Cecho, J. J. (2013). *Apache Sqoop cookbook: Unlocking hadoop for your relational database*. O'Reilly Media, Inc.

Trappey, A. J. C., Trappey, C. V., Hareesh Govindarajan, U., Chuang, A. C., & Sun, J. J. (2017). A review of essential standards and patent landscapes for the Internet of Things: A key enabler for industry 4.0. *Advanced Engineering Informatics, 33*, 208–229. https://doi.org/10.1016/j.aei.2016.11.007

Ullah, S., Higgins, H., Braem, B., Latre, B., Blondia, C., Moerman, I., Saleem, S., Rahman, Z., & Kwak, K. S. (2012). A comprehensive survey of wireless body area networks. *Journal of Medical Systems, 36*(3), 1065–1094. https://doi.org/10.1007/s10916-010-9571-3

Vora, M. N. (2011). Hadoop-HBase for large-scale data. In *Proceedings of 2011 international conference on computer science and network technology, ICCSNT 2011* (Vol. 1, pp. 601–605). https://doi.org/10.1109/ICCSNT.2011.6182030

Waxer, N., Ninan, D., Ma, A., & Dominguez, N. (2013). How cloud computing and social media are changing the face of health care. *Physician Executive, 39*(2), 58–62.

Weyrich, M., & Ebert, C. (2016). Reference architectures for the Internet of Things. *IEEE Software, 33*(1), 112–116. https://doi.org/10.1109/MS.2016.20

White, T. (2012). *Hadoop: The definitive guide*.

Wirth, R., & Hipp, J. (2000). CRISP-DM: Towards a standard process model for data mining. In *Proceedings of the 4th international conference on the practical applications of knowledge discovery and data mining* (Vol. 1).

Zaharia, M., Xin, R. S., Wendell, P., Das, T., Armbrust, M., Dave, A., Meng, X., Rosen, J., Venkataraman, S., Franklin, M. J., Ghodsi, A., Gonzalez, J., Shenker, S., & Stoica, I. (2016). Apache spark: A unified engine for big data processing. *Communications of the ACM, 59*(11), 56–65. https://doi.org/10.1145/2934664

Zhang, Z., Wang, H., Wang, C., & Fang, H. (2013). Interference mitigation for cyber-physical wireless body area network system using social networks. *IEEE Transactions on Emerging Topics in Computing, 1*(1), 121–132. https://doi.org/10.1109/TETC.2013.2274430

Zhang, X., & Xu, F. (2013). Survey of research on big data storage. In *Proceedings – 12th international symposium on distributed computing and applications to business, engineering and science, DCABES 2013* (pp. 76–80). IEEE Computer Society. https://doi.org/10.1109/DCABES.2013.21

CHAPTER

Application of computational intelligence in visual optimization tools to improve the performance of medical MIoT platforms

10

Siham Beloualid, Ilham Morino, Abdelhadi El Allali, Salma Ait Oussous, Anass Barodi, Abderrahim Bajit

Laboratory of Advanced Systems Engineering (ISA), National School of Applied Sciences, Ibn Tofail University, Kenitra, Morocco

10.1 Introduction

During the COVID-19 pandemic, several solutions have been proposed to limit the spread of the virus: artificial intelligence (AI) data analysis systems to control the flow in companies, controlled disinfection robots to maintain the hygiene of closed spaces (Nosirov et al., 2020; Shi et al., 2021), connected hydro alcoholic gel distribution systems (Objenious, 2020), and real-time tracking applications (Sun et al., 2021).

Access control to private or public spaces reduces contamination from COVID-19 and ensures health prevention for vulnerable people. Priority entry to these areas is reserved for those vaccinated with a current sanitary pass, for those for whom vaccination is contraindicated, and for those who have a negative PCR test less than 48 h old.

Each person vaccinated against COVID-19 has a unique numerical identifier that attests to the availability of a complete vaccination schedule. The fraudulent use of QR codes and fake passes presents a backdoor solution that many nonvaccinated individuals use to gain access to poorly controlled locations. Multiple websites and cybercriminals also offer stolen or fake sanitary passes at affordable prices; fraudsters manage to obtain a real QR code illegally, entitling the pretenders to the same privileges as a vaccinated person. The state curbs this type of unaccountable act with penalties ranging from huge fines to years in prison. This is the reason why many cases of contamination appear despite the country's efforts to limit this virus.

The difficulty of controlling access to a space is a challenge in the face of large numbers of people seeking access, such as entrances to stadiums, cinemas,

Computational Intelligence for Medical Internet of Things (MIoT) Applications
https://doi.org/10.1016/B978-0-323-99421-7.00004-0

conferences with many guests, or even in public transport. This difficulty is exacerbated during peak hours when many people try to enter at the same time, just minutes before the event starts. Data management is more complicated in terms of control time and the quality of information sent to the processing service (Baddi et al., 2022; Ghosh et al., 2021). IoT developments to control the propagation of the COVID-19 virus were considered early on, such as this system (Bindu et al., 2021) proposing to control access to a construction site. A similar strategy (Qin & Zhang, 2021) uses a RFID reader system to control the movement of schoolchildren on the bus, which generates an authenticated authorization of the child.

During access control, the person is asked to present his or her QR code, which requires verification of the code's validity and identification of its bearer. This requires real-time facial recognition, fast sending, processing of the image, and optimization of the quality and size of the data.

To authorize access to the QR code presentation at the reception, a double verification is needed to confirm the identity of the person and fight against any fraud or false document. This can be done through an IoT node that must send the recognized image of the person for a real-time identity check while managing the huge flow behind it. Our work consists in using two types of image coding: visual coding (Liu & Wang, 2008) for the scanned QR codes, and foveal coding (Wang & Bovik, 2001) for the images of people at the entries received from the cameras.

This paper is organized as follows: The MIoT platform architecture based on CoAP protocol, ECC encryption, and mesh topology is presented inSection 10.2. In Section 10.3, we study psychovisual and foveal image coding and evaluate the quality and runtime of this type of coding. These encoded/decoded and encrypted images are processed by AI to detect and recognize the face of the person, in Section 10.4, which will be sent to a decision system for processing and final action. Section 10.5 presents all the comparative results between the different types of image encoding/decoding and their performance in terms of quality and execution time.

10.2 MIoT platform access control

Due to the obvious COVID-19 epidemic, an infectious condition caused by this virus spreads when tiny liquid particles are released through the mouth or nose when an infected person coughs, sings, or breathes. Several questions have been raised concerning the steps that need to be taken to eradicate it and stop it from spreading, such as what health measures are required in addition to the vaccine and medications that researchers are looking for.

For this, we have proposed our solution, which is an intelligent, secure, and synchronized MIoT health platform to ensure health prevention for frail, elderly, or immunocompromised people. This platform, as shown in Fig. 10.1 allows managing access to public or private spaces. Access to these places requires the respect of several conditions.

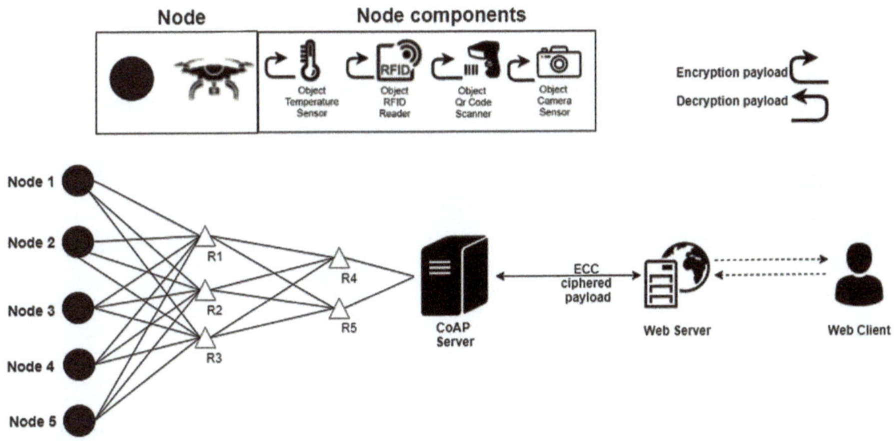

FIGURE 10.1

Intelligent control access platform MIoT architecture.

At the entrance of the space, there is an RFID node for data identification and a temperature node to monitor the temperature of the citizen. A camera sensor to detect faces and a QR code scanner to read QR bars. These IoT devices are connected to the internet via the CoAP protocol.

We use the camera sensor for the validation of the QR code of the vaccine and the facial recognition of its property to verify if it is the same person. If the visitor is not vaccinated, we check in a second step his negative PCR test certificate which should not exceed 48 h, then we proceed to facial recognition. If the visitor has neither his vaccine nor his PCR test, we check if he is already registered by his RFID (UID) in the database, and if so, we proceed to facial recognition. Access is then denied in the negative case of these tests.

To avoid that, the system blocks during the processing of the sending or the citizens take a long queue, we used the visual coding for the QR code and the foveal coding for the images of the citizens as shown in Fig. 10.2. The latter is used to compress the size of the image, which facilitates its sending and receiving in a favorable time compared to sending normal images with low bandwidth and keeping good quality.

Then, to guarantee confidentiality, integrity, and data availability during the sending and receiving, we have implemented the ECC security algorithm.

At the entry of the controlled place, our system has to check both the validity of the QR code and the identity of its holder through facial recognition to avoid any fakes. Two types of identification of people have been established. The first one is scanning the QR code of the sanitary pass or the PCR test of fewer than 48 h, and the second one is facial identification to prove the identity of the individual.

Once the picture of the individual is taken, a foveation is applied to get a face picture with a higher resolution. The image and the QR code are then encoded

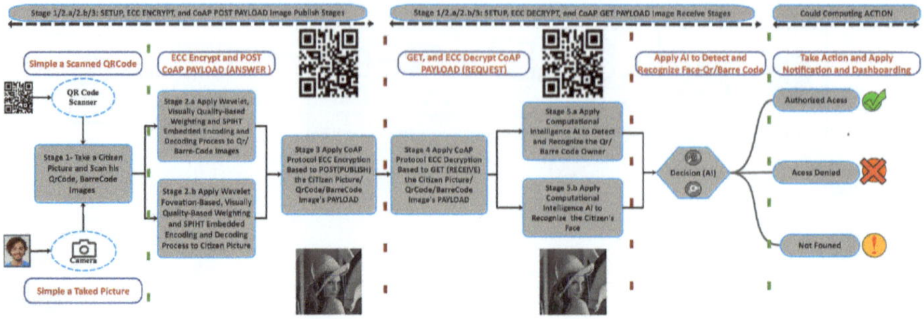

FIGURE 10.2

Artificial intelligence block diagram of platform.

and decoded, encrypted by ECC, and transmitted to the web server using the CoAP protocol. When the server gets the data, decryption is necessary to read the information and compare data with those existing in the database. A decision-making system gives or denies the person access to the area.

10.3 Psychovisual foveal coding and evaluation of the coding quality

The use of the QR code scanner, the RFID reader, and the camera allow obtaining more information about the person wishing to enter the controlled area. After the data acquisition, the transmission of the information is required for a check and verification with the database. For that purpose, an encoding/decoding and a secure image are performed, as shown in Fig. 10.3.

Facial recognition is used to control access to the MIoT platform (Kumar et al., 2020), verifying individual identities. When a human observes in a real field, the human eye focuses on an area surrounding the point of fixation, while collecting data

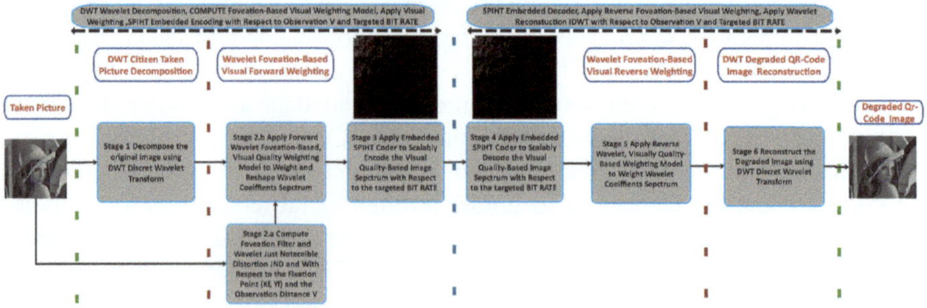

FIGURE 10.3

Foveation based visual encoding/decoding citizen's picture.

from this area with higher accuracy. The image viewed is sampled with the highest density and therefore viewed with the highest constraint sensitivity.

Each image contains a multiplied redundancy of high-frequency information in the peripheral regions, which is why we chose to compress the image using the foveal method. The advantage of this type of visualization is the fast encoding/decoding of a high-resolution image.

The foveal model chosen for this processing is the MEVIC model presented in Bajit et al. (2019), in different steps. The first step consists in removing more redundancies to keep only the most important face information. The second step consists in removing invisible contrasts while elaborating a calculation according to perceptual thresholds. The third step allows having an image with a more compatible resolution. This is done through different calculations that allow matching the resolution of the image and the given rate.

After that, we want to resolve more and more the quality of the resulting image. The application of the contrast sensitivity filter allows the elimination of imperceptible frequencies depending on the spatial frequency. The definition of the three parameters: The JND threshold of the just detectable distortions, the light, and the contrast will serve for the elaboration of an image of good quality, as show in Fig. 10.4.

After the foveally coded psychovisual face image and the QR code are extracted, the data to be sent to the Web server is prepared. For that, the security of data by ECC is imperative to keep the credential of the information of the people (Rajeswari & Thilagavathi, 2009).

Elliptical cryptography ECC is a wall crypto system used for encryption in SSL/TLS certificates. It is an alternative to RSA for devices with low resources. RSA requires much longer key lengths, this is not practical as it would require more computing power. Whereas ECC cryptography operates on points belonging to an elliptic curve. ECC has two important advantages: security and small key length. The computational speed and low power consumption, as well as the memory and bandwidth savings, are advantageous features for the use of ECC on mobile devices (Oussous et al., 2021).

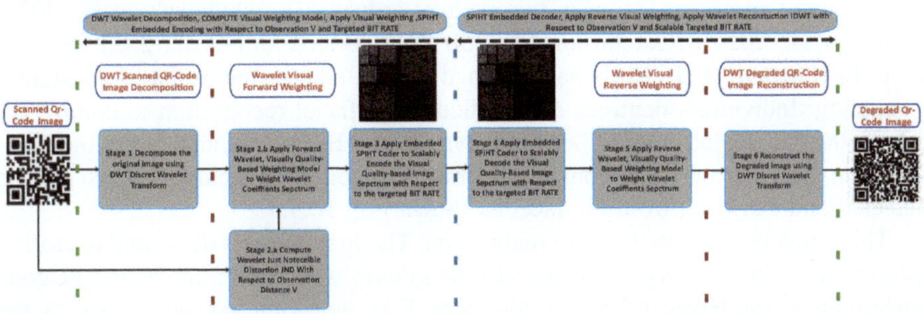

FIGURE 10.4

Visual encoding/decoding QR code image.

Any theory discovered in the RSA or ECC environment cannot be used directly; instead, standards for data structures and algorithms to process the information must be defined. ECC crypto operations are adopted and standardized by NIST, ANSI, IEEE, and the Internet Engineering Task Force. In cryptography, ECC is currently used in three applications. Elliptic curve integrated encryption system (ECIES) is a cryptographic scheme that uses elliptic curves to encrypt data, elliptic curve digital signature algorithm, elliptic curve Diffie-Hellman (ECDH) algorithm. We use the communication protocol CoAP to send the payload to the server once the payload security has been established. CoAP is based on the exchange of compact messages, which are sent via UDP by default (each CoAP message occupies the data section of one UDP datagram). A basic binary format is used for CoAP messages. A message is made up of a four-byte fixed-size header, a variable-length token, a CoAP option sequence, and the payload. Furthermore, CoAP has a client/server architecture comparable to HTTP. A client sends a request to the server that includes a method code, such as GET, PUT, POST, or DELETE. The server answers with a payload and a response code after receiving a request. Furthermore, CoAP is made up of two layers: communications and request/response. For redundancy and consistency of any message, the messaging layer is accountable while maintaining connectivity and communication is a request/response layer task. CoAP also permits multicast communications and supports asynchronous message exchange: Confirmable (CON), Non-Confirmable (NON), Acknowledgment (ACK), and Reset (RST) (Naik, 2017).

The data received is in the form of a payload. It contains the data from the QR code scanner and the person's face. Once the payload is received, it must be decrypted to be read. To decrypt the data we use ECC decryption, this requires a private key that is associated with the public key set for encryption. The result is the decrypted message.

10.4 Description of the realized recognition platform using AI

In recent years, AI (Artificial Intelligence) has become one of the most successful disciplines of computer vision in the medical industry (Przybylowski et al., 2021; Rathee et al., 2019). Recognition (Barodi, Bajit, Benbrahim et al., 2021; Barodi, Bajit, El Harrouti, et al., 2021) has spawned a multitude of studies that is constantly expanding. Individual identities are verified using facial recognition to control access to the MIoT platform (Miller & Brown, 2018). Before authenticating the identification, the relevant facial components for the recognition technique must first be detected and extracted from the face, as shown Fig. 10.5.

This study is composed of five main steps. The first phase is dedicated to storing information when adding a new user to the system with detection of the QR code performed by the Faster-RCNN architecture. Face detection was performed by the MTCNN architecture, and the learning step was based on FaceNet. The training is carried out on a database that brings together some people, each of whom is

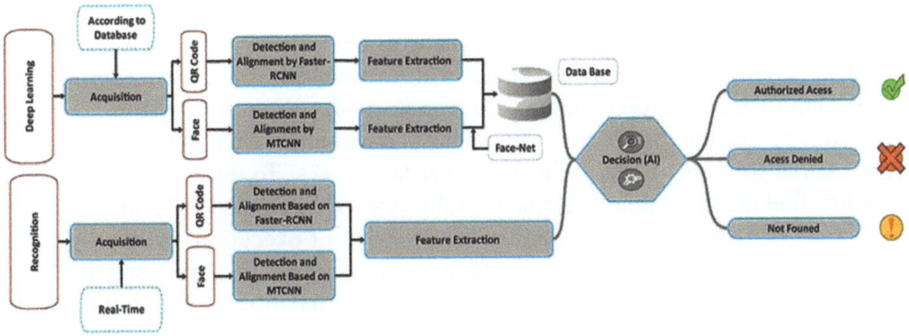

FIGURE 10.5

Description of the realized recognition platform.

associated with a good number of images, as well as the dedicated FaceNet architecture for face recognition.

The learning phase is carried out for the two models Faster R–CNN and MTCNN. The MTCNN model learns distinctive features of faces and produces face images as input. For each face image, the model produces a fixed-length embedding vector as a unique facial feature. Each person has several different images to generate their similarity vectors. These embeddings are used to understand the degree of similarity between two faces using Euclidean distance metrics or cosine similarity.

The learning process follows the recognition process, namely: image acquisition, detection and feature extraction. In our case, the acquisition of images or frames for video sequences is made from images and videos captured in deferred time. Then, preprocessing is performed. It consists of resizing the input images and normalizing them by removing the average pixel value. Thus, all detected regions of interest (ROI) are scaled to fit the CNN input. Finally, the extraction of the characteristics (characteristic vectors) is carried out. These are stored in the database to be subsequently used in the feature comparison phase.

Then, the detection phase is based on the MTCNN model. Its principle is to detect face bounding boxes in an image and five landmarks called "Landmarks." It includes three processing steps to simultaneously perform the detection of faces and that of facial landmarks. For the first processing block, multiple candidate windows through a shallow CNN (P-Net block) and then a second, more complex CNN that consists of refining the windows to reject a large number of windows that do not contain a face (block R-Net). In the third processing block, a robust CNN is used to polish the result and display the positions of the facial landmarks.

Recognition process is based on FaceNet and Feature extraction. For FaceNet, it is a facial recognition system, with unified integration for facial recognition and clustering. It's a system that, given an image of a face, extracts high-quality features of the face and predicts a 128-element vector representation of those features, called a face inlay. FaceNet directly learns a scene (images or video) from face images to a compact Euclidean space where distances correspond directly to a measure of face similarity. The classifier model used takes a face embedding as input and predicts the face identity which is stored and used as input to our recognition system.

However, Feature Extraction Alignment is a technique that applies a standardized rotation to the face that relies on facial landmarks. To do the alignment, you must first find the facial landmarks and for this, we used two models from the library. The model of facial markers is higher in the speed of execution. While the facial structure accuracy. This model is used to process the image to extract only the characteristics (the eyes, the contour of the face, the nose, the mouth, etc.) in the form of a vector, which can then be used in the comparison phase. characteristics to come out with a decision.

For Faster-RCNN Model (QR code), our approach explores the relevance of using features extracted from a CNN to detect QR codes. Faster R–CNN is composed of two branches that share convolutional layers. The first branch is a region proposition network that learns a set of window locations, and the second is a classifier that learns to label each window as one of the classes in the training set. In several works (Aslam & Curry, 2021; Parvathi & Tamil Selvi, 2021), our goal is to extract an image representation that contains a QR code. These images are processed by the convolution layers and also work faster. To construct a global image descriptor from faster R-CNN layer activations, we use all network layers that work with object propositions and extract features from the convolutional layers. Given the activations of an extracted convolutional layer for an image, we aggregate the activations of each filter to construct an image descriptor of the same dimension as the number of filters in the convolutional layer.

Faster-RCNN is an object detection method based on CNN and uses basic layers of conversion, composed of a feature extraction network to extract feature maps from the input image. Meanwhile, convolution layers don't change the image size, so usually adopt a size kernel, with pad and stride set, and each clustering layer shrinks the image half the original size. Therefore, there are multiple relationships between the size of the original input image and the feature map. Commonly used feature mining networks include Mobilenet VGG and Resnet (Shibly et al., 2020).

The relevance of this technique based on the Faster R–CNN method allows us to obtain better feature representations for the detection or else extract objects from images, and improves the performance of spatial analysis and reanalysis. To achieve this, we choose to tune Faster R–CNN to detect request objects to be retrieved by our platform.

Finally, for decision phase when access will be authorized, denied, or object not found, the extracted features are compared to those stored in the faces and QR codes database by averaging a similarity metric; in our case, we opted for the Euclidean distance. After exploring MTCNN face detectors, including a FaceNet facial recognition pack, for verified access. After receiving the payloads, the system starts to process the received information by comparing it with the existing database: Image of the person requesting access and image of the real QR code owner.

Once the system compares the received data with the existing one, the system decides whether to give access to the guest or not. If the person presented has a valid QR code and is the real holder of the pass or test, he/she is allowed to enter the space. If the person is exempt from the sanitary pass and his temperature does not exceed 37 degrees, the access is accepted.

If the person has a valid QR code but the image does not match the one already provided or cannot be found in the database, access is denied. If the person has an out-of-date QR code, a positive PCR test or, a PCR test that is over 48 h old, access is denied.

10.5 Discussion and results

Sending the image of the QR code and/or the face is more complex and much more voluminous. It is therefore necessary to find a solution for data transmission while preserving the relevant information for processing. We think to encode and decode the image with scalable encoders such as SPIHT. The integration of lossy and lossless coding is a concern in our approach. Indeed, the use of SPIHT allows encoding uniformly the whole image, which generates a loss of binary budget on the background of the image which contains less useful information.

A more improved version is to use EFIC and EVIC for coding based on the interest area and not on the whole image. These encodings are based on the characteristics of the human visual system (HVS), which allows to extract the region of interest without losses and to eliminate the nonperceptible area. In the case of an EFIC coding for the image of the person, this consists in decreasing the binary budget of the background, and increasing it for the face, which is beneficial in the clarity of the image and the quality of the data. For all these types of encoders, we notice that as long as the bit budget decreases, the quality, execution time and memory consumption decreases. We have compared the EFIC and SPIHT encoding in Fig. 10.6 and the EVIC and SPIHT encoding in Fig. 10.7. We remark that the

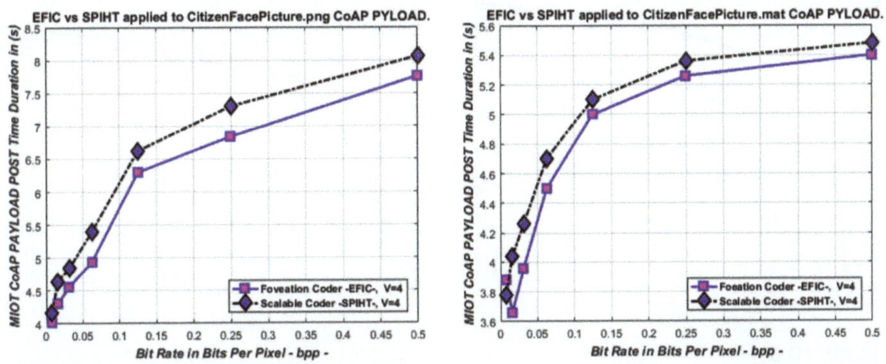

FIGURE 10.6

EFIC versus SPIHT applied to Citizen Face Picture.png and Citizen Face Picture.mat.

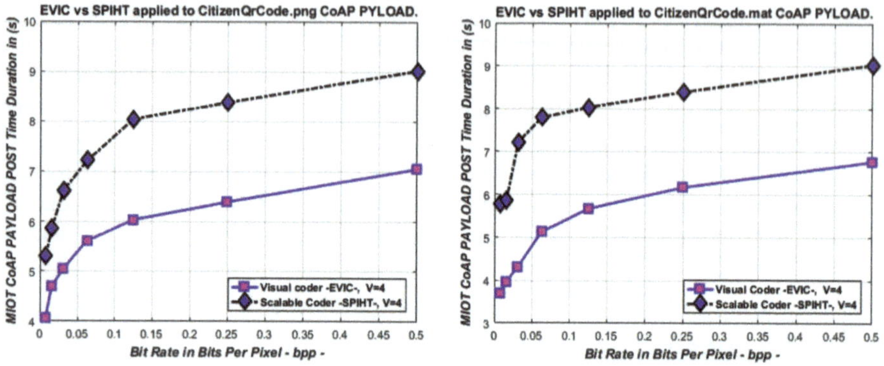

FIGURE 10.7

EVIC versus SPIHT applied to Citizen QRCode.png and Citizen QRCode.mat.

parameters such as: time, memory, and quality are much lower compared to SPIHT. This is due to the characteristics of EFIC and EVIC which are based on the region of interest and not on the whole image.

Fig. 10.8 shows Citizen Face picture Quality Metric (EFIC vs. SPIHT) and Citizen QR code Quality Metric (EVIC vs. SPIHT).

Fig. 10.9 shows QR Code EVIC visual coding images versus the SPIHT coding images and Lena EFIC visual coding images versus its optimized version SPIHT with their quality scores PS using visual WVDP assessor given for varying bit rate and fixed observation distance.

When we send the image captured from the camera or the QR code through the CoAP protocol to the server, the transmission time is much longer especially with the security layer, which makes the system slower. For this reason, we decide to encode and decode the image, which allows us to gain in terms of transmission

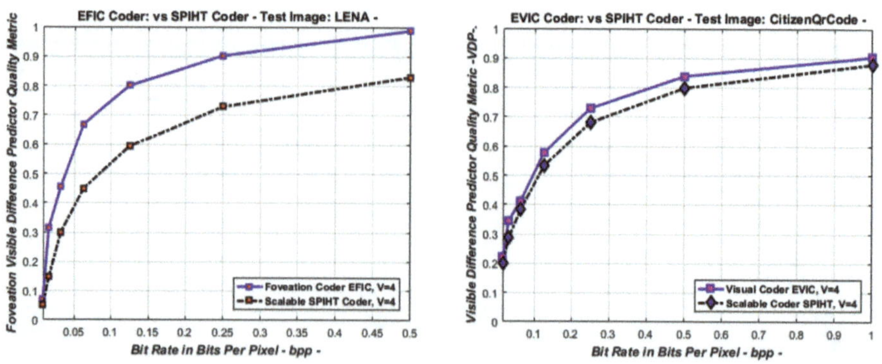

FIGURE 10.8

Citizen Face picture Quality Metric (EFIC vs. SPIHT) and Citizen QR Code Quality Metric (EVIC vs. SPIHT).

FIGURE 10.9

QR code EVIC visual coding images versus the SPIHT coding images and Lena EFIC visual coding images.

time. In Table 10.1 and Table 10.2, a calculation of the gain of execution time of the EFIC and the EVIC compared to SPIHT for two types of images mat and png. For a bit budget lower than 16:1 for png image, the execution time is faster.

The subjective quality in the foveation regions shown in Fig. 10.8 increases with the bit rate. It turns out that at bit rates lower than 16:1 bpp, EFIC and EVIC coding cannot produce an image of acceptable quality. Fig. 10.9 shows a comparison of the image quality between EFIC and SPIHT for the LENA test image, and EVIC and SPIHT for the QR code test image. Three types of bit rates are shown: high bit rates that give an excellent perceptual quality, medium bit rates that give an acceptable to good quality, and low bit rates that give poor and weak quality. The EFIC features

Table 10.1 Execution time gain Citizen QRCode (EVIC) and Citizen face (EFIC) pictures for the png image type.

Bit rate (bpp)	128:1	64:1	32:1	16:1	8:1	4:1	2:1
EVIC % SPIHT in (%)	23.01%	19.79%	38.22%	38.36%	45.27%	49.88%	57.20%
EFIC % SPIHT in (%)	−2.88%	1.29%	−15.70%	−19.96%	−0.30%	0.82%	3.72%

Table 10.2 Execution time gain Citizen QRCode (EVIC) and Citizen face (EFIC) pictures format image type.

Bit rate (bpp)	128:1	64:1	32:1	16:1	8:1	4:1	2:1
EVIC % SPIHT in (%)	−2.64%	9.40%	7.04%	4.25%	1.96%	1.86%	0%
EFIC % SPIHT in (%)	35.98%	32.42%	40.16%	34.10%	23.13%	26.42%	25%

that allow focusing on the face in an image and the facial recognition provides a more efficient result. The visual coding is then better than a scalable coding, in terms of perceptual quality (Bajit et al., 2019). The results of EFIC and EVIC coding in Fig. 10.9 demonstrate this.

10.6 Conclusion and perspectives

In this paper, we have applied computational intelligence (AI) in a visually optimized image's payload either in their communication through medical IoT managing the constrained applicative protocol CoAP and the light ECC encryption keying. Also, computational intelligence worked extremely well in the face object detection and recognition of the MIoT payloads in pre-IoT and post-IoT platform stages. These visual optimization tools, based on the human visual cortex properties and quality criterion, were adopted to upgrade the performances of the MIoT platform. Enhanced results have been observed either in terms of execution time, bandwidth, storage space, energy consumption and memory occupation. The psychovisual quality coding reshapes the payload spectrum, eliminates huge redundant contents, and keeps interesting information to be communicated to the cloud machine with minimum resource's consumption. Also we deployed the CoAP protocol for payload communication and the ECC to payload publication security within the MIoT platform. Modeling via this MIoT platform allowed us to perform the platform for several people with an updated sanitary pass while respecting a minimal delay for the control and saving time and platform resources in case a large number of people tried to access multiple public areas simultaneously. Our MIoT platform provided an interesting performance in terms of execution time reduction and saved the MIoT platform resources, which consequently allows the presented solution as a comprehensive security system that prevents the spread of viruses during pandemics.

References

Aslam, A., & Curry, E. (2021). A survey on object detection for the Internet of Multimedia Things (IoMT) using deep learning and event-based middleware: Approaches, challenges, and future directions. *Image and Vision Computing, 106*, 104095. https://doi.org/10.1016/j.imavis.2020.104095

Baddi, Y., Gahi, Y., Maleh, Y., Alazab, M., & Tawalbeh, L. (2022). Big data intelligence for smart applications. In *Springer studies in computational intelligence* (Vol. 994) Switzerland: Springer Nature.

Bajit, A., Najid, M., Tamtaoui, A., & Lassioui, A. (2019). A perceptually optimized embedded image coder and quality assessor based both on visual tools. *Advances in Science, Technology and Engineering Systems Journal, 4*(4), 230–238. https://doi.org/10.25046/aj040428

Barodi, A., Bajit, A., Benbrahim, M., Tamtaoui, A., Abouchabaka, J., Bourekkadi, S., Omari, O., & Slimani, K. (2021). Improving the transfer learning performances in the classification of the automotive traffic roads signs. *E3S Web of Conferences, 234*, 00064. https://doi.org/10.1051/e3sconf/202123400064

Barodi, A., Bajit, A., El Harrouti, T., Tamtaoui, A., & Benbrahim, M. (2021). An enhanced artificial intelligence-based approach applied to vehicular traffic signs detection and road safety enhancement. *Advances in Science, Technology and Engineering Systems, 6*(1), 672–683. https://doi.org/10.25046/aj060173

Bindu, P. V., Al-Hanawi, K. D., Al-Abri, A. M., & Mahadevan, V. (2021). IoT based safety system for school children: A contactless access control for post covid school conveyance. In *2021 2nd international conference for emerging technology, INCET 2021*. Institute of Electrical and Electronics Engineers Inc. https://doi.org/10.1109/INCET51464.2021.9456314

Ghosh, U., Maleh, Y., Alazab, M., & Pathan, A. S. K. (2021). *Machine intelligence and data analytics for sustainable future smart cities*. Springer.

Kumar, K., Kumar, N., & Shah, R. (2020). Role of IoT to avoid spreading of COVID-19. *International Journal of Intelligent Networks, 1*(1), 32–35. https://doi.org/10.1016/j.ijin.2020.05.002

Liu, L. X., & Wang, W. W. (2008). A wavelet image coding algorithm based on human visual system characteristics. In *Proceedings of the 2008 international conference on wavelet analysis and pattern recognition* (Vol. 1, pp. 113–117). ICWAPR. https://doi.org/10.1109/ICWAPR.2008.4635760

Miller, D. D., & Brown, E. W. (2018). Artificial intelligence in medical practice: The question to the answer? *American Journal of Medicine, 131*(2), 129–133. https://doi.org/10.1016/j.amjmed.2017.10.035

Naik, N. (2017). Choice of effective messaging protocols for IoT systems: MQTT, CoAP, AMQP and HTTP. In *2017 IEEE international symposium on systems engineering, ISSE 2017 - proceedings*. Institute of Electrical and Electronics Engineers Inc. https://doi.org/10.1109/SysEng.2017.8088251

Nosirov, K., Begmatov, S., Arabboev, M., & Medetova, K. (2020). Design of a model for disinfection robot system. In *2020 international conference on information science and communications technologies, ICISCT 2020*. Institute of Electrical and Electronics Engineers Inc. https://doi.org/10.1109/ICISCT50599.2020.9351370

Objenious. (2020). *500 Distributeurs de gel hydroalcoolique connectes arrivent dans les transports en commun bordelais*. https://objenious.com/presse/500-distributeurs-de-gel-hydroalcoolique-connectes-arrivent-dans-les-transports-en-commun-bordelais.

Oussous, S., Hamza, F. Z., Beloualid, S., allali, A. E., Bajit, A., & Tamtaoui, A. (2021). *Green smart city intelligent and cyber security based IoT transportation solutions for combating the pandemic COVID-19, computational intelligence techniques for green smart cities*.

Parvathi, S., & Tamil Selvi, S. (2021). Detection of maturity stages of coconuts in complex background using Faster R-CNN model. *Biosystems Engineering, 202*, 119–132. https://doi.org/10.1016/j.biosystemseng.2020.12.002

Przybylowski, A., Stelmak, S., & Suchanek, M. (2021). Mobility behaviour in view of the impact of the COVID-19 pandemic—public transport users in gdansk case study. *Sustainability, 13*(1), 364. https://doi.org/10.3390/su13010364

Qin, J., & Zhang, K. (2021). Face recognition construction site access control system based on open source computer vision. In *Proceedings - 2021 international conference on artificial intelligence, big data and algorithms, CAIBDA 2021* (pp. 1–4). Institute of Electrical and Electronics Engineers Inc. https://doi.org/10.1109/CAIBDA53561.2021.00008

Rajeswari, P. G., & Thilagavathi, K. (2009). A novel protocol for indirect authentication in mobile networks based on elliptic curve cryptography. *Journal of Theoretical & Applied Information Technology, 6*(1).

Rathee, G., Sharma, A., Kumar, R., & Iqbal, R. (2019). A secure communicating things network framework for industrial IoT using blockchain technology. *Ad Hoc Networks, 94*, 101933. https://doi.org/10.1016/j.adhoc.2019.101933

Shibly, K. H., Dey, S. K., Tahzib-Ul-Islam, M., & Rahman, M. M. (2020). *COVID faster R-CNN: A novel framework to diagnose novel coronavirus disease (COVID-19) in X-ray images*. medRxiv. https://doi.org/10.1101/2020.05.14.20101873

Shi, M., Yang, H., Liao, X., Chen, Y., Xiao, S., & Wu, J. (2021). Research on strategy of intelligent disinfection robot based on distributed constraint optimization. In *2021 IEEE international conference on artificial intelligence and computer applications, ICAICA 2021* (pp. 82–85). Institute of Electrical and Electronics Engineers Inc. https://doi.org/10.1109/ICAICA52286.2021.9497927

Sun, R., Wang, W., Xue, M., Tyson, G., Camtepe, S., & Ranasinghe, D. C. (2021). An empirical assessment of global COVID-19 contact tracing applications. In *Proceedings - international conference on software engineering* (pp. 173–174). IEEE Computer Society. https://doi.org/10.1109/ICSE-Companion52605.2021.00074

Wang, Z., & Bovik, A. C. (2001). Embedded foveation image coding. *IEEE Transactions on Image Processing, 10*, 1397–1410. https://doi.org/10.1109/83.951527, 10.

SECTION

3

Computational Intelligence for Medical Internet of Things (MIoT): Security and Privacy

CHAPTER

Edge intelligence case study on Medical Internet of Things security

11

Xiaohua Feng

School of Computer Science and Technology, University of Bedfordshire, Bedfordshire, Luton, United Kingdom

11.1 Introduction

Edge computing is computing that is near the source of the data, instead of relying on the cloud to do all the processing. It does not mean the cloud computing will disappear. It brings the cloud to you. Edge computing runs fewer processes in the cloud, and moving those processes to local places, such as on a user's computer, a MIoT device, or an edge server. Edge produced big data in real time (RT). Gartner (n.d) defines edge computing as "a part of a distributed computing topology in which information processing is located close to the edge." When edge device evolved to edge Intelligence, there are more threats of edge data governance faced, especially in data security.

Edge intelligence (edge artificial intelligence or edge AI, in other words) is a further development, it is easier to use and more secure. Edge nodes are at the edge to provide advanced data or big data analysis, scene perception, real-time decision-making, self-organization and coordination, and so on. At network edge which near the MIoT data source, offer a converged network, calculation, storage, application core competence open platform, such as robotics, AI devices, autonomous vehicles (AVs), Raspberry Pi, and so on.

The Medical Internet of Things (MIoT) has many applications, from public health to healthcare data management. One of application of MIoT examples is the Raspberry Pi in healthcare informatics applications; they are designed to produce many data. These data have potential to be carried out data analytics process to make predictions for our society. MIoT via wireless connect patients, medicine, treatment activity and all kinds of related treatment facilities. MIoT Pi is the useful tool for Healthcare provider and Healthcare staff to see the patient's develop trend and effectively respond the data. MIoT could also be used to notify patient individually alignment treatment. The device could be shown at Fig. 11.1. Raspberry Pi is a cost-effective, pocket size computer with a convenient size. It could perform MIoT functions as good as a simplified personal computer, as discussed in later sections below.

Robot as another one of MIoT edge intelligence devices would be discussed here. It developed rapidly, especially under the current pandemic. Recently it faced many

Computational Intelligence for Medical Internet of Things (MIoT) Applications
https://doi.org/10.1016/B978-0-323-99421-7.00003-9

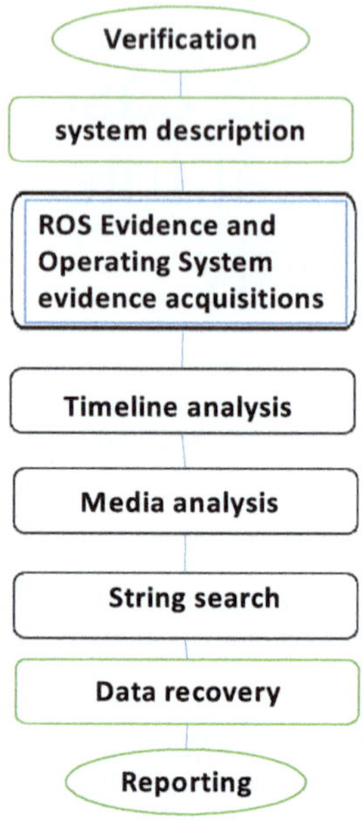

FIGURE 11.1

A primary framework of edge forensics investigation on ROS (Robot operating system).

more challenges, especially in edge security. A computer security and forensics laboratory had investigated some threats the edge intelligence devices facing. Observing robot and the working of robot operating systems had been carried out. And simulated robot security breach had been done. Research literatures were reviewed. A comparison of robot security and computer security had been investigated. An action of forensics framework for robot as edge device had been proposed for edge intelligence security (Abeykoon et al., 2021; Alexakos et al. n.d.). In order to perform RT data process properly, the robust infrastructures linked to the cloud are required with sufficient bandwidth and enough traffic capacity circumstances. The recent enforced Data Security Law should also be satisfied. If the condition is in doubt, it would be better to process the edge device produced data at edge, near the data source. If there were still data security threat, as Alexakos et al. discussed, some security frame works had been developed as Figs. 11.1 and 11.2 demonstrated (Alexakos et al., n.d.). Blockchain technology and Raspberry Pi served for healthcare informatics also performed MIoT functions significantly (Feng et al., 2017). Detailed discussions also demonstrated in Section 11.3 Case Studies.

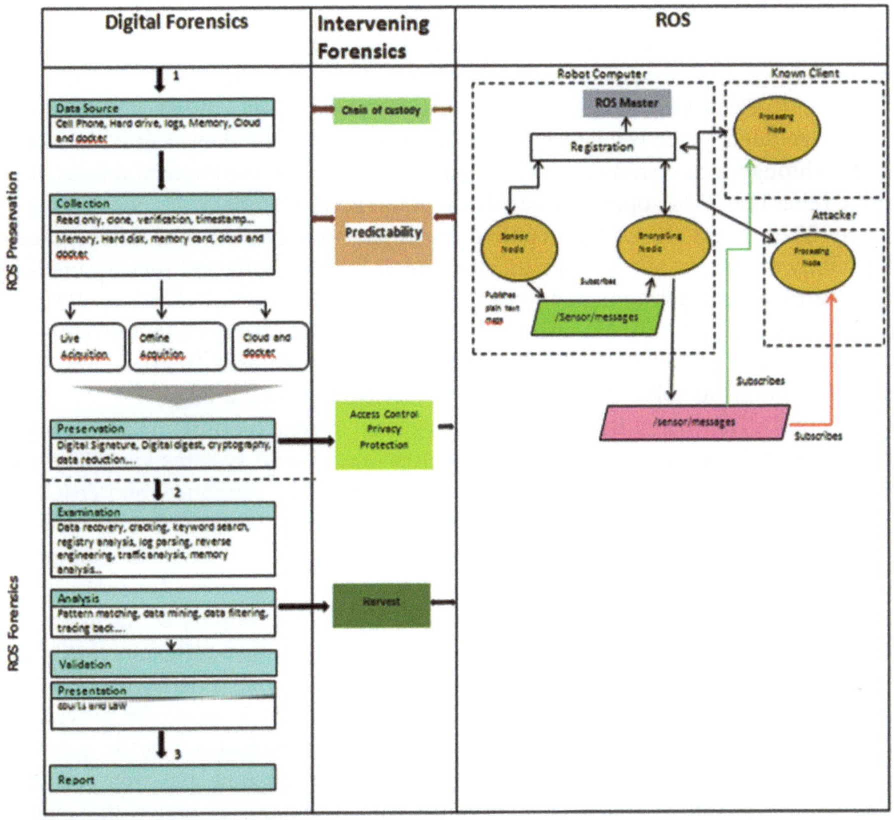

FIGURE 11.2

Forensics framework for edge robot healthcare data (Abeykoon et al., 2021).

11.2 Literature review

11.2.1 Recent edge computing development

Edge computing is defined as computing that is near the source of the RT data, instead of relying on the cloud to do all the process (Miller, 2018). It does not mean the cloud will disappear. It made the cloud is coming to you. While in its strictest connotation by NIST (National Institute of Standards and Technology), digital forensics is the application of computer science and investigative procedures involving the examination of digital evidence - following proper search authority, chain of custody, validation with mathematics, use of validated tools, repeatability, reporting, and possibly expert testimony (NIST, n.d).

The devices available at the edge have some limited amount of computing resources which can be utilized and incorporated with ML (machine learning) or DL (deep learning). AI algorithms could perform RT data analytics (IGI, n.d.).

Edge Intelligence or edge AI is one of the noticeable new areas in AI. Its aim and objectives are to support user to run AI near the source and ignore data transmission latency, congestion issues and privacy impacts.

In 2018, Plastiras et al. (2018) discussed, for a wide range of emerging applications edge intelligence is a necessary evolutionary need, and thus to provide a summary. Through a case study regarding computer vision for commercial drones, they argued that how these opportunities threat could be a potential.

By 2020, Xu et al. (2020) identified the key components of edge device issues, especially the recent of edge intelligence growing, robot collected sensory big data from surrounding environment day and night and provided various kinds services for users (Feng et al., 2020). Meanwhile, there were more concerns about privacy and security issues behind the uploaded data. Pushing intelligent frontiers would be one of solutions to solve these problems to release big data at edge.

Similarly, Bertin and Banerjee (n.d.) suggested, research efforts focused on specific application should be encouraged, with an end-to-end systems view. The tensions and trade-offs between safety, security, privacy, performance, and cost. The support of collaborative multi-disciplinary research between AI, MIoT systems, robot and so on applications. A recent healthcare edge AI blockchain example is also proposed by Linn & Koo, 2016 discussed later at Section 11.2.1. As a few edge intelligence threat were identified facing the future, Skirelis & Navakauskas, 2020 explored into different topology etc. have not provided sufficient clarity, on which parameters had a considerable impact on overall system performance.

Customer-oriented services were proposed by edge intelligence for provided a wider range of customer services than ever. Because organizations in the commercial sectors used intelligence computing in order to expand and improve their core services as well as create an opportunity to achieve more revenue with the latest effort edge intelligence worked to provide these companies with enhanced situation awareness and ability to access data and statistical analyzes in addition to reporting incidents and sending alerts and notifications when necessary. Because of its ability to provide unified communication capability between employees, edge intelligence had become a very attractive solution. The role of the 6G network served for robot is to define the right set of network technologies required to deliver robotics applications etc. (Gupta et al., 2021). There were many more gaps were discussed in Section 11.2.3.

11.2.2 Edge AI application for healthcare MIoT scenario

Edge AI provides high-performance application management. Edge AI could make AI technology broadly used in many field over the world. Edge AI could running on many edge devices, to expand advanced smart intelligence, on MIoT and data collection and analytics etc. Smart intelligence application in lightweight approach from the cloud down to the edge intelligence devices deployment. It integrate intelligence into edge computation structure, including computational intelligence for MIoT system applications. Edge AI could make user concentrate AI process but neglect privacy or data transmission speed impact. ML and DL methods could support on edge cache-aside pattern, edge computation, and the whole edge resource balancing and scheduling, in order to optimize edge computational intelligence system effect. Edge AI user only need to connect adapt device, it can drive intelligence application function performance: because of edge AI is able to provide embedded RT system functions, it could speed up MIoT processing time efficiently (Linn & Koo, 2016).

The MIoT of NHS (National Health Service) cyber security solutions with robots, blockchain, and Raspberry Pi were discussed in Chapter 3 in detail. Furthermore, robotics as its widely used MIoT edge intelligence device had more demands. Hence, the research is discussed in Section 11.3.2.1 below for work details.

11.2.3 Critical analysis edge intelligence

To compare edge computing and the cloud computing, the cloud computing offer computation process services through public Internet. While edge computing running process in their internal configured devices rather than connected to the cloud computing platform. These internal configured devices could be edge computing server, robot, internal configured device or MIoTs. The based on the cloud platform process would be constrained by the bandwidth and network latency, but edge does not.

Edge intelligence combine AI and edge computing technologies to make AI algorithm running on the edge-computing capable devices. Because the edge Intelligence devices could process data in RT, no need to connect to the cloud platform. Most of advanced AI process were processed in the cloud because of large amount of computation capability were required. But these AI would easily be affected by network latency even faulty.

Because of edge intelligence run on edge devices, the necessary big data could be processed locally, which save time. And DL algorithms could run on the data source device itself. In AI technology ML method in recent years were widely employed to many fields to assist knowledge gaining and decision-making tasks and so on. DL with ML algorithms growth and big data emerging, developed fast. DL as one of the most cutting-edge fields of science and technology currently, it could play an important role in guiding scientific and technological progress in the near future. DL will be applied in more fields of human life. In terms of explain data, DL worked like human brain mechanism, which were the reason that DL could be used on MIoT, AV, and robots (Alexakos et al., n.d.). Edge computing technology could learn generating data by deep learning on the cloud, but at data source, edge device inference and prediction of execution model data process and storage.

Advantages of edge intelligence computing:

- Bandwidth, edge device processed temporary data, no need to transmit all of the data to the cloud, to reduce bandwidth requirement (that way also reduce computation and storage resource need).

- Timing, when edge Intelligence device was given information process tasks, big data are processed RT and low latency and transmit the most important information locally, protect big data security, reduce big data transmission amount and maximum extent reduced communication interrupt possibility.
- Latency, data processed near data source end, reduced system latency, improve service responding time. Economic, execute computation at edge would cost less. Reliability, application maybe need operating continuously, but the cloud connection is not always reliable.
- Protect privacy, some sensitive data application still need processed locally. After discussing attacks, the paper has suggest solutions based on the literature review, like edge computing provides storage infrastructure for key sensitive data use. That enhanced big data security etc.

Disadvantages of edge intelligence:

- Edge facilities are varies. Some edge devices were rely on the cloud advanced configurations previously, did not consider the transmission issues, had not thinking of to enhance their own facilities technically in process capability, speed, storage, security, and so on.
- The environment condition might not be satisfactory to run intelligence algorithms; especially in NHS, well trained staff are in demand for MIoT intelligence.

11.3 Edge intelligence miot case study issues

11.3.1 Edge challenge facing

After an investigation and scientific research literatures review, a conclusion had been reached that big data security is one of the edge issues. Conventionally, because of the cloud powerful process and robust storage capability, big data produced from edge were send to the cloud to process. Nevertheless, with 6G technology in fast development, MIoT network created large amount of big data (Gupta et al., 2021). To send to the cloud to computation consume network bandwidth, affect traffic and caused response latency. In particular, for edge devices like Raspberry Pi, AV, smart phone or robot, RT response should be necessary. Network latency could lead to a disaster. Therefore, edge computing growth, some of computational functions had been moved to the edge, close to the data source. Edge computing saved transmission cost. It also decreased the cloud computation load. More importantly, it reduced RT response latency, reduced bandwidth demand, reduced network stream traffic, reduced network congestion and faulty possibility and reduced data breach caused privacy information protection during transmission security risk.

For instance, in order to support robot security as an edge intelligence device, a cyber security framework was proposed (see Fig. 11.2). Fig. 11.2 edge intelligence device security framework had been approved working efficiently in laboratory simulation (Abeykoon et al., 2021).

11.3.2 Security case study

Edge Intelligence is one of new area of AI applications for MIoT. The purpose is let user to run AI process near the data source but not worry impacts of privacy or big data transmission latency. Edge Intelligence could make AI used more widely. To make edge devices responded input faster, without rely on access to the cloud computing. Edge Intelligence needs still exploration in depth. In order to employ Data Security Law 2021, data security should be considered in edge device. In terms of apply Data Security Law to edge device, we taken Alexakos et al. (n.d.) suggestions, proposed some framework for robot security solutions as demonstrated in the following figures. These could be treated as application examples of Health informatics security.

11.3.2.1 Robot edge intelligence examples

Now, exploration edge intelligence applications will be carried out. Robot as a good healthcare assistant is investigated. Edge intelligence applications include almost all the real life examples to run the edge created MIoT big data analysis at the devices themselves, more efficiently than via the cloud platform. After big data process at the data device, there is no need to send the results to the cloud, which would benefit to reduce network traffic and ensure data privacy protection. For instance, edge Intelligence on robot, AV, edge Intelligence work for MIoT, edge Intelligence on smart phone application and edge Intelligence robots as well.

11.3.2.2 Framework developed for edge security

In order to serve cybersecurity for edge device, a forensics framework for edge robot had been developed in the edge intelligence mechanism as Figs. 11.1 and 11.2 shown. Abeykoon et al. simulated the framework implementation, proved the UCI (user computer interface) of it. This framework could work on other edge intelligence devices, such as AV in Fig. 11.1 shown. Further works were in progress at Computer Security and Forensics Lab. Take Abeykoon et al. (2021), Alexakos et al. (n.d.) works into account, edge intelligence security could be achievable. It is only the matter of time.

Figs. 11.1 and 11.2 for a robot produced every second big data proposed computer forensics frameworks proposes that the most appropriate process for the robot forensics investigation data security framework. The forensic investigation procedure is partitioned into stages, which in the procedure were related with each other. When these were completed, the results of the investigation had finished. And further investigation for another case procedure could be carried out. This robot forensics framework provided a valuable contribution for robot as the edge intelligence device security digital forensic investigations. It also may be used in MIoT backgrounded edge intelligence field because it presented a holistic way that is capable to integrate the aspects of handling investigations. The procedures included in the framework were capable to cover the procedures of the current models, which appeared that the proposed one was comprehensive sufficient to cover the processes. The benefits of the proposed framework were perceived how to extract relevant digital evidence forensically from robot operating systems so as to improve admissibility useful.

Nowadays, since the robot create RT data all the time, the data of robot operating system was not stored in cloud storage. It is the research focus that the framework would make new opportunities to the robot security and forensics community by supporting the cyber security and forensics specialists, law enforcement parties and robotics practitioners to introduce new method for robot operating systems investigation. These are the core advantages of the proposed framework (Abeykoon et al., 2021), which is appropriate to edge intelligence robot security, such as healthcare sensors (MIoT), security issue could be pin down. Consequently, new legislation for consumers would be considered.

11.3.2.3 Edge intelligence (edge AI) medical blockchain case study

The emerging technologies offer manifold advantages to healthcare sectors in different ways (Xu et al., 2020). Blockchain is based on opens source software, commodity hardware, and open APIs (application programming interfaces). These homogeneous components promote easier and faster interoperability between the systems and can adeptly scale to handle larger volumes of health data and more blockchain users. The blockchain architecture has in-built cryptography and data encryption technologies which are currently widely accepted and applied as industry standards. The healthcare blockchain technology would be designed and developed as open-source platform. AI and blockchain technology have the potentials to considerably impact the healthcare industry as a whole and specifically to providers, patients, and payers regarding clinical trials, drug traceability, data management, and research. In any case, blockchain technology for the healthcare industry would necessarily be designed to be public and would further have to involve efficient technological solutions for three major elements such as scalability, patients and general health data privacy, and access security. Fig. 11.2 depicts a typical blockchain technology based healthcare information technology (IT) solution showing the potential roles of AI and blockchain for healthcare industry. In Fig. 11.3, the health blockchain encompasses the totality of health records and data collected throughout a patient's life period, and a health record repository called data-lake stores all medical data. In the data lake, each blockchain transaction stores the specific location of the health data it references.

A Case Study was carried out in University of Bedfordshire (Feng et al., 2020). A sample of physical public blockchain for NHS was in progress (Xu et al., 2020), which could demonstrate patients' electronic medical records stored in blockchain under the decentralized, transparent, immutability antifraud feature security protection. In order to solve the faulty node, or compromised node, a practical Byzantine fault tolerance algorithm to defense malicious attack and tempt in the CS consideration (Bertin & Banerjee, n.d.; Feng et al., 2020).

Health information generated from health providers and specialists (doctors) such as prescriptions, laboratory results, MRI (magnetic resonance imaging), ECG (electrocardiogram) and pathology results, and data from personal devices

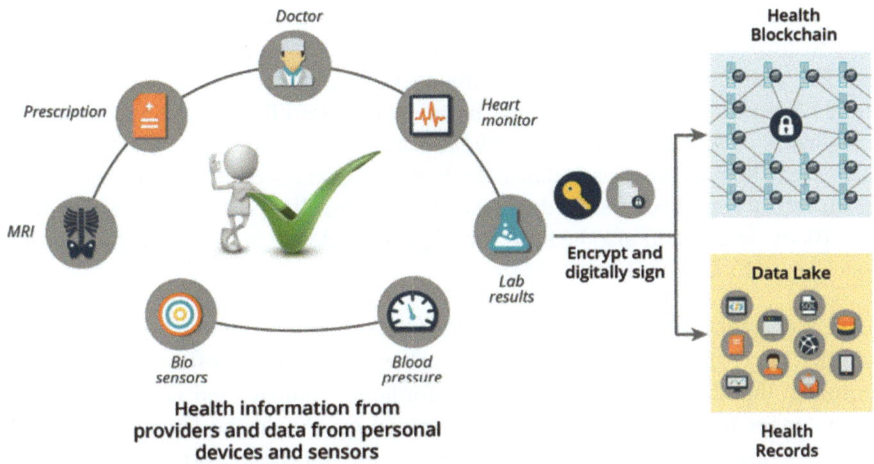

FIGURE 11.3

A typical blockchain technology based healthcare IT solution (Linn & Koo, 2016).

and sensors (Linn & Koo, 2016) such as bio sensors and blood pressure devices would be encrypted and digitally signed prior to storing in health records and health blockchain as illustrated in Fig. 11.3. Unlike the data lake, health blockchain (see Fig. 11.3) would work by applying a similar working principle like books library card catalog where the card catalog holds the metadata about the books and the locations where the books can be located. Like bitcoin blockchain systems, each transaction in the different blocks would contain the patient's unique identifier and timestamp showing when the transactions were created, and an encrypted link to the health record.

Linn & Koo (2016) make use of blockchain feature, to use free software, service hardware, and open APIs (apps. programming interfaces). These components promote easy and fast interoperability between the systems and can handle health big data and many blockchain users. The blockchain architecture has in-built cryptography and data encryption which are currently widely accepted (Feng et al., 2020).

Access control permissions could be a cyber security issue of MIoT on access permissions. The user could setup a detailed transactions particularly about who had accessed right at the agreed time for access and the particular types of data which could be accessed. At any permitted time the user might alter the set of permissions. Access control policies would also securely be stored on a blockchain, only the particular user should be allowed to make statement about which. This provides an environment of transparency and allows the user to make decision about what data could be collected and how these data could be shared, on the decentralized ledgers (Linn & Koo, 2016).

The healthcare blockchain can be designed and developed as a free platform. AI and blockchain technology have potentials to impact healthcare to providers, patients, and clinical trials, drug traceability, data management, and research.

Blockchain for healthcare would necessarily be designed to be public and would have to involve efficient solutions for three elements such as scalability, patients and PII (personal identifiable Information) data privacy, and access security. Fig. 11.3 demonstrated a blockchain based healthcare IT solution showing the potential roles of AI and blockchain for healthcare industry. In Fig. 11.3 shown, blockchain cover health records and data collected throughout a patient's life period, and a health record repository called data lake stores all medical data and evidence detection. Blockchain could also be used for edge AI evidence in data security (Bertin & Banerjee, n.d.; Linn & Koo, 2016).

11.3.2.4 More MIoT of NHS security issue

Another MIoT device application, the Raspberry Pi as a cost-effective, pocket size computer, the idea about developing an affordable, compact and yet programmable computer for little children was first conceived in 2006 at the University of Cambridge's Computer Laboratory when Upton et al. (DFRWS, 2001) in 2014 started growing concern about the decline in figures of aspiring Computer Science candidates and the level of their computer programming skills. This decline which they attributed to the expensive and obscure nature of current computers led to the design and development of a tiny and affordable computer with programming capability for children. This idea became a reality in 2008. It was mass produced and peaked at two million in sales within 2 years of production (Feng et al., 2017).

11.3.2.4.1 The progress

Later on, people found Raspberry Pi could do many things for MIoT. They could form a cluster in MIoT systems. Then to carry out a layered hierarchy for MIoT to process medical data at edge, to perform a regional center for MIoT system. With millions of units of the device already sold and still selling and also with promising and prospective uses yet to be realized, it is safe to assume that the Raspberry Pi device will play a role within computer security and digital forensics investigation in the near future. Also, digital forensics has been termed by some as a reactive science; saying that study and research in the field are most times as a result of the need to react to the occurrence of an event. Therefore, it is imperative that the Raspberry Pi device be studied in order to identify any cyber security threat that may arise as a result of its widespread popularity and to also establish evidential information that are recoverable from it in the case of non-conventional usage or compromised state. The outcome of the study will form a basis for reference when the need arise for a forensic investigation to be carried out on the device. This technique is now an important part of sensing data. Various fields of forensic science, like Forensic Medicine, Forensic Odontology, etc. (Feng et al., 2017), especially when data at the cloud environment, then digital forensics preparation becomes crucial.

The proliferation of digital electronic devices and our dependency on them in this information age has given rise to a new form of crime that can be categorized as computer crimes or computer-related crimes. This new wave of crime through the years has risen and is growing bigger with significant impact on government, business and individuals. This became a growing challenge for law enforcement agencies as they found themselves in situations where they have to retrieve or confiscate one digital device or the other from a crime scene which needs to be analyzed to solve a crime. Also several businesses and government need to investigate why and who attacked their critical infrastructure/intellectual properties. The need to investigate this new form of crime with its new form of digital forensics evidence led to the passing of new legislative laws and the birth of the new science known as Digital Forensics Science, and there is an event of organization DFRW (Digital Forensic Research Workshop).

11.3.2.4.2 Digital Forensic Science using Raspberry Pi

Digital Forensic Science was defined at the first Digital Forensic Research Workshop held in Utica, New York on August 7–8, 2001 as "The use of scientifically derived and proven methods toward the presentation, collection, validation, identification, analysis, interpretation, documentation and presentation of digital evidence derived from digital sources for the purpose of facilitating or furthering reconstruction of events found to be criminal or helping to anticipate unauthorized actions shown to be disruptive to planned operations" (DFRWS, 2001). The aim and objectives had been shown in Fig. 11.4 below (DFRWS, 2001). Each party use different approach to investigation, this is largely due to their varying objectives.

For example, law enforcement will not embark on an investigation until there exist sufficient information and fact that a crime has been committed whereas business and industry or military can move into investigation as soon as the slightest hitch is discovered so as to ensure availability of service, continuity of operations, protection against critical infrastructure and intellectual properties or protection against data/information theft but can still be after the fact in some cases as well for example as part of incidence response and disaster recovery. Digital forensic is a relatively mature but new field of study whose maturity can be said to be as a result of need; i.e., prominence and increased rate of computer crimes through the years prompted the need for a platform of investigation to address the issue. This is why compared to other forensic science field like DNA fingerprinting which came as a result of years and years of studying and experimentations, digital forensics seems to still lag behind in some aspects. However, like every other forensic science field, digital forensic science consists of four intertwined components regarding to the cybercrime, the evidence investigation, the digital forensics science and the computer law.

Area	Primary Objective	Secondary Objective	Environment
Law Enforcement	Prosecution		After the fact
Military IW Operations	Continuity of Operations	Prosecution	Real Time
Business & Industry	Availability of Service	Prosecution	Real Time

FIGURE 11.4

Parties involved in digital forensic science (DFRWS, 2001).

Digital Forensics Investigation Process Models were adopting the existing DFRW paradigm used in the handling of physical documentary evidence in legal cases, proposed a digital investigation process model as shown in Fig. 11.4 (DFRWS, 2001). Participants at the Digital Forensics Research Workshop which consisted of practitioners of the science, researchers in computing field, law enforcement agency, business, military, and so on agreed on the model shown in Fig. 11.5. The established that the Presentation, Collection, Examination and Analysis phases are the core processes in a digital forensics investigation process. But depending on the environment and parties involved, it is safe to say other phases are equally relevant as well. For instance, the identification is a core process in the case of incidence response in organizations, and also the presentation is crucial in both criminal case and incidence response as the investigator is responsible for interpreting observations and results in an understandable manner to decision makers (Judge, Jury or Management of law enforcement).

To take the DFRW recommendations into account, experiment has been carried out at the Computer Security and Digital Forensics Laboratory, University of Bedfordshire. The output results were discussed at Section 11.3.2.4.4.

Identification	Preservation	Collection	Examination	Analysis	Presentation	Decision
Event/Crime Detection	Case Management	Preservation	Preservation	Preservation	Documentation	
Resolve Signture	Imaging Technologies	Approved Methods	Traceability	Traceability	Expert Testimony	
Profile Detection	Chain of Custody	Approved Software	Validation Techniques	Statistical	Clarification	
Anomalous Detection	Time Synch.	Approved Hardware	Filtering Techniques	Protocols	Mission Impact Statement	
Complaints		Legal Authority	Pattern Matching	Data Mining	Recommended Countermeasure	
System Monitoring		Lossless Compression	Hidden Data Discovery	Timeline	Statistical Interpretation	
Audit Analysis		Sampling	Hidden Data Extraction	Link		
Etc.		Data Reduction		Spacial		
		Recovery Techniques				

FIGURE 11.5

Investigative process model for digital forensics (DFRWS, 2001).

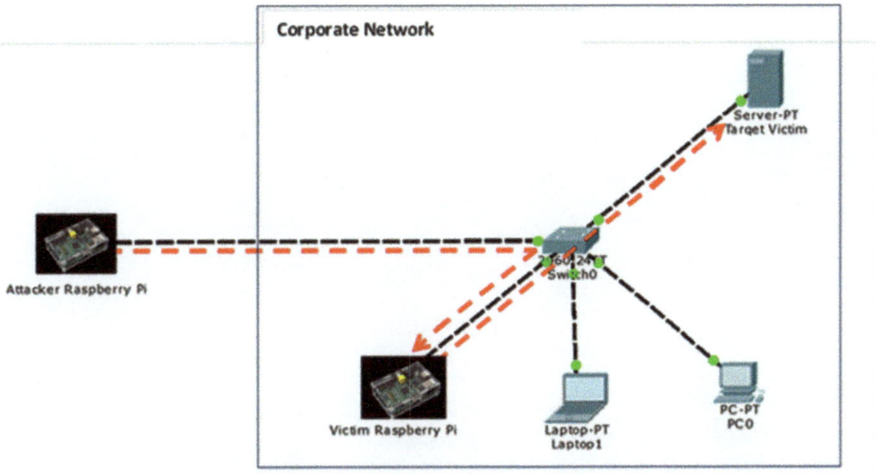

FIGURE 11.6

Case study scenario setup.

11.3.2.4.3 MIoT security scenario setup

The MIoT scenario depicted in Figure below was setup; an attacker compromised a Raspberry Pi device on the corporate network and used it violate a policy on the corporate server.

Security Issue, such as, the Raspberry Pi operating system has SSH (secure shell protocol) opened on port 22, secure shell is a protocol used for establishing remote log on. This port should be closed in situations where remote access to the device is not required. Another security issue observed on the device was that the Raspberry Pi operating system comes preinstalled with a default setting for beginning to use.

The bigger picture here is that with millions of Raspberry Pi devices in millions of places, the devices could be hijacked and turned into an army of botnets that can be used to participate in a mass email spamming or DDoS (distributed denial-of-service) attacks (Smith, 2016, pp. 209–223). Therefore it is recommended that a policy should be put in place to enforce changing the password after installation. Also port 22 should be filtered using a firewall or closed when remote log on would not be required.

Operating System Fingerprinting, was observed that the MIoT Raspberry Pi device does not give as much footprints in network scanning using tools like Nmap as does the computer or notebook platform; an operating system scan was performed on the network using the command Nmap (see Fig. 11.7), but the results of the scan indicates that the Raspberry Pi device does not return any information about the operating system it is running. This is a good thing as it makes it challenging for an attacker to determine the existence of the device on a network. The result of the Nmap—A command, however, gave a guess about the operating system, but this is only a guess as the kernel version of the operating system was not

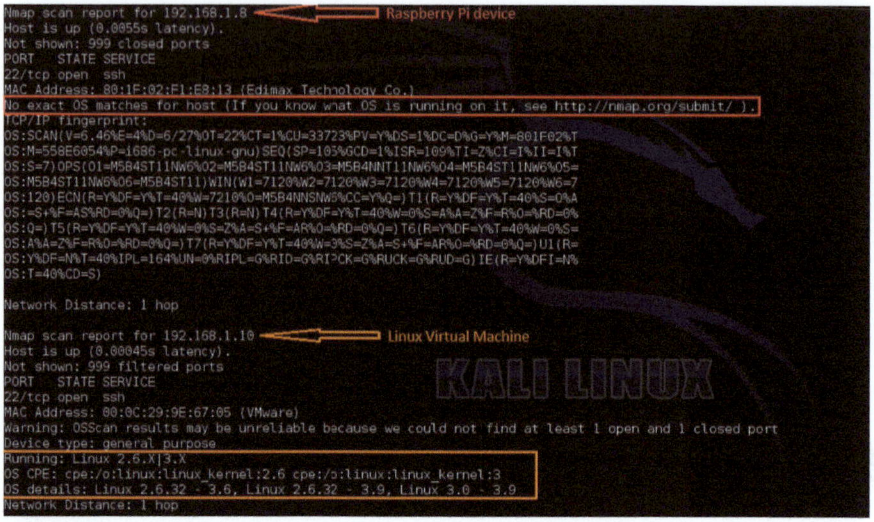

FIGURE 11.7

Result of the Nmap command to query for operating system.

revealed. This can still pose a challenge for an attacker because most network equipment like switches and routers run operating systems that are Linux kernel based.

This is when the Raspberry Pi as a device as a botnet attacker, to compromise the MIoT system circumstances experiment screenshot.

11.3.2.4.4 Analysis

The approach of evaluation was through comparison to established platform, standards, and related works on other platforms. The elements of this work being evaluated are via the approach to device's storage medium research. Qualitative method of approach had been used to attain numerous achievements through the manner of approach that was observed during the course of this work will be likened to stages involved in scientific method in an effort to evaluate and justify if it was worthwhile and meets its objectives.

- Observation: This work was conceived as a result of the observation of the global popularity of the Raspberry Pi computer as a MIoT result of its cost effectiveness and potentials. This observation led to questions and the need to provide answers to these questions led to the initiation of this work.
- Evidence need: does this global popularity of the Raspberry Pi device raise any security issue? This led to a research being initiated.
- Research: This research of the basic operations and structure of the Raspberry Pi device as a MIoT end device was conducted using various approaches, methods, models and so on in an effort to establish possibilities of answers to the identified questions.

- Hypothesis: The output of the research of the structure and operation of the device shed some lights which led to making strong assumptions about a possible security issue and the need for a MIoT Raspberry Pi forensics research in the field of digital forensics.
- Experiment: In order to test assumptions in an effort to confirm or discard hypothesis, a scenario was setup to simulate a real life situation. Attacks were attempted and the investigative process was observed which served as a baseline research for MIoT Raspberry Pi forensics investigation.
- Analysis: The laboratory experiment results analyzed which shown confirmed hypothesis and recommendations could be made.

To summarize above, the work had been verified, the possibility of how the MIoT Raspberry Pi device could be compromised due to a weak (default) configuration, a potential security threat that may arise if it should occur and the recommendations to ensure cyber secure usage of the device. These have also been identified, possible evidential information available for the purpose of digital forensic investigation of the MIoT device. Through this research, an investigation cyber security issues and evidential information recoverable from the Raspberry Pi devices as a MIoT had been carried out. The device as a botnet attacker and as an attack target are both tested for Digital Forensics Investigations.

11.3.3 Suggestions

In health informatics, MIoT dealt with many complicated aspects continuously. Edge intelligence issue was only one of aspect among them (Feng et al., 2020; Upton, 2014). More health informatics research still need to be carried out, in order to make MIoT systems to perform smoothly. Current smart phone apps provided many health measurement functions to monitor patient heart-beat rate, blood pressure, breath and so on. These should also be researched in the MIoT category.

Relevant computer law consideration, on the cyber legal aspect, from law theory of cyber science to a practical design application (Smith, 2016, pp. 209–223), GDPR 2018, Data Protection Act 2018, and Data Security Law 2021, etc. motivated research on data governance (Feng et al., 2016; Hawthorn et al., 2015; Maleh et al., 2017, p. p209), including MIoT data, from the cloud computing to edge intelligence. Further work on edge device should be required, such as PKI deployment, enhanced edge device RT big data process power, robust storage, security technology applications, etc. (Hawthorn et al., 2015).

Since 2019, machine learning technologies in recent times are widely applied in various areas to assist knowledge gaining and decision-making tasks and healthcare is one of the important area among these tasks. In this paper, we proposed a process to identify reliable health data from online resources and process the data to enable being used by the edge DL technologies (Maleh et al., 2017, p. p209). In addition, this proposal might also to be applied to healthcare services, due to they used a large amount of robot there.

11.4 Evaluation

11.4.1 Technical discussion

As shown in Figs. 11.1–11.7, the Smart data analysis needs safety and security protection solutions to be implemented for MIoT (Feng et al., 2016). Furthermore, PII (personal recognizable information) data need to be take into consideration. These should not be in the normal data hubs unless there is a consent in place. Therefore, the data storage in the cloud, authority access and process will be an issue (Maleh et al., 2017, p. p209). The data monitoring and analysis could be a daily task, also needs to pay attention to. Perimeter access control and extra host based access control should be applied to these data storage. Robust cryptography using modern PKI cryptography technique etc. could be applied (Washington, 2017).

Edge intelligence run the edge created big data process at the devices them self (the data source). Edge intelligence technology become more and more important, because more and more devices and facilities need to use AI technology when unable to access the cloud. Such as, automatic robot, MIoT Raspberry Pi, smart phone GPS (Global Positioning System) applications and so on. At those kind of applications, data transmission latency could cause disaster impact. When MIoT Raspberry Pi, or robot test the path, people and other obligations, they cannot be affected by latency. Due to immediate respond time is so important, use edge intelligence system is necessary (Audrey & Feng, 2021; Wang et al., 2020). Edge intelligence allows RT analysis and classify computer vision images locally rather than rely on visit the cloud (Muhammad Imran, 2019).

11.4.2 Challenges analysis

Based on the present work, to take these outstanding issues and suggestions into account, in the near future, a consideration design and execute comfortable and well-served societies for citizens in the world is possible. In terms of move many of RT big data process work uploaded to the cloud computing to local edge devices is a trends. Especially with smart city, MIoT widely application, 6G development (Gupta et al., 2021), edge intelligence become necessary in the future. The built generalized solution should also be extent possible. Therefore, to update edge devices become urgent to cooperate the trends for DL, RT, accuracy, cyber security, privacy protection, and so forth (Feng et al., 2016; Skirelis & Navakauskas, 2020).

11.4.3 Research limitations

For the time being of this investigation, research limitations and obstacle constrained further achievements (CSO, 2020; Cybersecurity, 2020; ICO, 2016). Nevertheless, the research scope of the aim and objectives were achieved. The rest could be left to future development of MIoT research on health informatics to be continued.

11.5 Conclusions

In this paper, we have discussed the recent cyber security threats and possible solutions for edge intelligence on health informatics. In order to governance MIoT data security, suggestions had been offered. Facing challenges in network transmission bandwidth, data response speed bottleneck, cyber security for big data, MIoT demands, AI expectation and so on, edge intelligence present require upgrade edge devices to current technology urgently. Here, a survey conclusion was demonstrated. A robot challenge, Raspberry Pi and blockchain in NHS case study as the edge devices had been represented with the proposed robot security framework and Raspberry Pi security testing for edge intelligence. The feasibility had been simulated too.

Moreover, future development suggested to pay attention to edge facilities and devices, like cooperative robotics on robot collaboration in services area. Because the devices need data to be processed locally but lack of updated present technology deploy properly. They are more in demand of modernization. Further work will be carried out in the computer security and forensics laboratory, University of Bedfordshire collaboratively with other academics. Nevertheless, MIoT information security governance is a continuous issue to be taking care of with cutting-edge technologies (Iredale, 2019; Vikram Dhillon, 2019). Scientists have been exploring a better trade-off between health informatics' performance and system cyber security consistently. A balanced compensation is maintained and will going on in the world.

Glossary

AI	Artificial Intelligence
API	Apps. Programming Interfaces
AV	Autonomous Vehicle
CS	Case Study
DDoS	Distributed Denial-of-service
DFIPM	Digital Forensics Investigation Process Models
DFRWS	Digital Forensics Research Workshop
DL	Deep Learning
DNA	Deoxyribonucleic Acid
ECG	Electrocardiogram
Edge AI	Edge Artificial Intelligence
GDPR	General Data Protection Regulation
IT	Information Technology
MIoT	Medical Internet of Things
ML	Machine Learning
MRI	Magnetic Resonance Imaging
NHS	National Health Service
NIST	National Institute of Standards and Technology

PII	Personally Identifiable Information
ROS	Robot Operating System
RT	Real Time
SSH	Secure Shell protocol
UCI	User Computer Interface

Acknowledgments

The author would like to appreciate the reviewers' constructive feedback comments to improve this chapter.

References

Abeykoon, I., & Feng, X. (2021). *Robotics security.* University of Bedfordshire. Submitted to IEEE Access.

Alexakos, C., lexakos, C., Katsini, C., Votis, K., Lalas, A., Tzovaras, D., Serpanos, D. (n.d.). Enabling digital forensics readiness for internet of vehicles. *23rd EURO work group on transportation meeting, EWGT 2020, Paphos, Cyprus. Transportation Research Procedia* (Vol. 52, pp. 339–346): ScienceDirect.

Audrey, A., & Feng, X. (June 2021). Content-based technical solution for cyberstalking detection. In *The proceeding of conference: 2021 3rd international conference on computer communication and the Internet (ICCCI), Nagoya, Japan.* https://doi.org/10.1109/ICCCI51764.2021.9486770

Bertin, E., & Banerjee, S. (n.d.). *Artificial intelligence at the edge*: A CCC-Quadrennial. https://cra.org/ccc/resources/ccc-led-whitepapers/#2020-quadrennial-papers computing. (Accessed 16 June 2021).

CSO. (2020). *Securing the edge*. CSO Online. (Accessed 16 May 2021).

Cybersecurity. (2020). *The impact of artificial intelligence on cyber security.* https://www.cybersecurityintelligence.com/blog/the-impact-of-artificial-intelligence-on-cyber-security-4946.html. (Accessed 16 May 2021).

DFRWS. (2001). Workshop 1 - a framework for digital forensic science. In G. Palmer (Ed.), *A road map for digital forensic research.* New York: DFRWS.

Feng, X., Onafeso, B., & Liu, E. (2017). *Investigating security issues and evidential information recoverable from a Raspberry Pi device for forensic investigation.* IRJES.

Feng, X., Onafeso, B., & Iron, A. (2016). Digital forensics smart city project with Raspberry Pi cluster. In *HEA 11th Workshop, UK.*

Feng, X., Conrad, M., Eze, E., Hussein, K. (2020). AI and blockchain for future cyber security applications. *IEEE the 5th international workshop on applications of AI, cyber security and economics big data (ACE-2021).*

Gartner. (n.d.). *Definition of edge computing.* https://www.gartner.com/en/information-technology/glossary/edge-computing. (Accessed 16 May 2021).

Gupta, R., Reebadiya, D., & Tanwar, S. (2021). *6G-enabled edge intelligence for ultra -reliable low latency applications: Vision and mission.* Elsevier.

Hawthorn, N. (2015). *White paper: How European Union data protection affects your data in the cloud.* Tthe new EU data protection regulations).

ICO. (2016). *Overview of the general data protection regulation (GDPR)*. https://ico.org.uk/for-organisations/data-protection-reform/overview-of-the-gdpr/. (Accessed 15 February 2021).

IGI Global. (n.d.). *What is edge intelligence*? https://www.igi-global.com/dictionary/role-of-edge-computing-to-leverage-iot-assisted-aal-ecosystem/97224. (Accessed 12 August 2021).

Iredale, G. (2019). *Blockchain for healthcare: Use cases and applications*. https://101blockchains.com/blockchain-for-healthcare.

Linn, L. A., & Koo, M. B. (2016). Blockchain for health data and its potential use in health IT and health care related research. In *ONC/NIST use of blockchain for healthcare and research Workshop* (pp. 1–10). Gaithersburg, Maryland: US ONC/NIST. Available online at: https://www.healthit.gov/sites/default/files/11-74-ablockchainforhealthcare.pdf. (Accessed 7 January 2021).

Maleh, Y., Sahid, A., Ezzati, A., & Belaissaoui, M. (2017). CAFISGO: A capability assessment framework for information security governance in organizations. *Journal of Information Assurance and Security, 12*(6), p209–217.

Miller, P. (2018). *What is edge computing*. The Verge.

Muhammad Imran, T. (2019). Agent based information security framework for hybrid cloud computing. Agent based information security framework for hybrid cloud computing. *KSII Transactions on Internet and Information Systems, 13*(1), 406–434. https://doi.org/10.3837/tiis.2019.01.023

NIST. (n.d.). Cybersecurity framework: Computer Security Resource Center. https://csrc.nist.gov/glossary/term/digital_forensics. (Accessed 16 September 2021).

Plastiras, G., Terzi, M., Kyrkou, C., & Theocharides, T. (2018). Edge intelligence: Challenges & opportunities of near-sensor machine learning applications. In *IEEE international conference on application-specific systems architectures and processors*.

Skirelis, J., & Navakauskas, D. (2020). Performance analysis of edge computing in IoT. *Elektronika ir Elektrotechnika*. https://doi.org/10.5755/j01.eie.26.1.23235

Smith, C. (2016). *The car Hacker's handbook*. Open Garages. Ch, 13 http://opengarages.org/handbook/ebook. (Accessed 23 June 2021).

Upton, L. (2014). *RACHEL-Pi – delivering education worldwide*. https://www.raspberrypi.org/rachel-pidelivering-educationworldwide/. (Accessed 8 May 2021).

Vikram Dhillon, J. B. (2019). *Blockchain in healthcare: Innovations that empower patients*. Connect professionals & improve care. Pristine Publishing.

Wang, X., Han, Y., Leung, V. C. M., Niyato, D., Yan, X., & Chen, X. (2020). *Edge AI: Convergence of edge computing and artificial intelligence*. Springer.

Washington, E. (2017). *Why data governance is crucial for big data environments*. Tdwi. https://tdwi.org/articles/2017/09/15/diq-all-data-governance-in-big-data-world.aspx. (Accessed 15 January 2021).

Xu, D., Li, T., Li, Y., Su, X., Tarkoma, S., Jiang, T., Crowcroft, J., & Hui, P. (2020). *Edge intelligence: Architectures, challenges, and applications*. Corpus.

CHAPTER

Data-driven intelligent Medical Internet of Things (MIoT) based healthcare solutions for secured smart cities

12

Anurag Mudgil[1], Kritesh Rauniyar[2], Raman Goel[1], Surendrabikram Thapa[2,3], Anvit Negi[4]

[1]*Media.Net Software Services (India) Private Limited, Mumbai, Maharashtra, India;* [2]*Department of Computer Science and Engineering, Delhi Technological University, New Delhi, India;* [3]*Department of Computer Science, Virginia Tech, Blacksburg, VA, United States;* [4]*Gas Authority of India Limited (GAIL), India*

12.1 Introduction

Data is ubiquitous, and a large volume of data is processed every second in the digital world we interact with. Every data point can give us some information. The information-rich data that surrounds us can be leveraged to make our lives easier. A smart city is defined as an advanced metropolitan region with technological advancements that collects data using various electronic technologies, voice activation methods, and sensors (Negi et al., 2021). The information gleaned is utilized to effectively manage a variety of services and resources and hence to enhance city operations. This data is made up of data gathered from people, places, and buildings, which is refined and analyzed for the purposes of planning and assessing traffic and cosmopolitan commuter rails, power production, utilities, public water infrastructures, disposal of waste, academic facilities, and health facilities (Jha et al., 2021).

The technology required for smart cities has to churn massive amounts of data, often dubbed as "big data," for proper functioning. Big data is characterized by three Vs as "increased volume, increased velocity, and increased variety information assets," which entails enormous data sets which are being processed rapidly and which utilize a variety of data sources, including integrating various data sets (Tsai et al., 2015). Artificial intelligence (AI) and big data are inextricably intertwined. AI refers to a variety of techniques for using a non-human machine that learns from these lessons and emulates human behavior. AI can effectively sort across large volumes of big data, generating data projections as well as cost-effective solutions to fuel smart city technologies.

Depending on whether the AI is supervised or unsupervised, the task of making data meaningful is performed in a variety of ways. Supervised learning employs a

Computational Intelligence for Medical Internet of Things (MIoT) Applications
https://doi.org/10.1016/B978-0-323-99421-7.00006-4

variety of data and target values for the purpose of training AI models on how to find actionable insights within the accumulated raw data. Following that, the AI will do routine duties and operations while also probing for better approaches and alternatives that may deliver improved outcomes than present solutions (Kumar et al.). Unsupervised learning utilizes unlabeled and unclassified data sets to train and query AI networks, which subsequently discover latent traits and unseen patterns within the data set. Some of the use cases of AI in smart cities are as follows:

12.1.1 Public transit

In a smart city, it is essential for people to have clean and efficient transportation of products and services. Numerous metropolises are looking toward smart technology to alleviate traffic bottlenecks and give users live information in order to improve mobility (Vakula & Raviteja). Cities with extensive public transportation infrastructure and systems can really enhance their system by using software applications that harmonize the user experience. Train, bus, and automobile passengers can submit real-time information on delays, breakdowns, and less crowded routes via their mobile apps. This would guide other commuters to tweak their travel routes, thereby alleviating future congestion. Gathering and analyzing data on public transport usage would also aid cities in making better-informed decisions regarding altering public transportation routes and schedules, as well as allocating more appropriate infrastructural or architectural budgets (Batty, 2013). To exemplify, Dubai recently carried out numerous smart city programs, including one that includes tracking bus drivers' health. Depletion and fatigue-related accidents decreased by 66% as a result of this monitoring.

12.1.2 Public safety

The safety of city residents is paramount in such urban areas. The development of smart cities enabled by AI empowers municipalities to proactively monitor their citizens through the use of CCTV cameras equipped with facial recognition (Vattapparamban et al.). Additionally, AI-based cameras which are capable of motion and smoke detection can be used for enhanced security monitoring. The same sensor and camera networks could also be employed to save lives and reduce crime. Emergency services can leverage traffic signals and congestion data to reach their terminus faster and safer (Isafiade & Bagula, 2020). Authorities might gather data on fatalities and some other variables in order to develop future predictive and preventive initiatives.

12.1.3 Smart building system

Devices can be installed strategically throughout a facility to collect data on energy consumption and anticipate consumer preferences (Snoonian, 2003). Store owners and merchants, for instance, may use sensors to figure out when most people visit and utilize their stores, as well as which parts of the store, attract the most interest. The data generated by AI can be used to make reliable forecasts and track regular and periodic variations.

12.1.4 Energy and waste management

The safety improvement and management of various power grids can be significantly improved by the use of AI (Calvillo et al., 2016). Existing grid network which incorporates electricity transmission networks, generating plants, etc., can be converted into smart grids by interception of AI-based systems in control and management of the network which in turn can collect and analyze enormous amounts of data in order to evaluate and forecast demand response and load clustering. Moreover, prediction models could be implemented to estimate the price and demand for energy at specified periodic intervals. According to the research, these models can outperform conventional approaches for estimating pricing and load. Likewise, in smart cities, the energy generation grid and intelligent water management are critical aspects in achieving low-pollution energy production. This practice also contributes to the provision of safe drinking water and the subsequent preservation of our natural environment.

12.1.5 Present challenges

Implementing an AI-based, full, functional smart city is not a straightforward undertaking due to several obstacles which are not only there on the development side of the project but are also present on the implementation side. Besides a lack of money and a lack of technical advancement, there are a few other factors to reason why developing such cities is challenging.

12.1.6 Infrastructure and financial implication

The majority of equipment and machinery deployed in smart cities make use of sensor technologies in order to collect and analyze data. Hence, a massive amount of data is collected periodically from cameras or sensors or any other security/surveillance system. Even the air quality index or the criminal record can contribute to humongous data sets (Lazarova-Molnar & Mohamed, 2016). The deployment of these sensors necessitates the establishment of a complicated and expensive infrastructure that is not very viable.

12.1.7 Concerns about data privacy/security

An additional difficulty in establishing such extensive systems is ensuring the protection and privacy of its inhabitants (Younus et al., 2019). As the data acquired from monitoring individuals or their actions rise with the usage of Internet of Things (IoT) and sensor technologies, it might be seen as difficult to assimilate and evaluate these large chunks of data.

12.2 Need of intelligent systems in healthcare

Healthcare is a pioneer modern success story. Average life expectancy has grown leaps and bounds with the subsequent advancements in healthcare systems which aid in early diagnosis and effective prognosis of even the most peculiar diseases (Adhikari et al., 2021). However, as life expectancy grows, healthcare systems confront increased demand, increasing expenses, and a staff that is straining to satisfy patient demands. Among the inexorable drivers, healthcare systems demand is majorly driven by a mixture of forces, namely: population aging, increasing patient expectations, lifestyle changes, and the unending cycle of innovation. To exemplify, it has been estimated that by the end of 2050, one in every four European will be over 65 in terms of age, hence putting serious pressure on the existing health systems to handle increasingly complicated patients. Managing such individuals is costly and necessitates a change from episodic treatment to proactive long-term care management.

Automation combined with AI has the potential which can be used to further advance healthcare and help alleviate some of the aforementioned major issues. AI can enhance medical outcomes by an increase in productivity and efficiency (Tanveer et al., 2020). Moreover, it can speed up life-saving therapies and fundamentally change the staff-patient equation resulting in an efficient and improved healthcare system. Although, concerns have been raised regarding the possible hazards of AI to patients, practitioners, and health systems and the ethical issues surrounding the use of AI and the data that powers it. However, AI has the potential to revolutionize healthcare delivery where the benefits far outweigh the potential cons associated with the introduction of such technology. A new analysis shows how the use of AI might enhance treatment results, the experience of the patient, and the contact with healthcare. It may improve care delivery productivity and efficiency, allowing healthcare institutions to serve more people better. AI may help healthcare providers spend more time with patients and less time on administrative tasks, reducing worker fatigue. All of which contribute to a significantly better experience as well as service.

Researchers have examined how automation and AI will influence the workplace in the long term. Almost all the employment across industries will be impacted by automated technology, however, the extent differs, and healthcare is one of the industries with the least possibilities for automation—35% of spending time is possibly automatable. Automation's potential is distinct from automation's possibility of adoption. When it comes to the healthcare sector, AI is an ever-expanding field that is highly adaptive to the changing needs of the patients it serves. In the past few years, AI has shown tremendous promise for improving medical care and alleviating the tremendous pressures that the medical industry is under (Thapa et al.).

12.2.1 Three phases of AI in healthcare

We are very much in the initial phases of understanding AI's role in modifying and its influence on healthcare (Jiang et al., 2017). It has been concluded that we can anticipate three stages of AI in healthcare based on recent studies. The first stage will be the introductory stage where AI will be introduced in administrative tasks and even the first level of diagnosis. Medical professionals spend a substantial amount of time doing regular, recurring, and primarily administrative chores, that can be addressed by AI-based solutions. AI can tackle mundane administrative tasks to allow medical professionals to focus on other more important tasks. This should improve the healthcare operations and increase the use of new technology. Imaging-based AI applications, such as those used in radiology, cardiology, and ophthalmology, would indeed be included in this introductory stage (Shah & Chircu, 2018).

Phase two might include further techniques and approaches that facilitate the transition from hospital to home care. Systems like remote monitoring, AI alerting systems, or virtual assistants are expected to be deployed in phase two as patients assume much more responsibility for their own health care. Natural Langugage Processing (NLP) systems in the hospital and at home might be used more widely, as well as AI can be used across a wider range of specialties including cancer, cardiology, and neuroscience, where improvements are already being achieved. In order for this to happen, it will necessitate a much greater level of involvement from organizations and health professionals. Well-designed and unified approaches are necessary to employ current technology in new situations. Deep learning, NLP, networking, and other technology advances, together with cultural shifts and the development of new capabilities inside enterprises will all contribute to this expansion of AI adoption (Jha et al., 2021).

Our expectations for the third phase of AI adoption in the healthcare industry are that we will see an increase in the use of AI solutions in the clinical setting, with an emphasis on enhanced clinical decision support (CDS) techniques. Respondents anticipate AI to be a vital component of everything from how we learn to how we diagnose and treat patients. However, the prerequisites for AI to prove its mettle in the field of healthcare are, namely, the inclusion of larger data sets throughout institutions, effective governance to enhance the quality of the data, and a sense of trust from organizations.

12.2.2 Diagnosis and treatment applications

In clinical diagnosis, AI aids in treatment planning, management, automation, administration, and numerous other operations (Han et al.). It may be deployed to identify cancer, triage crucial discoveries in medical imaging, highlight acute abnormalities, assist radiologists in prioritizing life-threatening patients, diagnose cardiac arrhythmias, forecast stroke outcomes, and aid in chronic disease management. AI is indeed a vast universe of data, techniques, statistics, supervised learning, neural nets, and discoveries that are continually expanding and adapting to the demands of the healthcare business and its patients.

For almost 50 years, healthcare has relied on AI for illness diagnosis and treatment. They could properly detect and provide treatment, even if the illness was not fully recognized in clinical practice. There was not a significant improvement in

AI-based diagnosis in comparison to the one done by humans majorly due to their noteworthy issue in integration with physician workflows and health record systems.

The use of AI in diagnostic and treatment plans might be challenging to integrate with clinical processes and electronic health record (EHR) systems. The difficulties in incorporation have hampered the use of AI in healthcare when we consider the suggestive accuracy of AI. Presently most of the medical software which uses or incorporates AI is utterly specific for the area of care. To fully use AI in healthcare, providers will need to either build their own AI-enabled EHR or hire third-party suppliers that can interact with their EHR (Khedkar et al., 2020).

There is a new emphasis in healthcare on pain management. With virtual reality and AI, the painkiller problem may be alleviated by creating a synthetic world that distracts people from their existing pain source. Techniques and results derived from AI may help enhance patient outcomes. This can reduce the side effects caused by the use of various drugs during the treatment.

12.2.3 Administrative applications

There are a number of practical uses of AI in healthcare. AI's function in hospitals is less revolutionary than inpatient care (Davenport & Kalakota, 2019). Yet, AI in-hospital management will save a huge amount of money. Claims processing, patient information, revenue cycle management, and clinical record-keeping are just a few of the uses of AI in healthcare. Millions of claims are verified every day by insurers and suppliers; false assertions and code mistake waste time, money, and energy for everyone. AI in healthcare can be used to match data from disparate databases using machine learning.

12.3 IoT, applications, and wearables for healthcare monitoring

Smart gadgets that can be worn as external items, incorporated in clothing and textiles, inserted in the body, or even bonded to or tattooed on the skin are all examples of IoT-enabled wearables. The wearable is also employed in the entertainment industry. Smartwatches, fitness bands, virtual reality glasses, and a variety of other gadgets are among the most regularly used wearables. We can now make the payment procedure incredibly simple by employing wearable gadgets (Drobot et al., 2019). The IoT will be fuel-efficient and suitable for a long-term plan in the industry as well as agriculture. Wearable sensors can be classified into four major classes (Pasluosta et al., 2015).

Biopotential-specific Sensor: Biopotential Sensors are galvanically separated, high-performance differential biological detectors designed (Brugarolas et al., 2014) to assess a broad variety of biological impulses including Electrocardiogram (ECG/EKG), Electromyography (EMG), Electrooculography (EOG), and Electroencephalography (EEG).

Motion sensor: A motion sensor (e.g., accelerometer and gyroscope) is a part of electronic equipment that detects and measures motion. Such sensors are commonly used in security systems for homes and businesses, but they could be seen in smartphones (Freedson & Miller, 2000), paper towel dispensers, and gaming systems.

Environmental Sensor: These sensors measure, monitor, and records environmental characteristics, such as temp, moisture, heat loss, and food deterioration detection utilizing gas sensors (Bader & Jagtap, 2020). These sensors are essential for ensuring that food is cooked or stored at the proper temperatures and that it is safe to eat.

Biochemical Sensor: A receptor and a biological ingredient, such as an enzyme, antibody, or nucleic acid, make up the device (Turner, 2013). The bio element interacts with the material being tested, and the converter converts the biological reaction into an electric pulse.

12.3.1 Cognitive IoT for healthcare monitoring

The cognitive computing system analyzes massive volumes of data in real-time to respond to particular questions and provide recommendations. In healthcare, the cognitive system connects people and machines functions, allowing the computer and the human brain to fully overlap to promote better decision-making (Behera et al., 2019). Cognitive computing can handle complicated tasks like NLP and classification, data mining, and knowledge management. Cognitive systems can handle complex work like relationship extraction from unorganized corpora, speech-to-text and text-to-speech converters, pattern recognition, computer vision, and machine learning (Coccoli et al., 2016). Reasoning, grasping fundamental concepts, forming hypotheses, and inferring and extracting ideas are all capabilities of cognitive computing systems. The system creates and quickens knowledge with each data set, interaction, and output, so it never ends learning.

Only with proper training can a cognitive system demonstrate its full potential. To do so, questionnaire pairs in natural languages must be created. It takes a lot of effort to generate a sufficient number of questionnaires. If certain standards are not followed, training cognitive systems can be arduous and ineffective. It is critical to establish clarity on roles between users and the system application in order to deploy cognitive applications successfully (Tarafdar et al., 2017). Although a cognitive system takes on some previously held functions, it also gives humans additional obligations, such as teaching and maintaining the cognitive application. Beyond verbal and visual comprehension, there are still significant obstacles to overcome. By identifying and retrieving content, it is crucial to grasp the contextual meaning and build deeper links among multimodal data.

In a variety of settings, cognitive systems can assist us in overcoming our limitations. The capabilities of cognitive systems are nearly limitless; their capacity to handle difficult tasks such as natural language processing (NLP), data mining, categorization (Adhikari et al., 2021), and knowledge management allows them to perform exceedingly complicated jobs and solve complex queries. Cognitive systems analyze large volumes of data in order to comprehend, reason, and adapt from it, as well as collaborate with healthcare providers to design better treatment or caring plans for patients.

12.3.2 Noninvasive methods for monitoring of vitals

When there is no interaction with the mucosa, skin tear, or interior body cavity beyond a naturally occurring body opening, it is considered noninvasive. The most appealing use in the IoT sector is interconnected health, which allows patients to be observed and cured remotely of their residences rather than going to clinics (Djelouat et al.). As the current situation is threatening due to the COVID-19 pandemic where the virus spreads in close contact with each other, so here the noninvasive method can be used to prevent the spread of the virus (Winck & Ambrosino, 2020). Noninvasive respiratory technology can be used by health workers to cure infected patients. Companies should be asked to provide safer interfaces, virus-proof circuitry, and latest generation noninvasive ventilators that integrate many therapies, provide customized tracking, and have all of the required safety features.

A noninvasive method for measuring diabetes is gaining popularity these days. Diabetes is among the deadliest diseases where Insulin is a hormone produced by a gland below and beneath the stomach (pancreas). The glucose concentration of the bloodstream is determined based on the intensity of the transmitted and reflected after an infrared Light-Emitting Diode (LED) is put over the fingertip to monitor blood glucose visually (Rahmat et al., 2017). After that, the input is filtered and enhanced before being supplied into the microcontroller, where it is shown on a display screen. Based on the voltages obtained and assessed, a person's glucose level is predicted. The glucose measurements also are relayed through Wi-Fi to a smartphone and presented via an Android app.

According to statistics, cardiovascular diseases (CVDs) are the leading cause of death. The electrocardiogram (ECG) is a frequently used tool for assessing a person's CVD. In the ECG process, there are several vital stages: first, the data acquisition is done using the ECG electrode and the data filtering takes place (Sahu et al., 2021). Then the average/peak data is captured and noise detection and unwanted distortion are removed. Finally, the time interval process is initiated where the PR interval and other vital factors are calculated. Eventually, ECG produces the result. Remote ECG can help the doctor as being their assistant and can help to correct their flaws. The remote ECG data can also be saved in the cloud and as per necessity, user can retrieve the data from the cloud.

12.4 Computer vision for medical diagnosis, prognosis, and treatment

Images are a major part of all multimedia. All the medical images are a product of digital imaging. The information is extracted and collected from the data set and images are manipulated by physicians with relevant tools. Thus, computer vision, a widely growing field, has a lot of usage in medicine (Song et al., 2016). An important concept in computer vision is digital imaging. A digital image is identified using a lattice. A lattice is typically a rectangular grid of n dimensions ($n > 1$). Here, n constitutes the spatial coordinates. In order to identify the changes with respect to ages, a new time coordinate can be added to the lattice.

12.4.1 Scope of computer vision in medicine

Analysis of multimodal data: This branch forms the part of diagnosis wherein any further possibility of image modalities is looked for. Analysis of images is done to find new patterns and insights, which might lead to a new anatomical structure (Colantonio et al., 2018).

Automation: Automation in medicine with help of computer vision is explored quite recently (Song et al., 2016). There are several advantages that can be traced to the advancement of automation. For an instance, guided vision surgery.

Prediction of accuracy: Computer vision can be used to precalculate accuracy using mathematical rigor. This is especially helpful when performing complicated surgery or radiation therapy (Esteva et al., 2019). A fair idea about the results of treatment can help in modifications in the treatment itself.

Understanding huge volume of data: As we advance in any field, data grows exponentially. Making sense from this huge amount of data in itself is a humongous task. Computer vision can help visualize this data in medicine and draw useful patterns (Thevenot et al., 2017). Thus, we can formulate a generic pipeline that can be used as a benchmark for all applications of computer vision in medicine.

12.4.2 Computer vision for early detection of diseases

Computer vision and image processing techniques can be used to detect several types of diseases at very early stages. There are many diseases like tumors, cancers, etc., which can pose a threat to the life of a patient if detected at any later stages. The chances of patient survival, in that case, might turn out to be sleek. Detecting early signs gives a high rate of survival. In these techniques, algorithms are trained with a huge amount of image data sets. Even the slightest abnormality can be a sign of disease. The algorithms are tuned to give a higher level of accuracy. Thus, professionals in the medical field can identify the patterns which would otherwise be missed.

Some research has already been done in this field. There are known and published algorithms that can be used to identify various diseases like respiratory diseases, diabetes, etc. (Jorquera-Chavez et al., 2021). Although there are established examples of using computer vision and image processing in medicine for the early detection of illness, there is still a huge scope for advancements. This is definitely a promising field. Applications of computer vision in detecting complicated and life-threatening illnesses like cancer can change the entire course of the medical industry. One of the examples for the overview of the identification of diabetes at early stage using image processing and computer vision is shown in Fig. 12.1 below.

12.4.3 Computer vision assisted diagnosis and identification of the diseases

There have been several efforts done to automate the medical diagnosis process and this has been an emerging target in the field of computer vision. There are several ways in which computer vision is used in the diagnosis and identification of diseases. Some of the major applications have been listed as follows.

Facial Medical Diagnosis: Face acts as an extremely useful sign for measuring health status. Several symptoms are evident from patients' facial abnormalities or typical features. There are several results that show the over 30 diseases that can be identified via facial diagnosis (Thevenot et al., 2017). Continuous efforts are being made in this field to arrive at more robust techniques.

Detection of Tumor: Deep Learning, Image processing, and computer vision techniques have been frequently used to detect tumors in patients (Zhao et al., 2018). The rate of spread of brain tumors to other parts of the brain is quite high. Early detection of the tumors can prove to be extremely beneficial in saving the life of the patient.

Monitoring and Rehabilitation: There are many instances where continuous monitoring is required once the patient is treated from a critical illness. On the other hand, there are also situations when the elderly need care and monitoring while being at home. Computer vision is proving to be an extremely useful technology in such cases (Thevenot et al., 2017). Since monitoring and rehabilitation can happen virtually, thus, these act as major areas where technology can play a significant role.

Medical Imaging: There has been a significant advancement in the field of medical imaging with the use of computer vision techniques (Thapa et al.). Nowadays, surgeons need not depend on traditional methods. Surgical platforms based on simulations have emerged out as a major area for the diagnosis of diseases.

Continuous efforts are being made in the field of computer vision along with deep learning and AI-based techniques to advance the future in medicine for the early detection, diagnosis, and identification of several diseases.

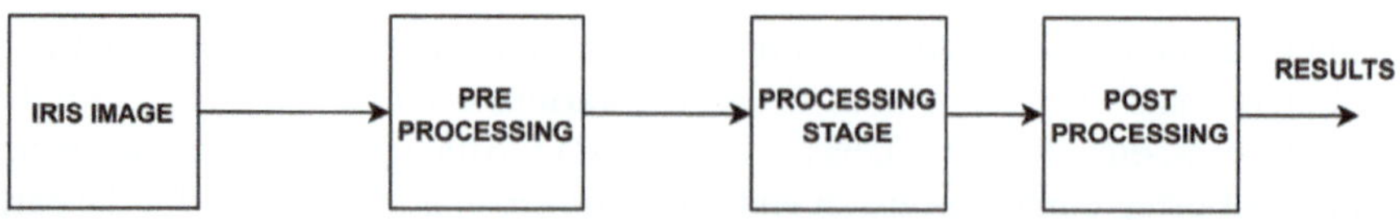

FIGURE 12.1 Identification of diabetes at an early stage using image processing and computer vision.

Identification of diabetes at an early stage using image processing and computer vision.

12.4.4 Computer vision assisted treatment procedure

Computer-aided diagnosis using computer vision assists in the treatment procedures of several major diseases. Computer vision techniques are processes to extract useful information from the raw image data. Several advanced techniques like magnetic resonance imaging (MRI) are used to assist professionals in the diagnosis and treatment of chest and abdomen-related issues (Thevenot et al., 2017). The methods called pattern recognition are used to process images and then draw useful patterns with the help of advanced machine learning and deep learning techniques. It is not possible to rely on manual procedures for this type of analysis. Other medical imaging techniques like CT scan, X-ray are also linked with computer vision techniques in the treatment of any disease (Kassania et al., 2021).

Image processing techniques like digital image processing, image segmentation, edge detection, selection of images on the basis of region of interest (ROI) are used for the image analysis part (Islam et al., 2018). Image segmentation is the process of breaking down images into several segments to extract information. These modules called segments are the further processes. Each segment contains a specific region for analysis. They are frequently used as a part of preprocessing the images before applying the machine learning algorithms.

Thus, it is quite evident that the computer vision techniques along with other computer-aided diagnosis methods like image processing, machine learning techniques, and other deep learning techniques form the future of medicine and can transform the entire course of the diagnosis and treatment procedure booting the average life expectancy. One of the generic workflow of application of computer vision in medicine is as shown in Fig. 12.2.

12.5 Harnessing the power of natural language processing for intelligent healthcare solutions

NLP blends statistical, machine learning, and deep learning techniques with computational lingual—rule-based analysis of human speech. Together, these technologies allow computers to "interpret" human communication in the form of textual or audio data, including the participant's or author's intention and emotion. Several NLP activities help the machine understand what it's absorbing by breaking down human text and speech input in ways that the computer can understand (Parihar et al.). The following are some of these responsibilities:

Speech Recognition: It is the task of consistently turning audio information into text information is known as speech-to-text (Abdel-Hamid et al., 2014). Any program that performs audio signals or responds to spoken questions requires voice recognition.

Part of Speech Tagging: It is the method to find out the pronunciation of a specific word or series of words depending on its use and situation (Naseem et al., 2021).

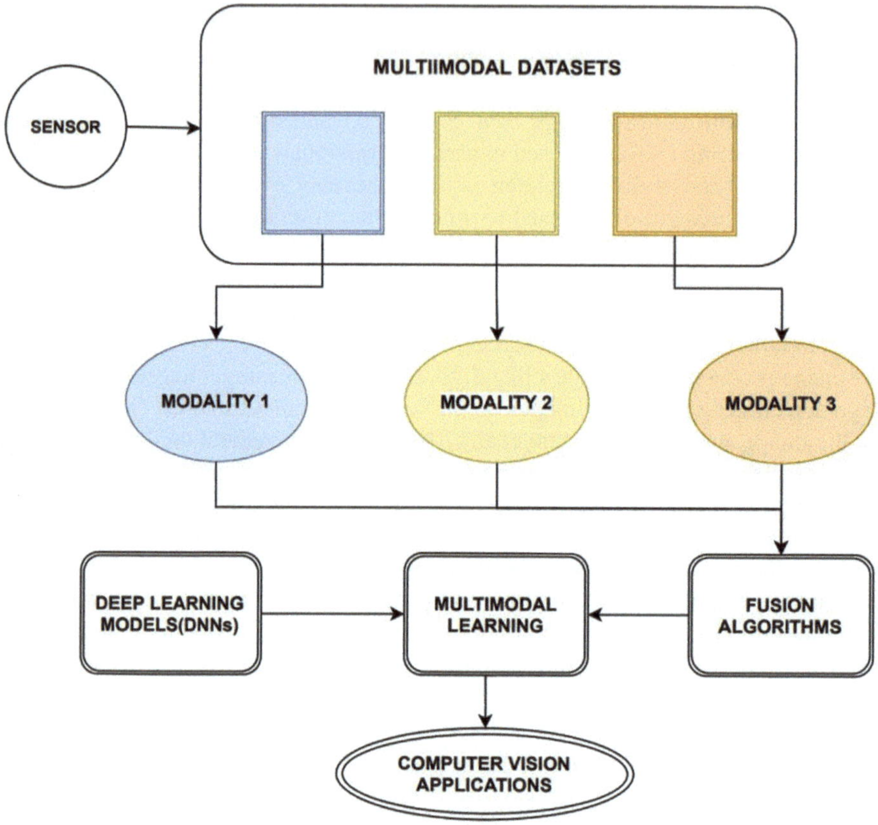

FIGURE 12.2 Generic workflow of application of computer vision in medicine.

Generic workflow of application of computer vision in medicine.

Word sense Disambiguation: It is the method of deciding the definition of a word with several meanings using a semantic procedure to discover which word makes more sense in the current scenario (Naseem et al., 2021).

Coreference Resolution: In this task, the process determines whether or not two words relate to the same item (Ng).

Sentiment Analysis: It seeks to obtain subjective aspects from text, such as opinions, reactions, humor, surprise, and doubt (Parihar et al.).

12.5.1 Handling clinical notes with natural language processing

NLP approaches must be developed in order to convert clinical material into structured medical data that can be handled immediately using ML algorithms (Thapa et al.). The use of NLP in the field of clinical is growing, with a wide range of applications such as the detection of biomedical ideas from radiology, nursing paperwork, and discharge instructions (Sheikhalishahi et al., 2019). To retrieve complex cancer characteristics from clinical text, NLP approaches are required. To identify the information of diseases, feature-rich methods require specialist expertise, such as linguistic, semantic, biological.

EHRs have been lauded for their ability to improve the quality of healthcare and serve as sources for rapid computerized patient identifying for research projects. Several diseases have been identified using NLP-based profiling algorithms, such as bowel syndrome, sclerosis, rheumatoid, asthmatic, and stomach cancer. To build and verify an NLP method for identifying critical limb ischemia (CLI) from clinical notes, researchers used a NLP algorithm (Afzal et al., 2018). They evaluated the CLI-NLP algorithm's performance on CLI-related ICD-9 itemized receipts. Human extraction of medical documentation from EHRs was the standard method for validation. The CLI-NLP method exhibited a better positive predictive value than billing codes.

12.5.2 Natural language processing for mental wellbeing

Inside AI in the field of biomedicine, NLP approaches have been identified as a key area of growth. Statistical difficulties, such as small sample size and recollection bias, have impeded suicide awareness studies. NLP methodologies have lately been utilized with EHR to improve extraction of information from text messaging comments as well as organized fields related to suicidal behavior (Fernandes et al., 2018), allowing access to considerably larger cohorts than previously allowed. Researchers can preprocess, identify, and assess classification models using NLP software for the Text Engineering platform. To assist with classification, preprocessing entails integrating tokenizers, sentence splitters, part-of-speech taggers, and semantic taggers to selected corpora.

Facebook demonstrated how modest tweaks to the Facebook news feed's filtering algorithm may have a big influence on users' moods. The experiment contrasted two filtering techniques, one of which reduced the number of positive statuses changes a person saw and the other being which suppressed negative Facebook statuses (Calvo et al., 2017). Much additional research uses Twitter to assess themes and feelings across whole populations in a similar way.

ML and NLP are AI techniques that allow for the effective examination of various data sets in order to uncover previously unknown trends and regularities. The first area of neuroscience to gain profit from the use of ML approaches to improve treatment plan was neuroimaging; lately, the use of ML methods to enhance motor function and language specification evaluation has shown promise in reducing the time it takes to perform patient evaluation.

12.6 Data-driven method for bioinformatics

As the amount of data generated in the biological sciences has increased at a very high pace with an increase in complexity, this is causing the research to move to a data-driven approach from a hypothesis-driven approach characterized by big data. Using data-driven approaches requires tools and computational methods that enable us to get the value and also create a new biological understanding. Bioinformatics is one such way to create new biological understanding (Larranaga et al., 2006). Bioinformatics is a field of computer science as well as biology that deals with collecting, handling, analyzing, and dissemination of biological data many times for DNA/RNA sequencing but also gene expressions and getting the information from protein. As the field of bioinformatics is growing rapidly it is a matter of immense interest that pace must be kept not just with getting new data but also generating new algorithms. There are four steps while solving a problem using bioinformatics. Search - This can be explained with the simple analogy of Google search. As we can search for information on topics on google which we want to know, we can similarly search to find biological identities like DNA, RNA, proteins, etc. We can also know more about diseases, compounds, drugs or metabolites, etc. Also, there are some databases like GenBank, ChEMBL, or PubChem that have chemical information, UniProt, and Protein Data Bank for information of protein, KEGG for biochemical pathways, etc. (Wratten et al., 2021).

Compare: Comparisons are a part of life and we compare just everything in our life. In bioinformatics, we need to compare genes or proteins and figure out how similar or different they are from each other (Pereira et al., 2020). Also, if they are similar then how so, etc.

Integrate and Curate: In the data science life cycle, a major portion is data collection and cleaning. We need to clearly define the research questions and then clean the data for subsequent data analysis to increase the reliability of the resulting analysis and model (Larranaga et al., 2006). In bioinformatics, one of the major challenges is to combine heterogeneous data sources and then remove the redundancy.

Model: A structural model is a two-dimensional or three-dimensional model of biological or chemical entities that are made up of virtual atoms that are joined to each other with chemical bonds. For example, the three-dimensional protein structure is made up of amino acids that are attached with peptide bonds. A predictive model using retrospective data is also built (Lai et al., 2018).

Now that we have seen the steps of bioinformatics, we will see what are the problems of bioinformatics that we can solve using AI.

12.6.1 DNA/RNA sequencing

To find the exact order among the nucleotides of a molecule of RNA or a DNA the method used is known as DNA/RNA sequencing. The order is among the four bases, i.e., guanine (G), thymine (T), cytosine (C), and adenine (A) in a DNA strand, This process can be used to find the individual genes sequence or the sequence in full chromosomes, or among entire genomes of an organism and is one of the most peculiar problems in biology.

To solve the problem of DNA/RNA sequencing many artificial intelligence-based approaches have come up in life science fields. For example, algorithms based on machine learning can be used for finding the patterns in RNA or a DNA sequence, for example accurately finding where the transcription start sites (TSSs) is located (Ohler et al., 2002). Also, they can be used in identifying the significance of the junk DNA in a genome and finding the untranslated regions (UTRs), exons as well as introns in eukaryotic chromosomes (Lai et al., 2018) Some more artificial intelligence-based methods are used to recognize, select, identify and classify the DNA sequences. Neural networks have come up as a very important AI algorithm for DNA sequence analysis because this method captures important features of intelligence which are not identified by the traditional symbolic and statistical methods. A classifier based on the neural network can also be used to identify genes in a DNA sequence (Anand & Huang, 2018).

Classifying the quality of DNA sequencing data as low quality or high quality is one of the most important tasks in the field of DNA sequencing. This can later be used so low-quality data can then later be reproduced. It can be seen as a two-class classification problem, i.e., low quality or high quality for which we can choose a support vector machine for classification. SVM gets trained on a training set and it learns the hyperplane and thus known as SVM learning. It is a really powerful technique to classify the data (Öz & Kaya, 2013). Promoters that are used to identify the genes can be predicted for a DNA sequence with the use of artificial neural networks and later their performance can be evaluated. SVM method can also be used to classify unlabeled inputs with the help of nonlinear kernel functions (Huang & Wang).

A hidden Markov model (HMM) is also a statistical model, which is very helpful for many of the tasks of biology. Sonnhammer et al., in 1998 (Sonnhammer et al.) and Boufounos et al., in 2004 (Boufounos et al., 2004) used the HMMs for DNA sequencing and developed a solution for the base calling problem of DNA sequencing. There are many more such examples where AI-based algorithms or models are playing a crucial role in DNA sequencing.

12.6.2 Extraction of information from protein

After the Human Genome Project and many efforts, data for DNA, RNA and proteins are getting collected at a very rapid pace. Mining these data to extract information is an essential step in genome processing. Many artificial intelligence-based techniques can help us to classify, extract information from a given protein data. Some of such techniques are:

Generative modeling of protein structure: GANs or generative adversarial network are neural networks that aim to learn the distribution of data. They can be used to artificially generate a data distribution. This technique of AI can be used to create protein structure for the prediction of an absent section of a manipulated structure of the protein. It uses a 3-dimensional protein structure that gets encoded as a 2-dimensional pairwise distance among the alpha-carbon also called 'maps'. Though this doesn't store the complete information and as the sequences are lost but it can be used for recovery of the structure (Huang & Wang).

Protein Homology Detection Based on MIL: Protein homology detection is the process of identification of similarities in protein sequence data based on its structure or function. One of the most important techniques for this is making n-grams and k-mers which are subsequences of consecutive symbols. So, when we represent it as a vector it shows the times the N-grams have appeared in a protein sequence. The value of N used here is small because a large value of N would lead to a long and sparse representation. Good results have been obtained by using multiple instance learning (MIL) for SVM-based discriminative techniques (Mensi et al.).

Protein Homology Detection Based on Profile: We can also detect the protein homology by creating a more descriptive representation of the sequence of protein data based on creating the feature vectors using a profile-based method with a position-specific frequency matrix (PSFM) for extracting the features which can remove noise from the profile by eliminating amino acids of low frequency (Liao et al.).

12.6.3 Analysis of gene expressions

Gene is the fundamental unit of all organisms. It holds the information to create and maintain the cells of an organism. When a gene is active it expresses a gene code also known as a gene expression. It is one of the most basic topics in cellular biology. It provides not only genetic characteristics of an organism but also physical or biochemical characteristics. Its analysis helps predict final protein products, helps cure disease by identification of abnormal cells, and also developing new drugs or vaccines (Raut et al.). With such a high-paced advancement in microarray technology gene expression data is getting generated in a very high throughput providing us the opportunity to apply machine learning models to analyze them.

Presently to classify genes we have two types of methods, i.e., supervised and unsupervised. In the former it is assumed that gene expression is mapped to a specific person and then this is used for the learning process while in unsupervised methods there is no such mapping; they are used to separate the expressions into classes by separating the unlabeled data into clusters. SVM, multilayer perceptron, and other supervised learning methods are more commonly used for the analysis of DNA microarray gene expression data (Furey et al., 2000; Valentini, 2002). In the unsupervised learning type most popular clustering algorithms used are hierarchical clustering, i.e., joining closest clusters after starting from a single cluster, K-mean clustering, and some other graph-based theoretic approaches like HCS (Hartuv & Shamir, 2000). As the gene is extremely high dimensional with very complex correlations it is a matter of great challenge to successfully apply these supervised and unsupervised learning methods. So, to get an intermediate solution of the twosome semisupervised algorithms are used that suggest using both labeled and unlabeled data for classification. It claims to have higher accuracy than the traditional supervised and unsupervised algorithms (Gong & Chen). There is still a huge scope of research in the field of bioinformatics which helps fight against diseases as well as for the manufacturing of new vaccines or drugs. With the generation of a large amount of biological data, it is become possible to use AI in bioinformatics. Soon we will be able to see lots of results in this field which will be very helpful to humankind.

12.7 Data-driven drug discovery and vaccine development

AI is proving to be one of the biggest assets in the field of health care. Not only it is capable to identify a pandemic, measuring the effectiveness of healthcare schemes, or detecting cancer but it is now also used for drug discovery and vaccine development. Using AI for drug discovery may seem a bit far-fetched but many effective drugs have been found with the help of AI. Many pharma companies have started to use AI for their R&D like Pfizer is using IBM Watson, an AI-based computer made by IBM to search for immunological drugs. They have also diagnosed a lady with leukemia using this. This AI-based approach can also be used for vaccine development. In the last few years, ML-based models when trained on certain biomolecules have presented cheap and quick implementation strategies for finding effective viral therapies. For a target biomolecule, these ML-based models can predict the inhibitor organism in a structured manner. If we could feed enough data to our model then it can help us to make a long-lasting and effective vaccine, even during COVID-19 pandemic, many researchers around the world proposed the vaccines developed using AI-based researches which assisted in the development of effective vaccines.

12.7.1 Data-driven drug discovery

Discovering a drug for a disease is similar to finding a lost key for a lock where in this case we are looking for a drug molecule that combines with the target molecule to perform a certain reaction. This looks similar to machine learning problems and thus artificial intelligence can be put to good use in this as the outcome of these reactions can be predicted by AI within a few seconds so we can try combinations of different compounds (Fleming, 2018).

There are two aspects of AI that are used. First is data mining, i.e., collecting research data, libraries on 3D molecular structure, properties of the molecule, etc. The second is using deep learning models to create binding profiles, e.g., convolutional neural networks can be used for this purpose which finds the best molecules under any set of parameters. Another deep learning is approach is based on using the network-driven discovery of drugs where instead of directly finding the effective molecule to the target molecule we try to find the ability of drug that can influence the network of disease. This is done using large databases and powerful computational methods (Lavecchia, 2019). Some current examples where AI is used for drug discovery are:

AtomNet: It is a deep convolutional network which is developed by a company named Atomwise. This network scrutinizes more than 100 million compounds each day and it has huge potential to find drugs for the disease Ebola (Wallach et al., 2015).

Exscientia: It is a pharmaceutical startup based out of Britain which created the first drug made with the help of AI, which is used to treat obsessive compulsive disorder (OCD) (Mullard, 2017).

There are many other companies that are working in this domain like Tubine.AI is a company working to find drugs for cancer patients. Antidote is a company trying to match researchers and patients for trials. A company named Insilco medicine made the headlines because it has developed a drug via its algorithm in just 45 days.

Major machine learning algorithms that are used for drug discovery are:

1. Random Forests: For the discovery of a drug these are mostly used for selecting features. They predict the affinity between the ligand molecule and the protein molecule by doing virtual screening with the help of molecular descriptors (Thapa et al.).
2. Naïve Bayes—based algorithms have shown high accuracy for the classification of biomedical data which are many times filled with noise, i.e., random information and data. They are also good at predicting ligand-target interactions (Thapa et al.).
3. Support Vector Machine: They are very important algorithms because they can be used in various scenarios. They have the power to distinguish between inactive and active compounds, they can be used to rank compounds in databases, they can also be used in training regression models, etc. (Thapa et al.).

12.7.2 Vaccine development with artificial intelligence

AI has started to play a major in drug discovery, likewise, it is also playing an important part in the field of vaccine development. To tackle with vaccine development problem, we first need to deal with the protein folding problem which means to predict the three-dimensional structure of the protein with amino acids as the sequence. So, we have to find the structure based on its amino acid sequence. Many companies are working in this domain as well for example a company named DeepMind launched a neural network-based framework known as Alphafold, which predicts the structure of a protein given its sequence of amino acids which was very accurate when compared with the actual structure. It used the ResNet deep learning algorithm was trained on 30K protein structures available in the protein database.

Once the structure of a protein is identified we can try to find an effective vaccine for it. Recently a group of scientists at MIT developed a vaccine using AI which used HLA haplotype frequencies to find the population coverage of potential vaccines (Liu et al., 2020). This vaccine provided 93.21% predicted population coverage with at least five vaccine peptide-HLA hits with all vaccine peptides perfectly conserved across 4690 geographically sampled people. Evaluation metrics used in this were EvalVax-Unlinked and EvalVax-Robust for the combinatorial optimization problem.

Using AI for vaccine development has proved to be very crucial and was used to develop the vaccine against the COVID-19 pandemic. One such vaccine developed was DeepVacPred, this vaccine used the in silico deep learning approach to multi-epitope the vaccine designs. This used the deep neural network architecture to find 26 fragments in SARS-CoV-2 spike protein and named them as vaccine subunit candidates. Then to develop the final vaccine linear B-cell epitopes, CTL epitopes, and HTL epitopes were predicted (Yang et al., 2021).

Various algorithms to analyze DNA and RNA sequences of the target pathogen to make effective vaccines have also been developed, e.g., Truncated Back Propagation Through Time (TBPTT) algorithm, which processes the viral sequence one step at a time, traits of the viral host can be predicted using the recurrent neural network (RNN). CNN can be used for the prediction of virus mutation (Kannan et al., 2020).

12.7.3 Artificial intelligence for antimicrobial resistance crisis

The amount of consumption of antibiotics has increased drastically in the last few years or so which is causing the problem of antimicrobial resistance (AMR) threatening global health. Various AI-based approaches have come up to tackle AMR and are crucial in preventing approx. 10 million deaths each year (Lv et al., 2021).

The commonly used AI approaches against AMR are:

1. **Naive Bayes:** This method is used to monitor the AMR. It was used by Rezaei-Hachesu et al. for the identification of resistance patterns as well as finding the important factors for the resistance (Rezaei-Hachesu et al., 2018). Also, Choisy et al. found the probabilities of ineffective treatment because of AMR with the help of a Naive Bayes—based approach (Choisy et al., 2019).
2. **Decision Tree:** Decision trees are very helpful in the decision-making of how to allocate medical resources so that the burden from AMR could be reduced. For example, Reynolds et al. used a decision tree model to find the cost of AMR and healthcare utilization finding that antibiotic selection is crucial and can provide considerable savings (Reynolds et al., 2014). To guide antibiotic use and shorten the treatment time a PCT (procalcitonin) -based decision tree model was used (Schuetz et al., 2012).
3. **Random Forest:** For the prediction of antibiotic combination this algorithm is used. For example, from chemogenomic data, A random forest model for the prediction of effective antibiotic combination therapies was developed by Chandrasekaran et al. (Chandrasekaran et al., 2016) Later Mason et al. used the molecular fingerprints as features to improve upon this model as the data developed was not sufficient in the former model (Mason et al., 2017).
4. **SVM:** To predict the phenotypes of AMR whether resistant or susceptible, SVM models are often used. For example, Her et al. (Her & Wu, 2018) used an SVM model to find that whether *E. coli* are resistant to antibiotics. Another use of the SVM model was to find the phenotype of five drugs (ampicillin, trimethoprim, tetracycline, enrofloxacin, and sulfisoxazole) (Her & Wu, 2018).
5. **Artificial neural networks:** Recently, a deep learning approach without any prior assumptions is developed to create new antibiotics using one of the artificial neural networks (Stokes et al., 2020).

AI is clearly playing a crucial role in our fight against AMR.

12.8 Epidemics and pandemics modeling with AI

12.8.1 Epidemic and pandemic modeling using AI

AI is playing a wide and important role in all the major industries. From driverless cars in the automobile industry to robots in the hospitality industry, AI had made things way too easy. On the same note, we should try to extend AI in the healthcare industry to prevent the lives of people. According to the various studies, it is believed that due to global warming and melting glaciers, more and more such pandemics can be seen in the near future (Nguyen et al., 2020). To prevent the losses of lives that we have witnessed during the COVID-19 can be stopped if we can prepare ourselves in advance, and AI models can be very helpful in this cause. It has been estimated that we could have saved more than 52%–90% of deaths in the United States if we had managed the COVID-19 cases more effectively. Considering all the fallbacks that we have witnessed in the current COVID-19 outbreak, we should develop more and more AI models to monitor the disease outbreaks, track the spread of the disease, avoid fake news during such pandemics.

12.8.2 Monitoring disease outbreaks with data and AI

In the recent decade, AI is playing a vital role in the healthcare industry, which is supported by the enormous amount of data we have. The health care researchers investigate the data collected from the physical world about the climate changes and various diseases people are getting in contact with around the words. Not only the data from the physical world but also the data in cyberspace which include the post made on social networking websites, various keywords searches help the researchers to investigate in the right direction (Zeng et al., 2021).

Now various AI and ML techniques help to depict the dependable variables such as when there can be a disease outbreak, what is the life cycle of the various disease-causing virus or bacteria. Now we will be discussing, how ML and AI techniques have been proved useful with physical data and cyberspace data.

12.8.3 AI techniques with the physical data

Based on the space-time data such as the economic status of the society, climate conditions, etc. collected from the physical world, ML techniques are applied to analyze the disease outbreaks.

In the past, we have witnessed the use of support vector machines (SVMs) (Vishwanathan & Murty) and random forests (RFs) (Thapa et al.) to prevent outbreaks of mosquito-borne diseases such as dengue and Chikungunya fever. The distribution of yellow fever mosquitoes was simulated using the SVMs and RFs which can be used to cut off the transmission path of these mosquitoes.

The risk of the ZIKV outbreak was predicted in the United States using the deep learning models which take the history of air travel volumes, vector distribution as input. In Taiwan, the AlexNet model (Yan et al., 2015) was constructed for examining the dengue hotspots in the town. This model was trained on the sea surface images along with the data on rainfall. The model had 100% accuracy.

12.8.4 AI techniques with the cyberspace data

Based on the data collected from the web such as the post made on social media, and keyword search, we can analyze the response to the infectious outbreak in different geographical locations. AI techniques are widely used for surveillance by detecting the sentiments from this data. Twitter has been proved highly effective in this task. Software that can track public sentiments can provide an early warning. The United Kingdom developed a similar software called DEFENDER that uses the SVM and Naive Bayes algorithm to integrate media news and tweets to detect outbreaks. Along with this Density-Based Spatial Clustering can be used to observe and track the behavior of the users. DEFENDER was also then integrated with the CNN and LSTM networks for further improvements. There exist many more such examples where data based on the physical world and cyberspace has been proved extremely useful and helped us to analyze the risk of disease outbreaks.

12.8.5 Intelligent techniques to track the spread

The best way to stop the spread of disease is to track the spread of the disease. The AI has been proved exceptional in tracking the spread of the disease. A Canadian company designed software that can predict infectious diseases. It also tracks the speed of the spread of the infection. It combines the epidemiologists' knowledge with AI. It analyzed the risk that various diseases pose and send the report to the health researchers (Nguyen et al., 2020).

Many apps were created during the recent COVID-19 outbreak, which tracked the covid infected patient and notify the persons that came in contact with the infected person. This helped the persons to quarantine themselves and stopped the spread. "AROGYA SETU" app is one of the examples of such an app (Kodali et al., 2020).

During the recent COVID-19 outbreak, Robots were used to provide food and medicines to the infected person so as to minimize contact with them and avoid cross-contamination. One of the examples is China, which used drones for contact-less delivery. The robots were also used in China to spray disinfectants. AI was also used to read the chest X-ray so as to reduce the load on the hospital staff (Reynolds et al., 2014).

AI was also used to avoid the spread of fake news. According to a study in Brazil, about 20% of the news spreading on Facebook or WhatsApp was fake, and because of all this, the Google search about the keywords related to fake news was increased by 34% (de Barcelos et al., 2021). In such cases, stopping the spread of fake news is one of the most important tasks to avoid panic. Many models using the NLP were constructed to avoid the spread of these news which played an important role in managing the COVID outbreak and also can be useful in future outbreaks.

12.8.6 Data-driven modeling of pandemics

As the pandemic continues, it becomes more and more important to model the statistics and learn lessons from the current situation to prevent any further destruction to lives and the same mistakes in the future. Any key pandemic model can be broken down into four stages. Each stage needs a different type of data, different tools, and has different challenges (Desai et al., 2019). We will now describe each stage in brief.

1. **Prepandemic:** This is the time when there are not so many people infected with the pandemic, and it is not yet declared as a pandemic. Here we basically need to understand the risk to different countries, symptoms of the disease. The data we need at this time includes travel restrictions, any data on similar kinds of viruses in the past, and the clinical investigations on the infected people (Ghimire et al.). Clinical investigations include the date of first symptoms observed, date of death/recovery, symptoms, etc.
2. **Acceleration:** When the disease covers the country, it comes in the accelerating stage. Here we need the data on how different regions are connected to each other, how countries are connected to each other so that we can minimize the acceleration of the epidemic. It also includes the data on the population of the country and the populations infected with the epidemic (Zeng et al., 2021).
3. **Mitigation:** Once the country is hit by an epidemic outbreak, the government tries to mitigate and control the spread. The key question in this model is what is the healthcare infrastructure needed, and what is the best intervention to stop the spread. As in the case of COVID-19, countries failed to predict the need for infrastructure and as a result, many persons have to lose their lives due to the lack of oxygen and other medical facilities. In this stage modeling we need data related to different strategies suggested and their impact on the virus, e.g., data on how social distancing helped during the COVID-19 spread or how PPE kits and masks helped to stop the spread (Nguyen et al., 2020).
4. **Suppression:** This stage involves different ways to control the outbreak. This includes contact tracing, apps like Arogya Setu can be used for this purpose (Kodali et al., 2020). This can help to isolate the infected person and maybe we can isolate the neighbors of the person or the in contact with the infected person in the last few days according to the mutation period of the virus.

12.9 AI for efficient healthcare resource management and in-hospital care

In many countries like the United States, healthcare services are where costly as well as cumbersome. The use of AI in this field can solve many of these problems like bed management, standing in long queues, resource management, etc. These same problems are also posed in traditional businesses and AI has provided a good solution for them so because such problems require pattern matching, optimization problems, or some intelligent search algorithms which all are the key solutions provided by artificial intelligence (Ghimire et al.). The only problem that could have come up because of the use of AI was data privacy which is a big concern when dealing with healthcare systems but the fact that operational difficulties do not involve much information regarding the patient like disease, diagnosis, etc. makes AI much more suitable to use (Adhikari et al.). The use of AI in this field should not only focus on profit-making but also on making the system easier for common people.

12.9.1 Use of AI for resource management

The concern with the use of AI is that it can only work with tasks that are defined well. It hasn't developed enough that it can replace doctors but still there are many places where it will find its good use. Such places can be:

1. **Bed management:** The biggest concern while admitting a patient to the hospital is to identify more critical patients and prioritize bed availability to them. Not limiting to this also managing the beds such that people with similar diseases are closer to each other. Not limiting to bed but also all the extra first aids and medicine with each bed is sufficient or not. These all problems can be easily solved with the help of AI. This can help by reducing the staff required and provides also provides an efficient way to manage the beds (Klumpp et al.).
2. **Data of patients:** Another important field of AI that is helpful is big data. In many countries like China, all the data regarding the patients was stored and each patient was provided with a QR code. This is also known as EHR. So, this made the system of patients easy that now they need not take the complete file of their reports, the doctor just needs to scan the QR code and the whole medical history of the patient was easily available (Devyania et al., 2020).
3. **Scheduling doctors:** AI can help to schedule and hence optimize the doctor's time for the patient and the doctor can devote more time for the critical patients. AI-based virtual assistants can be developed who will be present with the patient all the time that can carry out some tasks and the doctor will need to visit only when he is needed (Ghimire et al.).

12.9.2 Use of AI in in-hospital care

Now that we have seen how AI can help us in tackling resource-related problems we will now look at more patient-oriented services that AI will provide. Some of the in-hospital services that AI provides are:

1. **Disease prediction and Diagnosis:** Though a large amount of research is ongoing in using AI in the healthcare sector still most of the research focuses on cancer, the nervous or the cardiovascular system. Chronic and infectious diseases are also getting decent attention and now it has been made possible to get an early diagnosis for many conditions. This can be done by, first, the quality of clinical insight should be improved, and later this insight should be fed to a well-trained system (Jiang et al., 2017). One of the examples of such an approach is FDA in

the United States using this to detect fracture of wrists in patients (Vakula & Raviteja). There were many instances of the use of AI to detect coronavirus based on the X-ray report of patients. Image heatmap pattern recognition reported 74% accuracy among patients tested for major depressive disorder.

2. **Treatment effectiveness and outcome prediction:** It is again one of the major fields where AI can prove to be very useful. A few years back only molecular information and information by on clinical trials was the basis for the prediction of the outcome of cancer in a patient but now with the development of imaging, genomic technologies new kinds of inputs are collected, and predictions are made through them, with a considerable amount of data collected it has been seen that these algorithms can increase the accuracy of the prediction by up to 15%–20% (Cruz & Wishart, 2006). A supervised machine learning model was also used to study congestive heart failure on 396 patients among which 46 were clinical variables. The phenotypic heat map proved to be much more accurate than traditionally used risk assessment tools (Noorbakhsh-Sabet et al., 2019).
3. **Epidemic prediction: The** pattern of distribution of any infectious disease has a distribution pattern among the groups of the population based on ecological and biological features of the environment. If these parameters are partially known then we can predict an upcoming epidemic, e.g., the outbreak of filovirus was predicted in Uganda relating to the distribution of the bat in the area and previous outbreaks (Nyakarahuka et al., 2017). The morbidity rate of dengue fever was accurately predicted in parts of central Thailand with the help of estimation of the infectious rate among female *Aedes aegypti* larva (Kesorn et al., 2015).
4. **Prediction of recovery time:** The recovery time of the patient can also be predicted with the help of machine-learning-based algorithms. The recovery time for patients suffering from COVID-19 was predicted. Boosted random forest-based classifier gave a very high accuracy in predicting recovery time among patients.

Though the use of AI is becoming very common in the health care sector still there are lots of challenges faced by this because the margin for error is very small and it is still difficult to gain the trust of both the clinicians and the patients. Data privacy is another big concern but with rapid advancement, in technology, the power of machine learning to change data into insight will help the field of healthcare, and soon we will be able to see improvements in the field with the help of AI.

12.10 Remote healthcare

Remote medical care is a telemedicine that enables continuous monitoring of a medical illness as well as prevention and control strategies examinations outside of healthcare facilities. The use of mobile devices that monitor vitals enables this standard of treatment. Remote healthcare is made up of hardware and software that allow for quick and easy measurements of a patient's vital signs (Battineni et al.). The basic operation of remote healthcare is ECG, saturation, blood pressure, weight, and temperature.

12.10.1 Chatbots for remote healthcare

Automatic conversation bots that run on a programming language or a type of AI interaction between users and computers with the assistance of NLP are known as virtual chatbots. Governments have struggled to provide enough medical specialists, funds, and technology to hospitals and healthcare centers because of the constant flow of patients (Battineni et al.). As a result, an AI medical chatbot can help relieve the strain on health systems by determining the severity of disease. It also includes all of the required precautions, such as contacts with live specialists.

12.10.2 AI-enabled remote patient monitoring

Large-scale diagnostic testing is not possible in today's medical systems due to a lack of resources. As a result, vital sign observation might be used as a criterion for prioritizing testing. Hospital stays for vital sign monitoring, on the other hand (Pramanik et al., 2019), can result in an increase in preventing the transmission. Deep learning algorithms for vision-based analytics have provided revolutionary productivity advances, paving the way for the creation of nonintrusive or contactless diagnostics. Such methods can be extremely valuable for early monitoring and detection of diseases that are easily transferred, such as COVID-19. For edge-based patient monitoring, blockchain based techniques have also been proposed (Rohmetra et al., 2021). Many of these jobs can be performed remotely using ML-based algorithms, however some may necessitate the usage of specific equipment.

12.10.3 AI-enabled telemedicine

Many possibilities try to enhance care efficiency, availability, and clinical outcomes through telemedicine, but there are numerous problems relating to technology compatibility, the digital divide, and usability. Telemedicine develops to enable continuum of care throughout the patient journey, incorporating multidisciplinary care teams and the smooth integrating of data into the healthcare setting (Sun et al., 2021). Telemedicine must allow for multi-party communication as well as safe data sharing across teams and contexts. During the virtual appointment, the telemedicine system should allow access to the patient's history and medicines, as well as capture and record important patient information.

12.11 Conclusion

There are numerous areas within the healthcare industry where AI can be used. These systems can especially be more useful at the times like pandemic where health workers have hard time handling the cases. From diagnosis to treatment and better management of the disease, AI has played phenomenal role. There are some challenges too when it comes to using AI in the healthcare industry. The problems like data privacy, bias in models, etc. might arise with inculcation of AI in the healthcare industry. Despite the drawbacks, there are a lot of advantages that would easily outweigh the drawbacks. Thus, the future is clear, it will have data-driven systems extensively used in the healthcare industry.

References

Abdel-Hamid, O., Mohamed, A.-r., Jiang, H., Deng, L., Penn, G., & Yu, D. (2014). Convolutional neural networks for speech recognition. *IEEE/ACM Transactions on Audio, Speech, and Language Processing, 22*, 1533–1545.

Adhikari, S., Thapa, S., & Ghimire, A. (2021). Soft computing techniques for medical diagnosis, prognosis and treatment. In *Advanced soft computing techniques in data science, IoT and cloud computing* (pp. 371–399). Springer.

Adhikari, S., Thapa, S., Singh, P., Huo, H., Bharathy, G., & Prasad, M. A comparative study of machine learning and NLP techniques for uses of stop words by patients in diagnosis of alzheimer's disease. In *Proceedings of 2021 international joint conference on neural networks (IJCNN)* (pp. 1–8).

Afzal, N., Mallipeddi, V. P., Sohn, S., Liu, H., Chaudhry, R., Scott, C. G., Kullo, I. J., & Arruda-Olson, A. M. (2018). Natural language processing of clinical notes for identification of critical limb ischemia. *International Journal of Medical Informatics, 111*, 83–89.

Anand, N., & Huang, P. (2018). *Generative modeling for protein structures*.

Bader, F., & Jagtap, S. (2020). Internet of things-linked wearable devices for managing food safety in the healthcare sector. In *Wearable and implantable medical devices* (pp. 229–253). Elsevier.

de Barcelos, T., Muniz, L. N., Dantas, D. M., DF, C. J., Cavalcante, J. R., & Faerstein, E. (2021). Analysis of fake news disseminated during the COVID-19 pandemic in BrazilAnálisis de las noticias falsas divulgadas durante la pandemia de COVID-19 en Brasil. *Revista Panamericana de Salud Publica= Pan American Journal of Public Health, 45*. e65–e65.

Battineni, G., Chintalapudi, N., & Amenta, F. AI chatbot design during an epidemic like the novel coronavirus. In *Proceedings of healthcare* p. 154.

Batty, M. (2013). Big data, smart cities and city planning. *Dialogues in Human Geography, 3*, 274–279.

Behera, R. K., Bala, P. K., & Dhir, A. (2019). The emerging role of cognitive computing in healthcare: A systematic literature review. *International Journal of Medical Informatics, 129*, 154–166.

Boufounos, P., El-Difrawy, S., & Ehrlich, D. (2004). Basecalling using hidden Markov models. *Journal of the Franklin Institute, 341*, 23–36.

Brugarolas, R., Dieffenderfer, J., Walker, K., Wagner, A., Sherman, B., Roberts, D., & Bozkurt, A. (2014). Wearable wireless biophotonic and biopotential sensors for canine health monitoring. In *Proceedings of SENSORS* (pp. 2203–2206). IEEE.

Calvillo, C. F., Sánchez-Miralles, A., & Villar, J. (2016). Energy management and planning in smart cities. *Renewable and Sustainable Energy Reviews, 55*, 273–287.

Calvo, R. A., Milne, D. N., Hussain, M. S., & Christensen, H. (2017). Natural language processing in mental health applications using non-clinical texts. *Natural Language Engineering, 23*, 649–685.

Chandrasekaran, S., Cokol-Cakmak, M., Sahin, N., Yilancioglu, K., Kazan, H., Collins, J. J., & Cokol, M. (2016). Chemogenomics and orthology-based design of antibiotic combination therapies. *Molecular Systems Biology, 12*, 872.

Choisy, M., Van Cuong, N., Bao, T. D., Kiet, B. T., Hien, B. V., Thu, H. V., Chansiripornchai, N., Setyawan, E., Thwaites, G., & Rushton, J. (2019). Assessing antimicrobial misuse in small-scale chicken farms in Vietnam from an observational study. *BMC Veterinary Research, 15*, 1–10.

Coccoli, M., Maresca, P., & Stanganelli, L. (2016). Cognitive computing in education. *Journal of E-Learning and Knowledge Society, 12.*

Colantonio, S., Coppini, G., Giorgi, D., Morales, M.-A., & Pascali, M. A. (2018). Computer vision for ambient assisted living: Monitoring systems for personalized healthcare and wellness that are robust in the real world and accepted by users, carers, and society. In *Computer vision for assistive healthcare* (pp. 147–182). Elsevier.

Cruz, J. A., & Wishart, D. S. (2006). Applications of machine learning in cancer prediction and prognosis. *Cancer Informatics, 2*, 117693510600200030.

Davenport, T., & Kalakota, R. (2019). The potential for artificial intelligence in healthcare. *Future Healthcare Journal, 6*, 94.

Desai, A. N., Kraemer, M. U., Bhatia, S., Cori, A., Nouvellet, P., Herringer, M., Cohn, E. L., Carrion, M., Brownstein, J. S., & Madoff, L. C. (2019). Real-time epidemic forecasting: Challenges and opportunities. *Health Security, 17*, 268–275.

Devyania, R. D., Jewanc, S. Y., Bansal, U., & Denge, X. (2020). Strategic impact of artificial intelligence on the human resource management of the Chinese healthcare industry induced due to COVID-19. *IETI Transactions on Economics and Management, 1*, 19–33.

Djelouat, H., Baali, H., Amira, A., & Bensaali, F. IoT based compressive sensing for ECG monitoring. In *Proceedings of 2017 IEEE international conference on internet of things (iThings) and IEEE green computing and communications (GreenCom) and IEEE cyber, physical and social computing (CPSCom) and IEEE smart data (SmartData)* (pp. 183–189).

Drobot, A., Lewis, E., & Stuttgen, H. (2019). IEEE 5th world forum on internet of things brings together 500 experts to discuss the future of IoT. *IEEE Internet of Things Magazine, 2*, 44–46.

Esteva, A., Robicquet, A., Ramsundar, B., Kuleshov, V., DePristo, M., Chou, K., Cui, C., Corrado, G., Thrun, S., & Dean, J. (2019). A guide to deep learning in healthcare. *Nature Medicine, 25*, 24–29.

Fernandes, A. C., Dutta, R., Velupillai, S., Sanyal, J., Stewart, R., & Chandran, D. (2018). Identifying suicide ideation and suicidal attempts in a psychiatric clinical research database using natural language processing. *Scientific Reports, 8*, 1–10.

Fleming, N. (2018). How artificial intelligence is changing drug discovery. *Nature, 557.* S55–S55.

Freedson, P. S., & Miller, K. (2000). Objective monitoring of physical activity using motion sensors and heart rate. *Research Quarterly for Exercise and Sport, 71*, 21–29.

Furey, T. S., Cristianini, N., Duffy, N., Bednarski, D. W., Schummer, M., & Haussler, D. (2000). Support vector machine classification and validation of cancer tissue samples using microarray expression data. *Bioinformatics, 16*, 906–914.

Ghimire, A., Thapa, S., Jha, A.K., Adhikari, S., & Kumar, A. Accelerating business growth with big data and artificial intelligence. In *Proceedings of 2020 fourth international conference on I-smac (IoT in social, mobile, analytics and cloud)(I-smac)* pp. (441–448).

Ghimire, A., Thapa, S., Jha, A.K., Kumar, A., Kumar, A., & Adhikari, S. AI and IoT solutions for tackling COVID-19 pandemic. In *Proceedings of 2020 4th international conference on electronics, communication and aerospace technology (ICECA)* pp. (1083–1092).

Gong, Y.-C., & Chen, C.-L. Semi-supervised method for gene expression data classification with Gaussian fields and harmonic functions. In *Proceedings of 2008 19th international conference on pattern recognition* pp. (1–4).

Han, C., Rundo, L., Murao, K., Nemoto, T., & Nakayama, H. Bridging the gap between AI and healthcare sides: Towards developing clinically relevant AI-powered diagnosis systems. In *Proceedings of IFIP international conference on artificial intelligence applications and innovations* pp. (320–333).

Hartuv, E., & Shamir, R. (2000). A clustering algorithm based on graph connectivity. *Information Processing Letters, 76*, 175–181.

Her, H.-L., & Wu, Y.-W. (2018). A pan-genome-based machine learning approach for predicting antimicrobial resistance activities of the *Escherichia coli* strains. *Bioinformatics, 34*, i89–i95.

Huang, Y.-F., & Wang, C.-M. Integration of knowledge-discovery and artificial-intelligence approaches for promoter recognition in DNA sequences. In *Proceedings of third international conference on information technology and applications (ICITA'05)*; pp. (459–464).

Isafiade, O. E., & Bagula, A. B. (2020). Series mining for public safety advancement in emerging smart cities. *Future Generation Computer Systems, 108*, 777–802.

Islam, S. M. S., Hasan, M. M., & Abdullah, S. (2018). *Deep learning based early detection and grading of diabetic retinopathy using retinal fundus images*. arXiv preprint arXiv: 1812.10595.

Jha, A. K., Ghimire, A., Thapa, S., Jha, A. M., & Raj, R. (2021). A review of AI for urban planning: Towards building sustainable smart cities. In *Proceedings of 2021 6th international conference on inventive computation technologies (ICICT)* (pp. 937–944).

Jiang, F., Jiang, Y., Zhi, H., Dong, Y., Li, H., Ma, S., Wang, Y., Dong, Q., Shen, H., & Wang, Y. (2017). Artificial intelligence in healthcare: Past, present and future. *Stroke and Vascular Neurology, 2*.

Jorquera-Chavez, M., Fuentes, S., Dunshea, F. R., Warner, R. D., Poblete, T., Unnithan, R. R., Morrison, R. S., & Jongman, E. C. (2021). Using imagery and computer vision as remote monitoring methods for early detection of respiratory disease in pigs. *Computers and Electronics in Agriculture, 187*, 106283.

Kannan, S., Subbaram, K., Ali, S., & Kannan, H. (2020). The role of artificial intelligence and machine learning techniques: Race for covid-19 vaccine. *Archives of Clinical Infectious Diseases*, 15.

Kassania, S. H., Kassanib, P. H., Wesolowskic, M. J., Schneidera, K. A., & Detersa, R. (2021). Automatic detection of coronavirus disease (COVID-19) in X-ray and CT images: A machine learning based approach. *Biocybernetics and Biomedical Engineering, 41*, 867–879.

Kesorn, K., Ongruk, P., Chompoosri, J., Phumee, A., Thavara, U., Tawatsin, A., & Siriyasatien, P. (2015). Morbidity rate prediction of dengue hemorrhagic fever (DHF) using the support vector machine and the *Aedes aegypti* infection rate in similar climates and geographical areas. *PloS One, 10*, e0125049.

Khedkar, S., Gandhi, P., Shinde, G., & Subramanian, V. (2020). Deep learning and explainable AI in healthcare using EHR. In *Deep learning techniques for biomedical and health informatics* (pp. 129–148). Springer.

Klumpp, M., Hintze, M., Immonen, M., Ródenas-Rigla, F., Pilati, F., Aparicio-Martínez, F., Çelebi, D., Liebig, T., Jirstrand, M., & Urbann, O. Artificial intelligence for hospital health care: Application cases and answers to challenges in european hospitals. In *Proceedings of healthcare*; p. 961.

Kodali, P. B., Hense, S., Kopparty, S., Kalapala, G. R., & Haloi, B. (2020). How Indians responded to the Arogya Setu app? *Indian Journal of Public Health, 64*, 228.

Kumar, V., Ghimire, A., Hoon, H.K. Machine Learning and IoT based solutions for detection of arrhythmia using ECG signals. In *Proceedings of 2021 5th international conference on trends in electronics and informatics (ICOEI)* (pp. 477−484).

Lai, K., Twine, N., O'brien, A., Guo, Y., & Bauer, D. (2018). Artificial intelligence and machine learning in bioinformatics. *Encyclopedia of Bioinformatics and Computational Biology: ABC of Bioinformatics, 55*, 272.

Larranaga, P., Calvo, B., Santana, R., Bielza, C., Galdiano, J., Inza, I., Lozano, J. A., Armananzas, R., Santafé, G., & Pérez, A. (2006). Machine learning in bioinformatics. *Briefings in Bioinformatics, 7*, 86−112.

Lavecchia, A. (2019). Deep learning in drug discovery: Opportunities, challenges and future prospects. *Drug Discovery Today, 24*, 2017−2032.

Lazarova-Molnar, S., & Mohamed, N. (2016). Challenges in the data collection for diagnostics of smart buildings. In *Information science and applications (ICISA) 2016* (pp. 941−951). Springer.

Liao, Q., Guo, M., & Liu, B. Protein remote homology detection based on profiles. In *Proceedings of international work-conference on bioinformatics and biomedical engineering*; pp. (261−268).

Liu, G., Carter, B., Bricken, T., Jain, S., Viard, M., Carrington, M., & Gifford, D. K. (2020). Computationally optimized SARS-CoV-2 MHC class I and II vaccine formulations predicted to target human haplotype distributions. *Cell Systems, 11*, 131−144. e136.

Lv, J., Deng, S., & Zhang, L. (2021). A review of artificial intelligence applications for antimicrobial resistance. *Biosafety and Health, 3*, 22−31.

Mason, D. J., Stott, I., Ashenden, S., Weinstein, Z. B., Karakoc, I., Meral, S., Kuru, N., Bender, A., & Cokol, M. (2017). Prediction of antibiotic interactions using descriptors derived from molecular structure. *Journal of Medicinal Chemistry, 60*, 3902−3912.

Mensi, A.; Bicego, M.; Lovato, P.; Loog, M.; Tax, D.M. Protein remote homology detection using dissimilarity-based multiple instance learning. In *Proceedings of joint IAPR international workshops on statistical techniques in pattern recognition (SPR) and structural and syntactic pattern recognition (SSPR)*; pp. (119−129).

Mullard, A. (2017). The drug-maker's guide to the galaxy. *Nature News, 549*, 445.

Naseem, U., Razzak, I., Khan, S. K., & Prasad, M. (2021). A comprehensive survey on word representation models: From classical to state-of-the-art word representation language models. *Transactions on Asian and Low-Resource Language Information Processing, 20*, 1−35.

Negi, A., Raj, S., Thapa, S., & Indu, S. (2021). Field programmable gate array (FPGA) based IoT for smart city applications. In *Data-driven mining, learning and analytics for secured smart cities* (pp. 135−158). Springer.

Ng, V. Learning noun phrase anaphoricity to improve conference resolution: Issues in representation and optimization. In *Proceedings of proceedings of the 42nd annual meeting of the association for computational linguistics (ACL-04)*; pp. (151−158).

Nguyen, T. T., Nguyen, Q. V. H., Nguyen, D. T., Hsu, E. B., Yang, S., & Eklund, P. (2020). *Artificial intelligence in the battle against coronavirus (COVID-19): A survey and future research directions.* arXiv preprint arXiv:2008.07343.

Noorbakhsh-Sabet, N., Zand, R., Zhang, Y., & Abedi, V. (2019). Artificial intelligence transforms the future of health care. *The American Journal of Medicine, 132*, 795–801.

Nyakarahuka, L., Ayebare, S., Mosomtai, G., Kankya, C., Lutwama, J., Mwiine, F. N., & Skjerve, E. (2017). Ecological niche modeling for filoviruses: A risk map for Ebola and marburg virus disease outbreaks in Uganda. *PLoS Currents, 9*.

Ohler, U., Liao, G.-c., Niemann, H., & Rubin, G. M. (2002). Computational analysis of core promoters in the Drosophila genome. *Genome Biology, 3*, 1–12.

Öz, E., & Kaya, H. (2013). Support vector machines for quality control of DNA sequencing. *Journal of Inequalities and Applications, 2013*, 1–9.

Parihar, A.S., Thapa, S., & Mishra, S. Hate speech detection using natural language processing: Applications and challenges. In *Proceedings of 2021 5th international conference on trends in electronics and informatics (ICOEI)*; pp. (1302–1308).

Pasluosta, C. F., Gassner, H., Winkler, J., Klucken, J., & Eskofier, B. M. (2015). An emerging era in the management of Parkinson's disease: Wearable technologies and the internet of things. *IEEE Journal of Biomedical and Health Informatics, 19*, 1873–1881.

Pereira, R., Oliveira, J., & Sousa, M. (2020). Bioinformatics and computational tools for next-generation sequencing analysis in clinical genetics. *Journal of Clinical Medicine, 9*, 132.

Pramanik, P. K. D., Pareek, G., & Nayyar, A. (2019). Security and privacy in remote healthcare: Issues, solutions, and standards. In *Telemedicine technologies* (pp. 201–225). Elsevier.

Rahmat, M. A., Su, E., Addi, M. M., & Yeong, C. (2017). GluQo: IoT-based non-invasive blood glucose monitoring. *Journal of Telecommunication, Electronic and Computer Engineering (JTEC), 9*, 71–75.

Raut, S.A., Sathe, S., & Raut, A. Bioinformatics: Trends in gene expression analysis. In *Proceedings of 2010 international conference on bioinformatics and biomedical technology* pp. (97–100).

Reynolds, C. A., Finkelstein, J. A., Ray, G. T., Moore, M. R., & Huang, S. S. (2014). Attributable healthcare utilization and cost of pneumoniae due to drug-resistant Streptococcus pneumoniae: A cost analysis. *Antimicrobial Resistance and Infection Control, 3*, 1–8.

Rezaei-Hachesu, P., Samad-Soltani, T., Yaghoubi, S., GhaziSaeedi, M., Mirnia, K., Masoumi-Asl, H., & Safdari, R. (2018). The design and evaluation of an antimicrobial resistance surveillance system for neonatal intensive care units in Iran. *International Journal of Medical Informatics, 115*, 24–34.

Rohmetra, H., Raghunath, N., Narang, P., Chamola, V., Guizani, M., & Lakkaniga, N. R. (2021). AI-enabled remote monitoring of vital signs for COVID-19: Methods, prospects and challenges. *Computing*, 1–27.

Sahu, M. L., Atulkar, M., Ahirwal, M. K., & Ahamad, A. (2021). IoT-enabled cloud-based real-time remote ECG monitoring system. *Journal of Medical Engineering & Technology*, 1–13.

Schuetz, P., Amin, D. N., & Greenwald, J. L. (2012). Role of procalcitonin in managing adult patients with respiratory tract infections. *Chest, 141*, 1063–1073.

Shah, R., & Chircu, A. (2018). IoT and AI in healthcare: A systematic literature review. *Issues in Information Systems, 19*.

Sheikhalishahi, S., Miotto, R., Dudley, J. T., Lavelli, A., Rinaldi, F., & Osmani, V. (2019). natural language processing of clinical notes on chronic diseases: Systematic review. *JMIR Medical Informatics, 7*, e12239.

Snoonian, D. (2003). Smart buildings. *IEEE Spectrum, 40*, 18–23.

Song, H., Nguyen, A.-D., Gong, M., & Lee, S. (2016). A review of computer vision methods for purpose on computer-aided diagnosis. *Journal of International Society for Simulation Surgery, 3*, 1–8.

Sonnhammer, E.L., Von Heijne, G., & Krogh, A. A hidden Markov model for predicting transmembrane helices in protein sequences. In *Proceedings of ismb*; pp. (175–182).

Stokes, J. M., Yang, K., Swanson, K., Jin, W., Cubillos-Ruiz, A., Donghia, N. M., MacNair, C. R., French, S., Carfrae, L. A., & Bloom-Ackermann, Z. (2020). A deep learning approach to antibiotic discovery. *Cell, 180*, 688–702. e613.

Sun, R., Blayney, D. W., & Hernandez-Boussard, T. (2021). Health management via telemedicine: Learning from the COVID-19 experience. *Journal of the American Medical Informatics Association, 28*, 2536–2540.

Tanveer, M., Richhariya, B., Khan, R., Rashid, A., Khanna, P., Prasad, M., & Lin, C. (2020). Machine learning techniques for the diagnosis of alzheimer's disease: A review. *ACM Transactions on Multimedia Computing, Communications, and Applications (TOMM), 16*, 1–35.

Tarafdar, M., Beath, C. M., & Ross, J. W. (2017). Enterprise cognitive computing applications: Opportunities and challenges. *IT Professional, 19*, 21–27.

Thapa, S., Adhikari, S., Naseem, U., Singh, P., Bharathy, G., & Prasad, M. Detecting Alzheimer's disease by exploiting linguistic information from Nepali transcript. In *Proceedings of international conference on neural information processing*; pp. (176–184).

Thapa, S., Singh, P., Jain, D.K., Bharill, N., Gupta, A., & Prasad, M. Data-driven approach based on feature selection technique for early diagnosis of Alzheimer's disease. In *Proceedings of 2020 international joint conference on neural networks (IJCNN)*; pp. (1–8).

Thevenot, J., López, M. B., & Hadid, A. (2017). A survey on computer vision for assistive medical diagnosis from faces. *IEEE Journal of Biomedical and Health Informatics, 22*, 1497–1511.

Tsai, C.-W., Lai, C.-F., Chao, H.-C., & Vasilakos, A. V. (2015). Big data analytics: A survey. *Journal of Big Data, 2*, 1–32.

Turner, A. P. (2013). Biosensors: Sense and sensibility. *Chemical Society Reviews, 42*, 3184–3196.

Vakula, D., & Raviteja, B. Smart public transport for smart cities. In *Proceedings of 2017 international conference on intelligent sustainable systems (ICISS)* (pp. 805–810).

Valentini, G. (2002). Supervised gene expression data analysis using Support Vector Machines and Multi-Layer perceptrons. In *Proc. Of KES'2002, special session machine learning in bioinformatics*.

Vattapparamban, E., Güvenç, I., Yurekli, A.I., Akkaya, K., & Uluağaç, S. Drones for smart cities: Issues in cybersecurity, privacy, and public safety. In *Proceedings of 2016 international wireless communications and mobile computing conference (IWCMC)* (pp. 216–221).

Vishwanathan, S., & Murty, M.N. Ssvm: A simple SVM algorithm. In *Proceedings of proceedings of the 2002 international joint conference on neural networks. IJCNN'02 (cat. No. 02CH37290)*; pp. (2393–2398).

Wallach, I., Dzamba, M., & Heifets, A. (2015). *AtomNet: A deep convolutional neural network for bioactivity prediction in structure-based drug discovery* arXiv preprint arXiv:1510.02855.

Winck, J. C., & Ambrosino, N. (2020). COVID-19 pandemic and non invasive respiratory management: Every goliath needs a david. An evidence based evaluation of problems. *Pulmonology, 26*, 213–220.

Wratten, L., Wilm, A., & Göke, J. (2021). Reproducible, scalable, and shareable analysis pipelines with bioinformatics workflow managers. *Nature Methods, 18*, 1161–1168.

Yang, Z., Bogdan, P., & Nazarian, S. (2021). An in silico deep learning approach to multi-epitope vaccine design: A SARS-CoV-2 case study. *Scientific Reports, 11*, 1–21.

Yan, L. C., Yoshua, B., & Geoffrey, H. (2015). Deep learning. *Nature, 521*, 436–444.

Younus, M. U., ul Islam, S., Ali, I., Khan, S., & Khan, M. K. (2019). A survey on software defined networking enabled smart buildings: Architecture, challenges and use cases. *Journal of Network and Computer Applications, 137*, 62–77.

Zeng, D., Cao, Z., & Neill, D. B. (2021). Artificial intelligence–enabled public health surveillance—from local detection to global epidemic monitoring and control. In *Artificial intelligence in medicine* (pp. 437–453). Elsevier.

Zhao, X., Wu, Y., Song, G., Li, Z., Zhang, Y., & Fan, Y. (2018). A deep learning model integrating FCNNs and CRFs for brain tumor segmentation. *Medical Image Analysis, 43*, 98–111.

CHAPTER

13 A secure and efficient two-factor authentication protocol (SET-AP) for body sensor networks in IoT-enabled healthcare systems

Krishan Pal Singh[2], Shubham Tomar[1], Tejpal Kumar[1]

[1]*Central University of Rajasthan, Ajmer, Rajasthan, India;* [2]*Jaipur National University, School of Computer and System Sciences, Jaipur, Rajasthan, India*

13.1 Introduction

IoT is all about networks, embedded devices, and data that enables embedded sensors with an internet connection to interact with other wireless sensors over different networks. IoT connects various networks with internet access across the world. An IoT network requires sensors and actuators, data aggregation, and data conversion systems along with Data analysis and management including information storage (Singh et al., 2021, pp. 319–332). The embedded wireless sensors functions with limited power and storage with low computability therefore Cloud is integrated with WSN (Maleh et al., 2018) to create a new CloudIoT paradigm of IoT applications such as healthcare IT applications.

Recent surveys of the American Medical Association (AMA) and various Healthcare IT News articles published in 2020 suggest a significant adoption growth of healthcare IT services in the past few years. According to these articles, remote monitoring of patients has increased to 22% from 13% during 2016–2019. The exponential growth of smartphone and embedded devices with an internet connection will further add-on to the prospects of the healthcare IT sector. As per the Mobile Economy 2020, the population of unique Smartphone connections is around 5.2 billion in 2019 and is expected to grow up to six billion in a decade. Further, Internet connectivity of devices has also increased from one-quarter of a billion to around 3.5 billion during 2018–19.

Internet connection to embedded devices has improved diagnosis and medicament of diseases with high p2d (patient to doctor) interactions to patient's satisfaction. This assimilation of various communication and information technologies leads to new paradigms of IT such as emergent agile systems, IoT, and cloud

Computational Intelligence for Medical Internet of Things (MIoT) Applications
https://doi.org/10.1016/B978-0-323-99421-7.00009-X

computing to provide such systems that add new dimensions to healthcare IT systems. CloudIoT-enabled healthcare infrastructures ensemble with e-health data and emergent agile solutions i.e., Biochip, smart-wearable, and astute software entities that demonstrate an unparalleled potential to provide smart, agile, automated, and sustainable healthcare services.

CloudIoT has huge prospects and will become an essential factor of an Individual's life. With that rapid growth, new threats will emerge every day thus security of vital information such as Identity, previous medical records, recent diagnosis details, etc., become the primary concern of healthcare applications. Also, confidentiality must be addressed to establish trust between the cloud server and the nodes. Various authentication mechanisms have been proposed to achieve these requirements for the CloudIoT environment. However, these mechanisms have certain limitations that must be resolved such as environments with storage and power constraints, which require optimal key length to achieve higher security (Maleh et al., 2016a).

Intent to resolve the above security issues and shortcomings of various researches has been presented in this paper. This mechanism establishes trust using two-factor authentication between the biochip and the mobile gateway based on the discrete-log problem of Diffie-Hellman algorithm. Here, we summarize the proposed SET-AP mechanism, to address several security threats, DLP (discrete logarithm problem) is used.

The SET-AP mechanisms adopt the concept of one-time authentication to verify the legitimacy of the connection request of the device to prevent replay, impersonation, and man-in-the-middle attacks (Maleh et al., 2016b).

To ensure Two-factor authentication and forward secrecy, a unique method to compute authentication code and secure session key is proposed. AVISPA is used to perform a formal security analysis of SET-AP. To address various security attributes (privacy, authentication, impersonation attack, replay attack, session key agreement, forward secrecy, insider attack, man-in-the-middle attack), an informal analysis of SET-AP mechanism is performed and compared with some existing mechanisms.

The remaining sections of this paper are assembled as follows. Section 13.2 describes the related work and Section 13.3 contains the Proposed SET-AP protocol, notations, and its phases. Formal analysis using BAN logic is the core of Section 13.4 whereas Section 13.5 focuses primarily on security analysis using SPAN + AVISPA, respectively. Section 13.6 outlines the comparison of the functionalities of SET-AP with various existing mechanisms. In Section 13.7, we conclude this paper and envision the future of this protocol.

13.2 Related works

Authentication has a prominent role in the successful conjunction of sensor-enabled devices with the cloud environment. The population surge and the decline of the health index places a serious strain on traditional healthcare. This affects various factors such as doctors and hospital resources to population ratio and the availability of medicament. Hence, the need to introduce an effective alternative were nigh. The smart healthcare system provides the ability to adapt and expand that traditional healthcare systems are lacking. CloudIoT-based systems facilitate remote live health status observation of a patient and transmit that data to cloud server. the server forward the information to the entity with legitimate access i.e., doctors, emergency services, caretakers, and health systems.

Smart healthcare systems are described as BeeNet with interactive sensor devices that access information dynamically, connects devices, objects, and healthcare institutes. It monitors, manages, and reacts to the Medical environment astutely. Authors in (Dimitrov, 2016; Fan et al., 2014; Kalra & Sood, 2015) have stated about device-to-device (D2D) communication of these sensors to collect and distribute the data between wireless sensors.

Authors in (Baker et al., 2017; Chang et al., 2016; Wolgast et al., 2016; Zhu et al., 2015) have denoted IoT-based healthcare systems as an alternative to traditional systems. The authors developed smart healthcare system for specific purposes such as ambient life assistance for patients, rehabilitation, drug management, and diabetes monitoring. Pasluosta et al. (2015) performed health monitoring of patients diagnosed with Parkinson's disease, using the existing IoT-enabled applications.

Several researchers (Olaronke & Oluwaseun, 2017; Zhou et al., 2017) integrated cloud computing to store and organize data in IoT-based healthcare systems and achieved a significant improvement in data processing performed by wearable devices with limited resources when integrated with the cloud. However, a drawback of cloud assimilation is its introduction of various security vulnerabilities thus the need to improve data security has become essential. A huge bunch of sensitive information being stored in a cloud brings forth several security threats along thus the need to monitor the communications, authentication of the end-users, and a potential requirement to reconfigure sensors on regular basis to ensure its accurate monitoring, and disconnection if the sensors run out of battery or cross the cellular range. Various access control mechanisms and encryption techniques have been proposed to increase security but each standard alone has been insufficient for IoT-enabled healthcare infrastructures. With relatively few limitations, remote health monitoring has prospered well in recent years (Singh et al., 2021, pp. 319–332).

Yang and Chang (2009) proposed mutual authentication and also featured a session key generation between the embedded device and the Cloud server. Yoon and Yoo (2009) observed that the protocol in fails to achieve perfect Forward Secrecy and is prone to impersonation attack thus they suggested an improvement in the protocol to improve security. A detailed study of by Islam et al. (Islam & Biswas, 2011) denoted its efficacy to provide perfect forward secrecy and to counter this issue the authors introduced an identity-based secure remote login mechanism that provides a three-way handshaking technique for challenge-response and resolves the clock synchronization issue and minimizes the cost of computation.

Abou-Nassar et al. (2020) proposed a decentralized, interoperable believe version that suffuses blockchain into healthcare IoHT. Their proposed framework is a resilient atmosphere that supports semantic annotations for health side layers in IoHT. They makes use of a nonpublic blockchain ripple chain to set up trustworthy communication channel by validating nodes based on their interoperable structure so that controlled verbal exchange required to remedy fusion and integration problems are facilitated thru one-of-a-kind zones of the IoHT infrastructure.

EL-Latif et al. (2020) had presented a novel quantum walks based image encryption mechanism for privacy retaining to the IoT-based healthcare systems with a view to secure the patients' privacy. The set of rules provided by the authors has two levels: substitution and permutation, which each are based totally on controlled alternate quantum walks (CAQW) and every of them have its own initial key parameters. Their results proved that the presented mechanism has high efficiency in addition to excessive security.

Chou et al. (2013) highlighted the lack of appropriate public-keys of protocols in Yang and Chang (2009), Yoon and Yoo (2009) and designed an ECC-based Session key agreement protocol using multiple Identities for mobile ecosystems. Farash and Attari (2014) found a vulnerability of Impersonation attack in protocol and proposed a solution of an advanced identity-based key sharing protocol, increasing the computational cost to achieve higher security than (Chou et al., 2013).

After observation of the above-mentioned literature, we deemed an introduction of a secure and efficient device authentication for IoT-based healthcare applications, essential. So, we propose a secure and efficient two-factor authentication protocol (SET-AP) for smart healthcare applications. Table 8.4 provides a summary of the merits and demerits of few standard authentication mechanisms with a comparison to SET-AP.

13.3 The proposed SET-AP protocol

In this section, we propose a SET-AP to establish a secure environment of communication between a biochip and a healthcare professional with intention of only providing access to genuine professionals who can access the data of a patient. This protocol is eligible for deployment in both homes and healthcare centers. The core belief of SET-AP is to register both biochip and mobile gateway to a hospital cloud server. Once the registration phase is successful, the mobile gateway receives an authentication code from the server and forward this authentication code along with a connection request to the biochip. If the biochip validates the authentication code then it responds to the connection establishment request and generates the session key. The gateway receives the acknowledgment and generates its key. The DLP for Diffie-Hellman protocol is used to generate the key between both the nodes with the belief that hospital cloud server is a trusted entity.

13.3.1 Discrete-log problem for cryptography

Let G be a group that represents multiplication as the group operation with 1 as the identity, has an element g. Now we denote an *n*th product of *g*, for $n \varepsilon I^{+}$ as g^{n}.

$$g^{n} = g*g*g*g \ldots \text{(n times)} = y\text{(assume)} \tag{13.1}$$

Then, Discrete Log of *n* is –

$$n = \log_{y} g \tag{13.2}$$

And, if $n = |g|$ then –

$$\text{Log}_{y} g = n \ (\text{mod } N) \tag{13.3}$$

Table 13.1 presents the notations used in the SET-AP model.

13.3.2 Registration process

In this phase, both biochip and mobile gateway register themselves on the hospital cloud server.

Biochip Registration – After deployment of the biochip, it initiates the proceedings by registering itself on the hospital cloud server. The biochip computes an authentication code and transmits it along with the ID and nonce of the biochip.

$$\textbf{(EB} \rightarrow \textbf{CS): \{\{ID}_{E}\textbf{, N}_{E}\textbf{, Auc\_code\}K'}_{E}\textbf{\}K}_{S}$$

Table 13.1 Notations used in the SET-AP model.

Notation	Description
EB	Embedded biochip
CS	Hospital cloud server
MG	Mobile gateway
ID_E, ID_M	Identities of biochip and mobile gateway
G	Discrete log generator group (large prime number)
h(.)	One-way cryptographic hash function
K_E, K'_E	Public-key and private-key of embedded biochip
K_M, K'_M	Public-key and private-key of mobile gateway
K_S, K'_S	Public-key and private-key of hospital cloud server
N_E, N_M	Nonce of biochip and mobile gateway
$\oplus$	X-or function
SK	Secure session key
E, P	Generators of EB and MG

Authentication Code(Auc_code) is a one-way hash function that includes X-or function of identity and nonce of biochip along with its generator X and the private-key. This Auc_code will work as one-time access to the biochip.

$$Auc\_code = h(ID_E \oplus N_E \oplus K'_E \oplus E)$$

Mobile Gateway Registration – The gateway device registers itself on the server using its identity encrypted with its private key and the public key of the server.

$$(MG \rightarrow CS): \{\{ID_M, N_M\}K'_B\}K_S$$

13.3.3 Authentication process

Here, biochip authenticates mobile gateway with the help of the cloud server. Biochip first verifies the authentication key, it received from the mobile gateway. Then it validates the identity of the mobile gateway received from cloud server and mobile gateway by comparing them. If the identity of mobile gateway is confirmed it shifts to key-gen phase.

$$(CS \rightarrow MG): \{\{ID_E, N_E, K_E\}K'_S\}K_M, \{\{ID_M, N_M, K_M, Auc\_code\}K'_S\}K_E$$

Mobile gateway decrypts the first part encrypted with K M and finds the identity and public-key of the biochip. So in the next message, it attempts to communicate with the biochip by forwarding the unreadable text of the previous message along with a message with its ID and generator.

$$(MG \rightarrow EB): \{\{ID_M, N_E, N_M, G^M\}K'_M\}K_E, \{\{ID_M, N_M, K_M, Auc\_code\}K'_S\}K_E$$

After receiving this message the Biochip confirms the origin of the messages and verifies the authentication code by recalculating the hash of $(\mathbf{ID_E} \oplus \mathbf{N_E} \oplus \mathbf{K'_E} \oplus \mathbf{E})$. If the New hash matches the hash it received from The Server via Mobile Gateway then it decrypts the remaining message and finds the generator of mobile gateway (G^M). Fig. 13.1 shows the flowchart of the SET-AP model.

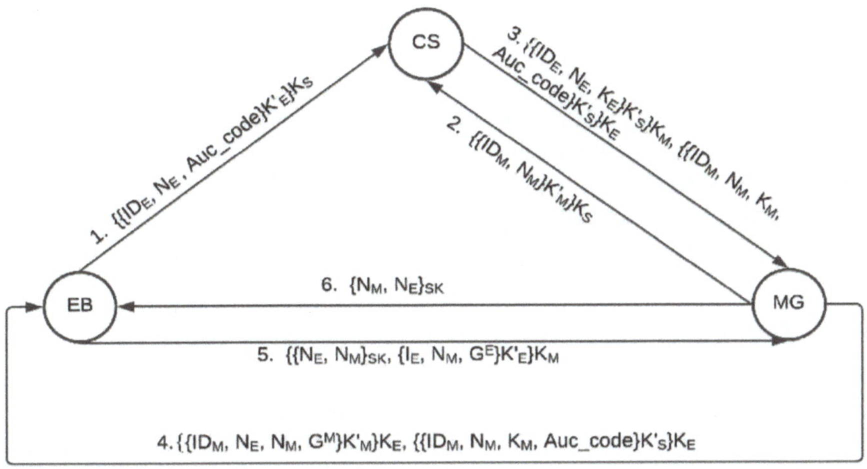

FIGURE 13.1

Flowchart of the SET-AP model.

13.3.4 Key-generation process

In this process, the biochip will generate a secure session key (SK) using the generator of mobile gateway. We select for a large primc number as G to ensure DLP can't bc solved easily using Pohlig–Hellman algorithm.

Key-Gen at Biochip: SK = $(G^M)^E$

Biochip then transmits a message to the mobile gateway, which contains the generator of biochip encrypted with K'_E and K_M, respectively.

(EB → MG): $\{\{N_E, N_M\}SK, \{ID_E, N_M, G^E\}K'_E\}K_M$

Mobile gateway receives this message and decrypts it to get G E after which it generates the secret session key and using that further decrypts the remaining message.

Key-Gen at Mobile Gateway: SK = $(G^E)^M$

(MG → GB): $\{N_M, N_E\}SK$

Here, biochip (EB) verifies the freshness of the nonce to enable the secure communication channel between the Biochip and the mobile gateway. SET-AP mechanism uses public-key cryptography to ensure the data security in the communication channel between agents.

13.4 Formal analysis of SET-AP using BAN logic

Formal analysis verifies the righteous and error-free modeling of protocol functions before the real-time performance analysis. Here, the description of the formal analysis is stated to verify the behavior of SET-AP using BAN logic. We provide a brief introduction to BAN logic in Sections 13.4.1 and 13.4.2 to demonstrate the analysis and authentication proofs of SET-AP using the BAN logic.

13.4.1 BAN logic

Burrows, Abadi, and Needham (BAN) introduced benchmark logic for formal analysis of security protocols (Burrows et al., 1871). In Table 13.2, we enlist a few standard notations used in BAN logic.

13.4.2 Formal analysis of SET-AP

In this section, we illustrate the behavior of the proposed authentication logic using BAN logic. SET-AP has three main principles: embedded biochip (EB), mobile gateway (MG), and hospital cloud server (CS). We use public-key cryptography and authentication Code (Auc_code) to exchange a secure session key (SK). The following postulates are used for formal analysis:

Table 13.2 Notation used in BAN logic.

Notation	Description
P believes X	Entity P believes verbatim on message X
P sees X	Only entity P can read encrypted message X
P said X	Entity P once sent a message that included X
P controls X	Entity P has authority over message X and must be believed because a trusted server always generates keys adequately
Fresh(X)	It prevents replay attack by ensuring the freshness of X during the protocol implementation
P K Q	K Is a secret session key exchanged between entities P and Q and K will not be revealed to anyone others than P and Q
$\{X\}_K$	Encrypted X with key K
$<X>_Y$	Combination of secret Y in formula X

SK, N_E, N_M, G, E, M : number

K_E, K_M, K_S : public_key

K'_E, K'_M, K'_S : private_key

Idealized Protocol:

$EB \rightarrow CS : \{\{N_E, Auc\_code\}K'_E\}K_S$;

Here, $Auc\_code = h(ID_E \oplus N_E \oplus K'_E \oplus E)$

$MG \rightarrow CS : \{\{N_E\}K'_M\}K_S$

$CS \rightarrow MG : \{\{N_E, K_E\}K'_S\}K_M, \{\{N_E, K_M, Auc\_code\}K'_S\}K_E$

$MG \rightarrow EB : \{\{N_E, N_M, G^M\}K'_M\}K_E, \{\{N_M, K_M, Auc\_code\}K'_S\}K_E$; $SK = (G^M)^E$

$EB \rightarrow MG : \{\{N_E, N_M\}SK, \{N_M, G^E\}K'_E\}K_M$; $SK = (G^E)^M$

$MG \rightarrow EB : \{N_M, N_E\}SK$

Belief:

$\{\{X\}K'_E\}K_S$

B1: EB believes EB CS

$\{\{X\}K'_M\}K_S$

B2: MG believes MG CS

$\{\{X\}K'_S\}K_M$

B3: CS believes CS MG

$\{\{X\}K'_M\}K_E$

B4: MG believes MG EB

{{X}K'$_E$}K$_M$

B5: EB believes EB MG

B6: EB believes fresh (N_E, G^E) ; B7: MG believes fresh (N_M, G^M)

B8: CS believes fresh (N_E, N_M)

Goal:

SK

G1: EB believes EB MG

SK

G2: MG believes MG EB

G3: EB believes fresh (N_M, G^M)

G4: MG believes fresh (N_E, G^E)

G5: EB believes Auc_code

Message 1: (EB → CS): {{N_E, Auc_code}K'$_E$}K_S

M1. CS believes EB said {{N_E, Auc_code}K'$_E$}K_S by message meaning rule using B1.

M2. CS believes fresh {{N_E, Auc_code}K'$_E$}K_S by freshness rule using B8, M1.

M3. CS believes EB believes {{N_E, Auc_code}K'$_E$}K_S by nonce verification rule using M1, M2.

M4. CS believes EB believes {{N_E, Auc_code}K'$_E$}K_S CS believes EB believes Auc_code by belief conjucatenation rule and using B6, M3.

Message 2: (MG → CS): {{N_M}K'$_M$}K_S

M5. CS believes MG said {{N_M}K'$_M$}K_S by message meaning rule using B2.

M6. CS believes fresh $\{\{N_M\}K'_M\}K_S$ by freshness rule using B8, M5.

M7. CS believes EB believes $\{\{N_M\}K'_M\}K_S$ by nonce verification rule using M5, M6.

Message 3: (CS → MG): $\{\{N_E, K_E\}K'_S\}K_M$, $\{\{N_M, K_M, Auc\_code\}K'_S\}K_E$

M8. MG believes CS said $\{\{N_E, K_E\}K'_S\}K_M$ by message meaning rule using B3.

M9. MG believes fresh $\{\{N_E, K_E\}K'_S\}K_M$ by freshness rule using B7, M8.

M10. MG believes CS believes $\{\{N_E, K_E\}K'_S\}K_M$ by nonce verification rule using M8, M9.

M11. MG believes CS said $\{\{N_M, K_M, Auc\_code\}K'_S\}K_E$ by belief conjucatenation using M10.

M12. MG believes fresh $\{\{N_M, K_M, Auc\_code\}K'_S\}K_E$ by freshness conjucatenation rule using B7, M11.

Message 4: (MG → EB): $\{\{N_E, N_M, G^M\}K'_M\}K_E$, $\{\{N_M, K_M, Auc\_code\}K'_S\}K_E$

$SK = (G^M)^E$

M13. EB believes MG said $\{\{N_E, N_M, G^M\}K'_M\}K_E$, $\{\{N_M, K_M, Auc\_code\}K'_S\}K_E$ by Message-meaning rule using B4.

M14. EB believes fresh $\{\{N_E, N_M, G^M\}K'_M\}K_E$, $\{\{N_M, K_M, Auc\_code\}K'_S\}K_E$ by freshness rule using B6, M13.

M15. EB believes MG believes $\{\{N_E, N_M, G^M\}K'_M\}K_E$, $\{\{N_M, K_M, Auc\_code\}K'_S\}K_E$ by nonce verification rule using M14(Goal G5).

M16. EB believes fresh $\{G^Y\}$ by freshness conjucatenation rule using B6, M15.

Message 5: (EB → MG): $\{\{N_E, N_M\}SK, \{N_M, G^E\}K'_E\}K_M$ $SK = (G^E)^M$

M17. MG believes EB said $\{\{N_E, N_M\}SK, \{N_M, G^E\}K'_E\}K_M$ by message-meaning rule using B5.

M18. MG believes fresh $\{N_M, G^E\}K'_E\}K_M$ by freshness rule using B7, M17.

M19. MG believes EB believes $\{N_M, G^E\}K'_E\}K_M$ by nonce verification rule using M18.

M20. MG believes fresh $\{N_M, G^E\}K'_E\}K_M$ by freshness conjucatenation rule using B7, M19(Goal G2, G4).

Message 6: (MG → GB): $\{N_M, N_E\}SK$

M21. EB believes MG said $\{N_M, N_E\}SK$ by message-meaning rule using B6.

M22. EB believes fresh $\{N_M, N_E\}SK$ by freshness rule using B6, M22.

M23. EB believes MG believes $\{N_M, N_E\}SK$ by nonce verification rule using M23.

M24. EB believes fresh $\{N_M\}$ by freshness conjucatenation rule using B6 (Goal G1, G3).

Here, we verify the establishment of a secure session between the biochip and mobile gateway by B5, M17, M20, M21, and M24. Furthermore, B3, B5, G5, S5, M14, M15, M17, and M20 ensure two-factor authentication of mobile Gateway to the biochip. Hence, we achieve the objectives of SET-AP: (1) to exchange a secure session key and establish a confidential environment between the biochip and the mobile gateway, and (2) to ensure the authenticity of the mobile device that requests access to the information captured by the biochip.

13.5 Security analysis and performance evaluation

13.5.1 Security analysis using SPAN

We analyzed Security of SET-AP using SPAN (Security Protocol Animator for AVISPA) to ensure security against various practical attacks (Baker et al., 2017; Viganò, 2006). AVISPA (Automated Validation of Internet Security Protocols and Applications) is a simulation tool for HLPSL with four back-ends (Chevalier et al., 2004). We designed the protocol with two composite and three basic roles as suggested in Table 13.3.

13.5.2 Performance evaluation

Here, we analyze the behavior of SET-AP by implementing various practical attacks and security attributes.

Table 13.3 Environment setup for security analysis.

Version	SPAN + Avispa v1.6
Language	HLPSL(High level protocol specification language)
Back-end	OFMC(On-the-fly model-Checker), CL-Atse(Constraint logic-based attack Searcher)
Composite role	Session and environment
Basic role	Role_EB, Role_MG and Role_CS

Replay Attack: An adversary (or an insider) may attempt to perform a replay attack by capturing the registration request, transmitted from mobile gateway to cloud server, and resend the captured transmission to cloud server. Once the server receives the request, it'll check for the mobile's id in the database. If the mobile is already a registered user, the server will assume an attempt of impersonation has been made based on reregistration and repeated freshness bit else it will respond using the public key of the mobile and the adversary cannot decipher the response it received. Hence, SET-AP is immune to replay attacks.

Impersonation Attack: Any attempt of impersonation on either the biochip or mobile gateway will not succeed as all the messages before key exchange are encrypted with the public key of the receiver and the private key of the transmitter. An adversary cannot pass the encryption layer without the private key of the receiver about which the adversary has no idea.

Information-Leakage: SET-AP facilitates two-level of encryption for each message featuring the public key of the receiver and the private key of the sender. Hence, even if an attacker eavesdrops, information cannot be deciphered or gathered.

Biochip Secret Guessing: In SET-AP, the biochip exchanges the key after authentication of the mobile gateway using Auc_code, forged using its private-key, Freshness bit, and a random generator. Except for the private key, both the bits change after each session thus impossible to guess for any adversary.

Confidentiality: Confidentiality is essential factor for data security. SET-AP has two layers of encryption at each message level to provide confidentiality and message integrity.

Two-factor Authentication: The Biochip first verifies Auc_code (forged using the hash of its ID, nonce, generator, and private-key), it received in message four by rehashing the same parameters again to ensure its integrity. Further, The biochip validates the ID of the mobile gateway, it received from the cloud server and mobile gateway itself to ensure the authenticity of the mobile device.

Secure Session Key: SET-AP provides an environment for session key sharing between the biochip and mobile gateway after two-factor authentication where both the entities generate a session key, respectively to begin a secure communication ecosystem without the cloud server.

Perfect Forward Secrecy: Forward secrecy that is not weathered even if an adversary exposes previous session keys is considered as perfect forward secrecy. In SET-AP, the session key [SK = $(G^E)^M$] is calculated using G^E and G^M. E and M are generated by the biochip and mobile gateway, individually. After each session both the entities exchange a new key calculated using new generator values and biochip only exchanges its generator once mobile gateway's two-factor authentication which also is generated using fresh nonce (N_E, N_M) and generator (E, M) value each time.

Hence, if an adversary knows previous session keys, it will not help to calculate or guess the next session key because the nonce and generator values have no static generation order therefore, SET-AP facilitates perfect forward secrecy.

13.6 Functionality analysis

In this section, we perform a comparative study of few related schemes with the proposed protocol, illustrated in Table 13.4. The formal and informal security analysis depicts that SET-AP is secure against various security threats. SET-AP also facilitates data integrity, confidentiality, two-factor authentication of the mobile gateway by the biochip, and a secure environment for key exchange.

Below is the HLPSL code for the proposed protocol.

Table 13.4 Comparison of SET-AP with other related schemes.

Functionalities	Le et al. (2011)	Das (2009)	Vaidya et al. (2010)	He et al. (2010)	Kumar and Lee (2011)	Kalra and Sood (2015)	SET-AP
Two-factor authentication	No	No	No	No	No	No	Yes
Secure session key exchange	No	No	No	No	No	Yes	Yes
Confidentiality	No	No	No	No	No	No	Yes
Protection to replay attack	Yes	Yes	Yes	Yes	Yes	Yes	Yes
Security against biochip secret guessing	Yes	No	No	No	No	No	Yes
Security against impersonation attack	No	No	No	No	No	No	Yes
Security against information-leakage	No	No	No	No	No	Yes	Yes

```
role role_EB(EB:agent, CS:agent, G:text, E:text, KE:public_key, KS:public_key,

SND, RCV:channel(dy), HF: hash_func)

played_by EB

def=

local State:nat,Auc:text,MG:agent,KM:public_key,M:text,NM:text,NE:text,SK:message

init

State := 0

transition

1.   State=0   /\   RCV(start)   =|>   State':=1   /\   NE':=new()   /\   E':=new()   /\
Auc':=HF(EB.NE'.inv(KE).E')

/\witness(EB,EB,auth_1,Auc')    /\witness(EB,MG,auth_2,NE')/\
SND({{EB.NE'.Auc'}_inv(KE)}_KS)

4.   State=1   /\
RCV({{MG'.NE.NM'.exp(G,M')}_inv(KM')}_KE.{{MG'.NM'.KM'.Auc}_inv(KS)}_KE)      =|>
State':=2

/\request(EB,EB,auth_1,Auc)__/\SK':=exp(exp(G,M'),E)/\
SND({{NE.NM'}_SK'.{EB.NM'.exp(G,E)}_inv(KE)}_KM')

/\ request(EB,MG,auth_3,NM')

6. State=2 /\ RCV(_SK) =|> State':=3
end role

role   role_MG(MG:agent,   CS:agent,   G:text,   M:text,   KM:public_key,   KS:public_key,
SND,RCV:channel(dy))

played_by MG
```

```
def=

local

State:nat,Auc:text,EB:agent,KE:public_key,E:text,NM:text,NE:text,SK:message

init

State := 0

transition

2. State=0 /\ RCV(start) =|> State':=1 /\ NM':=new() /\ witness(MG,EB,auth_3,NM')

/\ SND({{MG.NM'}_inv(KM)}_KS)

3. State=1 /\ RCV({{EB'.NE'.KE'}_inv(KS)}_KM {{MG.NM.KM.Auc'}_inv(KS)}_KE') =|>
State':=2

/\ request(MG,EB,auth_2,NE') /\
SND({{MG.NE'.NM.exp(G,M)}_inv(KM)}_KE'.{{MG.NM.KM.Auc'}_inv(KS)}_KE')

5. State=2 /\ RCV({{NE.NM}_exp(exp(G,M),E').{EB.NM.exp(G,E')}_inv(KE)}_KM) =|>
State':=3

/\SK':= exp(exp(G,E'),M) /\ SND(_SK')
end role

role role_CS(EB:agent, MG:agent, CS:agent, KE:public_key, KM:public_key,
KS:public_key, SND,RCV:channel(dy))

played_by CS

def=

local

State:nat,Auc:text,NM:text,NE:text
```

```
init
State := 0
transition
1. State=0 /\ RCV({{EB.NE'.Auc'}_inv(KE)}_KS) =|> State':=1
2. State=1 /\ RCV({{MG.NM'}_inv(KM)}_KS) =|> State':=2
/\ SND({{EB.NE.KE}_inv(KS)}_KM.{{MG.NM'.KM.Auc}_inv(KS)}_KE)
end role
role session1(KE:public_key, E:text, EB:agent, MG:agent, CS:agent, G:text, M:text,
KM:public_key, KS:public_key, HF:hash_func)
def=
local
SND3,RCV3,SND2,RCV2,SND1,RCV1:channel(dy)
composition
role_MG(MG,CS,G,M,KM,KS,SND3,RCV3)
/\ role_CS(EB,MG,CS,KE,KM,KS,SND2,RCV2)
/\ role_EB(EB,CS,G,E,KE,KS,SND1,RCV1,HF)
end role
role environment()
def=
local
```

```
key3:public_key,server:agent,alice:agent,key1:public_key,const_1:text,bob:agent,i:agen
t,g:text,

key2:public_key,key4:public_key,auth_1:protocol_id,auth_2:protocol_id,auth_3:protocol
_id,sk:protocol_id,

auc:protocol_id,hf:hash_func

intruder_knowledge =

composition

session1(key1,const_1,alice,bob,server,g,const_1,key3,key2,hf)

/\session1(key1,const_1,alice,i,server,g,const_1,key3,key4,hf)
end role
```

Figs. 13.2 and 13.3 shows that the execution of HLPSL code of SET-AP model on SPAN + AVISPA is safe on multiple states with bounded number of Sessions which signifies that the protocol is secure from numerous potential intrusions and only legitimate user can access the network. A detailed study of results has been discussed in Section 13.6.1.1 and Table 13.4.

13.6.1 Discussion

Here, we summarize the overall analysis of the proposed mechanism.

SET-AP achieves Two-factor authentication between the biochip and mobile gateway. SET-AP attains enhanced security than related schemes in (Chang et al., 2016; Das, 2009; He et al., 2010; Kalra & Sood, 2015; Le et al., 2011; Vaidya et al., 2010). SET-AP achieves perfect forward secrecy using a secure session key exchange between EB and MG which is not feasible in the related protocols.

In SET-AP, EB generates Auc_code and verifies the mobile gateway using the same thus consume a little time for computation.

13.7 Conclusion and future scope

Biochip enables remote health observation of patients and offers a huge help to critical patients. Smart healthcare systems also resolve traditional issues of the p2d ratio. But as the data over the cloud increases, we need to ensure the security and

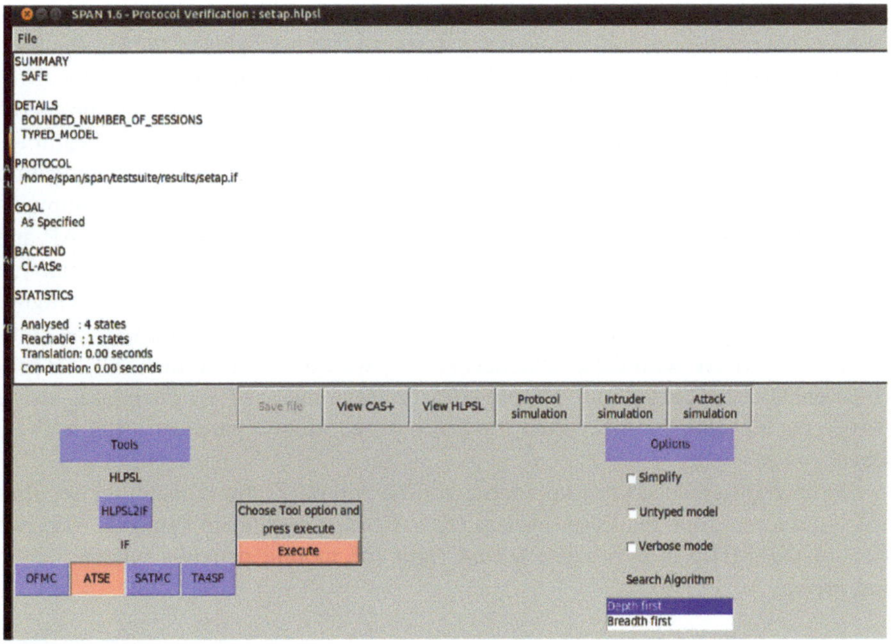

FIGURE 13.2

Execution of SET-AP with CL-Atse back-end.

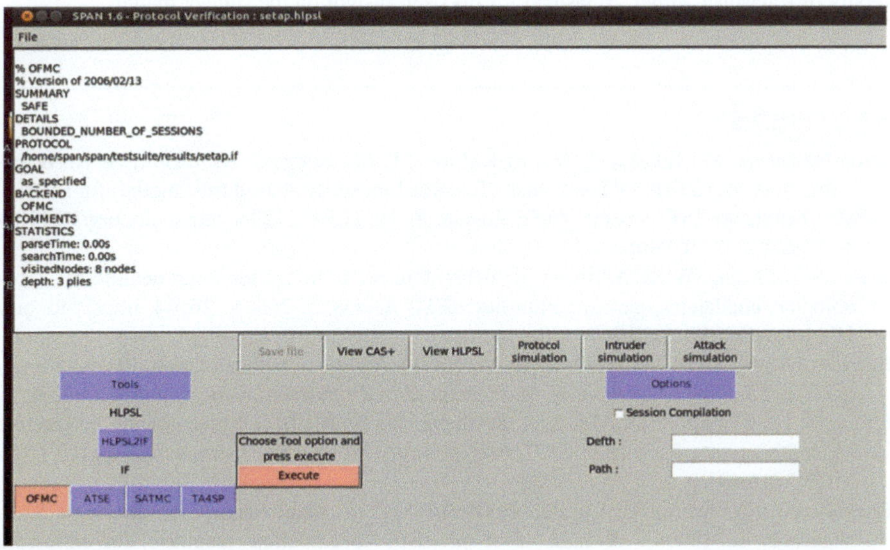

FIGURE 13.3

Execution of SET-AP with OFMC back-end.

confidentiality of the information. This situation leads to various research problems such as data protection, authentication of users, and access rights of the information.

In this paper, we proposed a DLP-based two-factor authentication protocol for the CloudIoT paradigm such as IoT-based healthcare systems. Existing protocols fell short to provide sufficient security of the sensitive information, i.e., health records of the patient. Our proposed protocol facilitates two-factor authentication and provides a secure environment to exchange a session key for further communication. Protocol simulation tool AVISPA is used for the analysis of SET-AP and executed on OFMC and CL-Atse back-end. The protocol is safe and immune from various potential threats. As informal analysis shows, SET-AP achieves higher security from existing schemes. Table 13.4 depicts a detailed summary of the comparison of SET-AP with these schemes. Hence, we can conclude that SET-AP provides enhanced security and is capable to improve message confidentiality using two-factor authentication between the biochip and mobile gateway using a cloud server.

We intend to reduce the computational time without compromising the security and build a real-time multiuser system for IoT-based healthcare systems. Also, we plan to use SET-AP to provide access right for mobile patient's authentication and privacy.

Acknowledgments

Authors express their deep gratitude to Dr. Muzzammil Hussain, Asst. Professor, Central University of Rajasthan Ajmer, Rajasthan for his deep insight on the subject matter.

References

Abou-Nassar, E. M., Iliyasu, A. M., El-Kafrawy, P. M., Song, O. Y., Bashir, A. K., & El-Latif, A. A. A. (2020). DITrust chain: Towards blockchain-based trust models for sustainable healthcare IoT systems. *IEEE Access, 8*, 111223–111238. https://doi.org/10.1109/ACCESS.2020.2999468

Baker, S. B., Xiang, W., & Atkinson, I. (2017). Internet of things for smart healthcare: Technologies, challenges, and opportunities. *IEEE Access, 5*, 26521–26544. https://doi.org/10.1109/ACCESS.2017.2775180

Burrows, M., Abadi, M., & Needham, R. M. (1871). A logic of authentication. *Proceedings of the Royal Society of London. A. Mathematical and Physical Sciences, 426*, 233–271.

Chang, S. H., Chiang, R. D., Wu, S. J., & Chang, W. T. (2016). A context-aware, interactive M-health system for diabetics. *IT Professional, 18*(3), 14–22. https://doi.org/10.1109/MITP.2016.48

Chevalier, Y., Compagna, L., Cuellar, J., Drielsma, P. H., Mantovani, J., Mödersheim, S., & Vigneron, L. (2004). A high level protocol specification language for industrial security-sensitive protocols. In *Workshop on specification and automated processing of security requirements-SAPS'2004*. Austrian Computer Society.

Chou, C. H., Tsai, K. Y., & Lu, C. F. (2013). Two ID-based authenticated schemes with key agreement for mobile environments. *Journal of Supercomputing, 66*(2), 973–988. https://doi.org/10.1007/s11227-013-0962-3

Das, M. L. (2009). Two-factor user authentication in wireless sensor networks. *IEEE Transactions on Wireless Communications, 8*(3), 1086–1090. https://doi.org/10.1109/TWC.2008.080128

Dimitrov, D. V. (2016). Medical internet of things and big data in healthcare. *Healthcare Informatics Research, 22*(3), 156–163. https://doi.org/10.4258/hir.2016.22.3.156

EL-Latif, A. A. A., Abd-El-Atty, B., & Venegas-Andraca, S. E. (2020). Controlled alternate quantum walk-based pseudo-random number generator and its application to quantum color image encryption. *Physica A: Statistical Mechanics and Its Applications, 547*. https://doi.org/10.1016/j.physa.2019.123869

Fan, Y. J., Yin, Y. H., Xu, L. D., Zeng, Y., & Wu, F. (2014). IoT-based smart rehabilitation system. *IEEE Transactions on Industrial Informatics, 10*(2), 1568–1577. https://doi.org/10.1109/TII.2014.2302583

Farash, M. S., & Attari, M. A. (2014). A secure and efficient identity-based authenticated key exchange protocol for mobile client-server networks. *Journal of Supercomputing, 69*(1), 395–411. https://doi.org/10.1007/s11227-014-1170-5

He, D., Gao, Y., Chan, S., Chen, C., & Bu, J. (2010). An enhanced two-factor user authentication scheme in wireless sensor networks. *Ad-Hoc and Sensor Wireless Networks, 10*(4), 361–371. http://www.oldcitypublishing.com/FullText/AHSWNfulltext/AHSWN10.4fulltext/AHSWNv10n4p361-371He.pdf.

Islam, S. H., & Biswas, G. P. (2011). A more efficient and secure ID-based remote mutual authentication with key agreement scheme for mobile devices on elliptic curve cryptosystem. *Journal of Systems and Software, 84*(11), 1892–1898. https://doi.org/10.1016/j.jss.2011.06.061

Kalra, S., & Sood, S. K. (2015). Secure authentication scheme for IoT and cloud servers. *Pervasive and Mobile Computing, 24*, 210–223. https://doi.org/10.1016/j.pmcj.2015.08.001

Kumar, P., & Lee, H. J. (2011). Cryptanalysis on two user authentication protocols using smart card for wireless sensor networks. In *2011 wireless advanced, WiAd 2011* (pp. 241–245). https://doi.org/10.1109/WiAd.2011.5983262

Le, X. H., Khalid, M., Sankar, R., & Lee, S. (2011). An efficient mutual authentication and access control scheme for wireless sensor networks in healthcare. *Journal of Networks, 6*(3), 355–364. https://doi.org/10.4304/jnw.6.3.355-364

Maleh, Y., Ezzati, A., & Belaissaoui, M. (2016a). An enhanced DTLS protocol for internet of things applications. In *Proceedings - 2016 international conference on wireless networks and mobile communications, WINCOM 2016: Green communications and networking* (pp. 168–173). Institute of Electrical and Electronics Engineers Inc. https://doi.org/10.1109/WINCOM.2016.7777209

Maleh, Y., Ezzati, A., & Belaissaoui, M. (2016b). DoS attacks analysis and improvement in DTLS protocol for internet of things. In *ACM international conference proceeding series*. Association for computing machinery. https://doi.org/10.1145/3010089.3010139

Maleh, Y., Ezzati, A., & Belaissaoui, M. (2018). Security and privacy in smart sensor networks. In *Security and privacy in smart sensor networks* (pp. 1–441). IGI Global. https://doi.org/10.4018/978-1-5225-5736-4

Olaronke, I., & Oluwaseun, O. (2017). Big data in healthcare: Prospects, challenges and resolutions. In *FTC 2016 – proceedings of future technologies conference* (pp. 1152–1157).

Institute of Electrical and Electronics Engineers Inc. https://doi.org/10.1109/FTC.2016.7821747

Pasluosta, C. F., Gassner, H., Winkler, J., Klucken, J., & Eskofier, B. M. (2015). An emerging era in the management of Parkinson's disease: Wearable technologies and the internet of things. *IEEE Journal of Biomedical and Health Informatics, 19*(6), 1873−1881. https://doi.org/10.1109/JBHI.2015.2461555

Singh, K. P., Tomar, S., Jain, U., & Hussain, M. (2021). *Simplified and secure session key sharing for internet of things (IoT) networks*. Springer Science and Business Media LLC. https://doi.org/10.1007/978-3-030-76736-5_30

Vaidya, B., Rodrigues, J. J., & Park, J. H. (2010). User authentication schemes with pseudonymity for ubiquitous sensor network in NGN. *International Journal of Communication Systems, 23*(9−10), 1201−1222. https://doi.org/10.1002/dac.1097

Viganò, L. (2006). Automated security protocol analysis with the AVISPA tool. *Electronic Notes in Theoretical Computer Science, 155*(1), 61−86. https://doi.org/10.1016/j.entcs.2005.11.052

Wolgast, G., Ehrenborg, C., Israelsson, A., Helander, J., Johansson, E., & Manefjord, H. (2016). Wireless body area network for heart attack detection [education corner]. *IEEE Antennas and Propagation Magazine, 58*(5), 84−92. https://doi.org/10.1109/MAP.2016.2594004

Yang, J.-H., & Chang, C.-C. (2009). An ID-based remote mutual authentication with key agreement scheme for mobile devices on elliptic curve cryptosystem. *Computers & Security, 28*(3−4), 138−143. https://doi.org/10.1016/j.cose.2008.11.008

Yoon, E. J., & Yoo, K. Y. (2009). Robust ID-based remote mutual authentication with key agreement scheme for mobile devices on ECC. In , *roceedings − 12th IEEE international conference on computational science and engineering, CSE 2009: Vol. 2. P* (pp. 633−640). https://doi.org/10.1109/CSE.2009.363

Zhou, J., Cao, Z., Dong, X., & Vasilakos, A. V. (2017). Security and privacy for cloud-based IoT: Challenges. *IEEE Communications Magazine, 55*(1), 26−33. https://doi.org/10.1109/MCOM.2017.1600363CM

Zhu, N., Diethe, T., Camplani, M., Tao, L., Burrows, A., Twomey, N., Kaleshi, D., Mirmehdi, M., Flach, P., & Craddock, I. (2015). Bridging e-health and the internet of things: The SPHERE project. *IEEE Intelligent Systems, 30*(4), 39−46. https://doi.org/10.1109/MIS.2015.57

CHAPTER

Pervasive m-health for chronic diseases

14

Rehab A. Rayan[1], Imran Zafar[2], Christos Tsagkaris[5], Andreas S. Papazoglou[3], Dimitrios V. Moysidis[4]

[1]*Department of Epidemiology, High Institute of Public Health, Alexandria University, Alexandria, Egypt;* [2]*Department of Bioinformatics and Computational Biology, Virtual University of Pakistan, Lahore, Punjab, Pakistan;* [3]*Athens Naval Hospital, Athens, Greece;* [4]*Hippokration University Hospital, Aristotle University of Thessaloniki, Thessaloniki, Greece;* [5]*Faculty of Medicine, University of Crete, Rethymno, Greece*

14.1 Introduction

Contemporary healthcare practice is challenged by many issues, including the shortage of healthcare providers and the rise in the incidence of chronic diseases (Tamura et al., 2009). Chronic diseases such as cardiovascular conditions, cancer, musculoskeletal pain, and respiratory conditions constitute the primordial causes of morbidity and mortality worldwide. The World Health Organization (WHO) reported that chronic diseases cause almost 82% of population mortality worldwide, where related deaths are expected to reach 52 million by 2030 (World Health Organization, 2014). Usually, uncontrolled chronic conditions lead to inferior quality of life, more financial load, and social issues (Dearden et al., 2010). There is a great demand to ensure access to cost-effective healthcare services for all, anywhere, and anytime to support and monitor patients and limit costly hospital admissions and chronic debilitation (Varshney, 2014).

Ubiquitous technology incorporates technology in the workplace and living environments in such a way that communication between people and devices such as wireless machines, wearables and immobile equipment becomes streamlined and ambient. Because of this, the user can achieve diverse types of data collection (Zhang et al., 2018). Healthcare apps embedded in smartphones or dedicated health devices can make the collected data easily accessible to the user, healthcare personnel, and caregivers. Mobile healthcare is taking steps toward the design, creation, and evaluation of technology that helps people to engage in their own treatment more closely and merge their treatment with their daily living activities. Common health problems including hypertension, arrhythmia, diabetes mellitus, and metabolic syndrome have so far visited healthcare providers as essential. Despite this, the monitoring of these conditions has relied on low-accuracy methods such as paper calendars where patients would insert regular measurements of values related to their condition (blood pressure, pulse, blood glucose levels, etc.). The compliance of patients with the collection of measurements is inversely associated

Computational Intelligence for Medical Internet of Things (MIoT) Applications
https://doi.org/10.1016/B978-0-323-99421-7.00014-3

with the number of measurements that patients were expected to perform daily Agar (Agarwal & Cappola, 2020). However, even in patients with elevated levels of adherence, it has not been possible to measure the full range of measurements variations for a long time. For instance, although Holter monitors can measure heart rhythm for several hours or days, arrhythmias occurring beyond the period of monitoring remain unnoticed. The same applies to glucose monitoring, where out-of-range glucose levels occurring during the night of sleep cannot easily be detected (Uniyal & Raychoudhury, 2014).

Pervasive healthcare (PH) is a novel field that comprises applying the existing computing techniques, such as biosensors, communication protocols, and smart solutions, to supply emergency and preventive healthcare services. PH could dynamically observe key patients' vitals, enabling preventive care and ongoing monitoring, hence enhancing both system efficacy and dependability. The key advantages involve its pervasive and assistive techniques, self-control of diseases, distant monitoring, better medical evaluations and healthcare services, and a critical decrease in the rising health expenses. The patients can thus enjoy ambient daily living conditions. Nowadays, many PH systems are applying mobile techniques for their great accessibility and different built-in sensors. Many studies have investigated pervasive mobile health (m-health) services (PMS), yet there is a greater need to explore late advances and existing opportunities and challenges for the future projection of this rising research field. This chapter summarizes PMS with a focus on their applications, challenges, and future opportunities.

14.2 Methods

The authors searched scholarly databases (PubMed, Scopus, Google Scholar) and gray literature (Legislation, Policy reports) with keywords (m-Health, pervasive m-Health, mobile health, digital health, privacy, confidentiality, data protection) and Boolean operators (where applicable) to identify content related to the characteristics and the applications of pervasive m-Health. Many official reports were considered. Resources in a language different from English, German, Arabic, and Greek were not considered. Because of the broad character of the topic and the informative character of the chapter, the search did not comply with any of the Preferred Reporting Items for Systematic Reviews and Meta-Analyses (PRISMA) extensions. Instead, it attempted to map the literature in the field and critically synthesize key findings and information from academic and official but nonacademic sources.

14.3 Characteristics of pervasive m-health

14.3.1 Architecture

Client-server, web-based, or autonomous seems to be the most common framework for building m-health. Technology that uses a client-server architecture or web-based system has three levels of identical architecture: Tier 1 (WBAN), Tier 2 (Access Point, AP), and Level 3 (Remote Server). Level 1 corresponds to the virtual interconnection of object sensor networks with AP, level 2 is often used to facilitate communication through related network architectures to the remote server and level 3 corresponds to the regional service that hosts time-sensing data. The smartphone is used as a transmitter and AP by the autonomous framework. The Committee of Experts addresses many performance issues in the market to improve the use of these structures in the development of the comprehensive m-health infrastructure.

14.3.2 Data protocols

Statistics are now transferred from existing m-health instruments via various network topologies, including high-speed technology 2G/3G, 3G/4G, Bluetooth, Wi-Fi, and UMTS, IEEE 802.15.4, ZigBee, UBS, and GPRS. They also facilitated object detection via the Internet or easy access of objects via HTTPS to the monitor station. Because m-health included multiple microsensors, smartphone communications, cloud servers, and the Internet, the consistency elements of the network protocol must be considered. Within the framework of all information exchanges, the connection possibilities must be dependable without intervention.

14.3.3 Technologies

In many intelligent decision-making studies, they are often used to build data mining and training models such as decision-making trees, redirected networks, probabilistic reasoning, the Hidden Markov chain model, and the support vector machine. Machine learning models, such as vector regression, Bayesian connectivity, and learning strategies, are used by Abbate et al. (2012), to create an insightful system for selecting activity algorithms. The Gaussian Process Regression (GPR) model was used (Juen et al., 2015) to migrate the treadmill, a three-layer artificial neural network (ANN) to reduce mean square errors using evolutionary algorithms and the naive Bayes framework, and 0.01 epsilons in indifferent missing function has been used.

The hidden Markov chain model (HMM) has been used as a proposed tool in combination with vector recognition technology to determine the number of effective health activities depending on several intervals for the experimental exercises. The previous researcher also used other data mining algorithms, such as hierarchical allocation techniques and design and adaptation of interactive multimedia, and transmission of high-speed data (Majeed et al., 2015). Liu also proposed a small processing machine that performs simple data collection operations and describes scalable data analysis. The processing logic includes an appropriate data collection, a conversion method for converting common data to a specified format, and an encryption protection activity.

14.4 Applications

M-health applications are suitable for pervasive health monitoring. Interconnected apps providing multiple faceted information for many patients can ease physicians, establish proper documentation of health and disease records, and decrease the cost and burden of healthcare via preventive interventions and early diagnosis and referral. Interconnection is facilitated via the open m-health framework, an open-source project established in platforms such as Google Fit and Fitbit (Majeed et al., 2015).

Vital signs (blood pressure, pulse rate, oxygen saturation levels) and other health-related measurements, such as blood glucose levels, can be documented regularly or continually. This information is compared with given normal values and is often adjusted for age, height, and nutrition or physical activity patterns (Al-Dowaihi et al., 2013; Liu et al., 2011; Nawka et al., 2011). Temperature sensors can inform patients, caregivers, and healthcare providers early about an infection in vulnerable patients with multi-morbidity. Oxygen saturation levels can similarly inform about an exacerbation of asthma or chronic obstructive pulmonary disease (COPD).

While we can describe many applications of PMS, diabetes, a multifaceted disease afflicting up to one out of 12 people globally, serves as an overarching example. Rapid diagnosis of complications such as hypoglycemia or diabetic ketoacidosis, continuous monitoring of treatment compliance and lifestyle modifications, and teleconsultations in the era of COVID-19 have been achieved with m-health means. Similar interventions in Sweden have emphasized self-care, providing patients or family members and carers with remote aid whenever necessary (Zhang et al., 2018).

At a central level, these applications can collect data comprehensively about patient-oriented databases where educational and communication resources are available, constantly updated patients' records for physicians, help at home services at a regular or an urgent basis, healthcare providers and community supportive services interoperability and finally labor division and organizational culture (Sannino et al., 2015; Triantafyllidis et al., 2015).

For instance, VSM1 and COMPASS are diagnostic tools based on a bracelet placed on the patient's forearm. Detectors in skin contact and pulse, body temperature, respiration, and effect in people suffering from COPD are continuously tracked (Hofer et al., 2015). Intelligent bracelets based on photoplethysmography were used to monitor, heart rate and oxygen saturation during sleep, sitting, standing, and physical activity (Postolache et al., 2011). Zephyr Bio-Harne is a portable multi-sensing tool for acute and hyperthyroidism clinics that regulate heart rate, movement, attitude, respiratory rates, and body temperature. It is based on a diverse set of detectors, including microcontrollers, ECG, electromyography (EMG), pulse and blood flow, EDA, and oxygen saturation sensors, which collect stimuli from high-risk patients (Horta et al., 2013). Jimenez et al. reported the use of CC2451 sensor tags to capture critical information about temperature, humidity, pressure, accelerometer, gyroscope, magnetometer, and smart system-type monitoring strap to track cardiac responses in patients (Abbate et al., 2012). Abbate et al. used the Shimmer sensor to track patients' body gestures and the Eno-bio sensor that measures rapid eye activity stimuli to monitor sleep phases and identify EEG indications to regulate neural function during sleep for patients such as neurological impairment, schizophrenia, or dementia (Abbate et al., 2012).

The case of chronic mental health conditions is better reflected in the contemporary PMS planning for depression. As a common mental health problem characterized by loss of interest in activities people normally enjoy, it is suitable for behavioral tracking. The withdrawal of a patient from a daily exercise routine may show deterioration of the disease, which can be managed effectively if communicated timely with their physician. The same applies to medication compliance, considering that depression medicines can take a long time to achieve therapeutic levels and clinical improvement. Pervasive monitoring can track discontinuations of the treatment and create alerts for the patients, their caregivers, and their physicians (Fanti, 2013; Jara et al., 2013).

Pervasive m-health has manifested a significant record in chronic diseases such as cancer and diabetes. The means of interventions span from mere phone calls or SMS to machine learning modalities. In the first case, the interface is user-friendly and accessible to elderly individuals with a low level of digital skills, while in the latter case the services' potential is skyrocketed. For example, a cancer treatment center in Spain has implemented a program with short—duration (3–5 min) telephone calls (Bielli et al., 2004). Making healthcare providers access to patients has decreased patients' visits to the center by up to 40%, decreasing the burden of care and easing both the patients and the physicians. Short calls and text messages (SMS) have also been used in Africa to deliver reminders about immunization coverage among residents of rural areas in Kenya (Wakadha et al., 2013).

According to the classical quality healthcare model of Avedis Donabedian personnel, infrastructures and organizational cultures are the pillars of an effective healthcare system (Glickman et al., 2007; Ramesh et al., 2012). M-health applications can bring healthcare personnel close to the patients regardless of the distance, use digital devices every day to healthcare infrastructure and keep track of the proper division of roles among specialties upholding the standards of the organization's culture.

14.5 Opportunities and challenges

Pervasive m-Health has a major potential to serve as a pillar of personalized and precision medicine in the future. At the clinical level, the expanded use of m-Health can improve the prevention and management of noncommunicable diseases (NCDs). This constitutes a priority for the international community following the disruption of NCDs care during the COVID-19 pandemic. Along the same lines, research and innovation can benefit from the effort to ameliorate pervasive health. The nature of the service and its challenges require multidisciplinary collaboration.

The need for a rapid reach of the devised solutions to the market enables the creation of entrepreneurial and intrapreneurial entities that can provide highly specialized technical solutions to a wide range of challenges. An overview of the challenges is provided in the following sections and described in Fig. 14.1.

14.5.1 Node-level challenges

14.5.1.1 Efficiency/energy consumption

Using energy in m-health sensors is a multilevel challenge. A recent study projected that current and power can be optimized to increase battery performance by approximately 6 h (Ramesh et al., 2012). The demand for electricity from portable devices is still a critical issue. Other systems use convenience to collect information that lowers the sensor's energy needs, making it compact and environmentally friendly. Acceleration sensitivity strategies also help minimize electricity consumption (Hofer et al., 2015).

Sophisticated sensors and continuous data collection and communication algorithms are energy intensive. The ongoing climate disruption calls for less sustainable devices, while the significant increase in the cost of energy can increase the indirect healthcare costs of patients using energy intensive m-Health devices. This can have a significant impact on the adoption and application of mobile health. Along these lines, the future acceptance of m-health means lies upon low-power monitoring sensors. The recent concept of green m-health investigates optimizing the functionality of the devices through improved performance and/or alternative sources of energy.

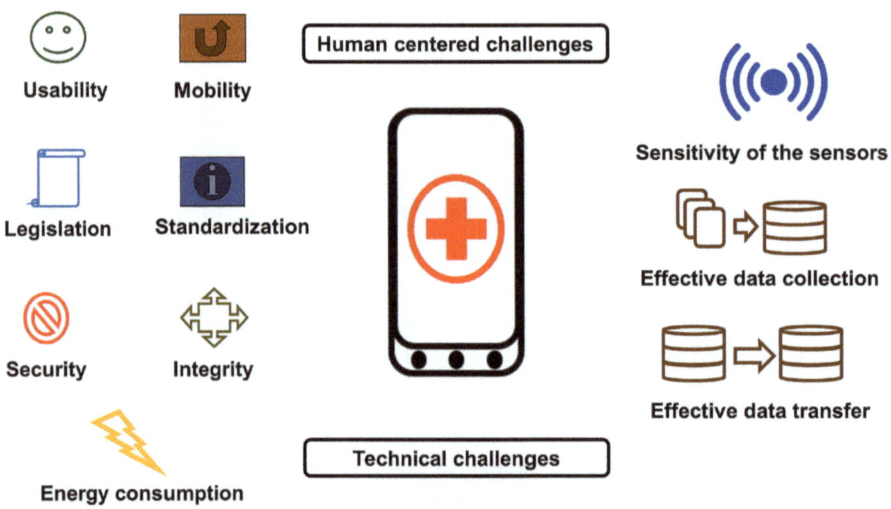

FIGURE 14.1

Technical and human-centered challenges for the wider use of pervasive m-health.

14.5.2 Network—level challenges

14.5.2.1 Effective data collection methods

Optimized data collection methods play a critical role in the management of patients. For efficient data collection, accurate movement, sound, temperature, and image acquisition and processing methods are used (Postolache et al., 2011). More research is necessary to improve the quality of data collection on detection devices. In addition, the timestamp and sequence of events are open problems when synchronizing different sensors. Regarding wearable devices, the accuracy of data collection is often subject to the compliance of the user. For instance, 24-hour pulse measurements cannot be reliable in individuals who intentionally or accidently use the device for less time than required. Similarly, environmental sensors providing input about temperature or humidity may become less functional because of prolonged exposure to adverse weather (Sheikh et al., 2021). The latter is particularly important in the context of climate health. In the context of climate adaptation and relevant health preparedness, m-Health devices providers should assess the usability of sensitive pieces of equipment such as gyroscopes, accelerometers, and barometric pressure sensors in prolonged periods of heat or cold.

14.5.2.2 Effective data transfer

A crucial factor in m-health is efficient data transfer. Detecting interrupted objects can lead to misdiagnosis, unnecessary care, and early decisions. Specific signal APIs have been used in the communication of sensor data covered in the response direction for accurate transmission of information. The precision of communication through simultaneous publishing and discovery in the unit is guaranteed by dynamic publishing/subscription mechanisms. Furthermore, low transmission intensity and small wireless sensor antennas lead to lower signal-to-noise ratios, thereby increasing the bit error rate and decreasing the reliable coverage area. Resolute data transfer must be analyzed, as it is still an issue of m-health.

14.5.2.3 Security

For efficient design and acceptance of m-health, protection is crucial through the collection and transmission of data from sensors into access points and access points to remote servers and certain systems (Moser & Melliar-Smith, 2015). Some systems have used wireless communication, mobile communication, and encrypted Internet communication through Bluetooth to ensure data security and to prevent potential interruptions in data usage. To increase the need for good mobile health, safety criteria such as NIST and HIPAA need to be met. Security requirements must be respected to do this. Moreover, little data protection encryption or encryption is used in systems, which is why their growth and development is still relevant. Authentication is assured in protocols like OAuth (Triantafyllidis et al., 2015) and other web applications with PHMS (Liu et al., 2011).

14.5.2.4 Integrity

Several research studies have been conducted to ensure that patient data confidentiality (Nawka et al., 2011). The physiological test protocol in Moser and Melliar-Smith is suggested to ensure the integrity of the patient (Moser & Melliar-Smith, 2015). Integrity is preserved in protocols like OAuth. Status warnings often notify patients, but they may also be expected to notify caregivers or healthcare providers. In this case, a secure connection is used to encrypt the content of this communication. The risk of external parties such as employers or insurance providers accessing this information limits the willingness of patients to adopt m-health because of inadequate security of privacy. Confidentiality mechanisms must be implemented to embrace m-health and ensure data confidentiality.

14.5.3 Human-centered challenges

14.5.3.1 Usability

User acceptance of technology is especially important for a successful implementation of m-health. It is, however, significant to increase usability among population groups with low levels of health literacy. Integrated technical assistance in the form of interactive instructions and in-app troubleshooting functionality is essential, but it needs to be complemented by help centers with human operators, who can guide users through the solution of their problems and increase their perceived safety. This has been identified as a major barrier for the access of elderly to m-Health healthcare services (Parker et al., 2013). Further, studies investigate the perceived usability of m-health technology and regular consultation of the industry with patients, caregivers, and healthcare providers is necessary.

14.5.3.2 Sensitivity of the sensors

The rapid increase in using m-health has rendered the sensitivity of the devices a critical issue. Sensitivity appears as a deeply technical issue with distinctive features in wearable and environmental (non—wearable) sensors (Begay et al., 2019). Nevertheless, linking technical sensor's sensitivity to the epidemiological notion of sensitivity can serve as a standpoint for the improvement of the existing concerns. In epidemiology, sensitivity refers to the ability of a test or a measurement to yield a positive result for a person who suffers from a given condition. Sensitivity is inversely related to specificity, which stands for the ability of the same to obtain a negative result for a person who does not suffer from the given condition (Shreffler & Huecker, 2020). In fact, increasing the sensitivity of a sensor of tachycardia can create false alarms by detecting increased heartbeat because of physical activity and not because of a pathological heart condition. This can jeopardize the quality of m-Health with patients being unwilling to use devices that make them feel insecure. Therefore, technical sensitivity should be limited to where it may detect more physiological than pathological signals. An additional crucial factor for consideration is the variability among patients and the variability within the same patient during a disease—which may involve the development of a comorbid disease (e.g., visual impairment on the grounds of diabetes mellitus). Because of this, m-Health devices need to include self-calibrating algorithms capable of personalizing the output of the device and detecting the "new normal" in the vital signs of a patient who recently suffered a condition that changed their daily living and physical activity.

14.5.3.3 Mobility

Mobility is significant for prolonged periods, particularly when mobile devices, tablets, intelligent watches, and sensors are used (Horta et al., 2013). To ensure that patients are connected to other devices, data centers and health facilities everywhere and always, a proper communication network is essential. M-Health improves patients more and makes routine, omnipresent and unrestricted monitoring possible. To facilitate versatility in the ad hoc and multihop sensors. Tracking mobility may be seen as a threat to the right of free movement, though. Certain types of mobility, such as travel by air or sea, pose challenges to the continuity of data transmission, which is essential for people with chronic health conditions such as heart failure and arrhythmia (Izadi et al., 2014).

14.5.3.4 Standardization

It is now critical that standardization is developed and enforced in every mobile health care system, for it to work interdisciplinary and independently with its suppliers. Open standards, such as Zig Bee's IEE-based E802.15.4, included in cheap and low-cost wireless networks. Open architecture is necessary if the emergency sensor services are to be easily integrated with the current health infrastructure (Jimenez & Torres, 2016). Standardization makes m-Health products more marketable as well because healthcare providers can easily integrate them into their patients' documentation system. A recent analysis of the German standardization model for healthcare apps described "Medication, Clinical, Diagnostics, Workflow, and Finance" as the principal domains to be standardized and emphasized the need to align standardization of digital health services with the prevalence of health conditions in local populations (Theilig et al., 2020). While this recommendation is reasonable, it questions the financial sustainability of standardized m-Health systems for rare diseases or diseases that are prevalent in low and middle-income countries (LMICs).

14.5.3.5 Interoperability

The constant stream of information between heterogeneous sensors over the network is important for opener systems. To ensure interoperability, common formats and protocols can be used. CDG (Continuous Development Guidelines) is in some cases used to restrict hardware. Medical Markup Language (MML) is also used to define physiology and health level seven international (HL7) representations. The interoperability question is also addressed by different programs and protocols, including the European Interoperability Framework, which provides 47 recommendations. The content of these recommendations spans from governance to streamlined processes and end-to-end data transfer (Ganck, 2019). Interoperability is still actively researched because of the grave implications of clinical decisions made based on unreliable data. For instance, transporting a patient to a hospital for a mistakenly suspected myocardial infarction compromises the patient's quality of life, increases the burden on the healthcare system, and increases insurance costs. Particularly during the COVID-19 pandemic, it increases the risk of infection in potentially vulnerable population groups. To ensure interoperability between health sensors, IEEE 11073–20601 specification, was used. The interoperability aspect of PHMS must therefore be discussed in the regular dissemination.

14.5.4 Legislative challenges

Pervasive m-Health is still debated among legislators worldwide. The risk of obtaining health-related data and exposing individuals' daily living is perceived in diverse ways across legislative systems. The matter has been widely studied in the context of the European Union, which adopts a strict approach to the matter based on the General Data Protection Regulation (GDPR), the same regulation, enables patients and healthy individuals to consent about the collection and use of their health data in an informed manner (Genovese et al., 2022). Further, the European Data Protection Regulation promotes data altruism, encouraging individuals to share their data for research and development purposes. This endeavor can be implemented through the European Health Data Space, an initiative of the European Commission seeking to create a transparent model of health data utilization and resolve the alleged conflict between the GDPR and the expanded utilization of health data from academic and industrial entities (Fadrique et al., 2020). On these grounds, it is important that countries and regions across the world should upscale their data protection regulations, with a framework for health data use and exchange.

14.5.5 Challenges with open research

M-health has significant potential for chronic disease surveillance. The rapid development of m-health may turn pervasive healthcare into a global paradigm in the following years. While further research on applications improving self-care, patients' safety, screening, and continuous monitoring can provide solutions to emerging operability issues, researchers need to constantly monitor the frameworks and policies regulating the field (Fadrique et al., 2020).

14.6 Conclusion

The chapter reviewed commonly applied PMS in health, emphasizing on applications and challenges. PMS are increasingly used in supplying intelligent healthcare for diverse patients. Experts are investigating technical interventions for improving healthcare parallel to the current services. Several PMS are used in enhancing the quality of life for patients; however, some major limitations are described to be considered in developing PMS. For future research, implementation, and user satisfaction could be considered. Frequent conditions like asthma, COPD, sleep disorders, cardiac diseases, hypertension, stress, cognitive impairment, dementia, Alzheimer's, falling risks, and other chronic diseases are highlighted principally for older patients.

Client-server and web-based models are the widespread options for PMS, where it applies different wireless communication protocols to send data from sensors to access points and distant servers. Different sensors gather the patient's vital signs to monitor conditions. Yet, there are many limitations need addressing at all levels, from sensor to network, and human levels. However, the future trend would comprise shifting the model of delivering healthcare from doctor-focused to patient-focused, from acute curative to ongoing preventive, and from sampling to monitoring. The growth of PMS could enhance the health status and life expectancy for many patients. The existing design limitations were highlighted, and so as the major domains of research for successful development, implementation, and smooth incorporation of PMS into patients' life.

References

Abbate, S., Avvenuti, M., & Light, J. (2012). Mims: A minimally invasive monitoring sensor platform. *IEEE Sensors Journal, 12*(3), 677–684. https://doi.org/10.1109/JSEN.2011.2149515

Agarwal, S., & Cappola, A. R. (2020). Continuous glucose monitoring in adolescent, young adult, and older patients with type 1 diabetes. *JAMA - Journal of the American Medical Association, 323*(23), 2384–2385. https://doi.org/10.1001/jama.2020.7058

Al-Dowaihi, D., Al-Ajlan, M., Al-Zahrani, N., Al-Quwayfili, N., Al-Jwiser, N., & Kanjo, E. (2013). mBreath: Asthma monitoring system on the go. In *International conference on computer medical applications, ICCMA 2013*. https://doi.org/10.1109/ICCMA.2013.6506169

Begay, C., Schenone, A., Dimitropoulou, L., Margolin, G., & Narayanan, S. (2019). Lessons learned: Recommendations for implementing a longitudinal study using wearable and environmental sensors in a health care organization. *JMIR mHealth and uHealth, 7*(12).

Bielli, E., Carminati, F., La Capra, S., Lina, M., Brunelli, C., & Tamburini, M. (2004). A Wireless Health Outcomes Monitoring System (WHOMS): Development and field testing with cancer patients using mobile phones. *BMC Medical Informatics and Decision Making, 4*(1). https://doi.org/10.1186/1472-6947-4-7

Dearden, A., Wright, P., Bowen, S., Rahman, F., Cobb, M., & Wolstenholme, D. (2010). Pervasive healthcare in lived experience: Thinking beyond the home. In *2010 4th International conference on pervasive computing technologies for healthcare, pervasive health 2010*. https://doi.org/10.4108/ICST.PERVASIVEHEALTH2010.8831

Fadrique, L. X., Rahman, D., Vaillancourt, H., Boissonneault, P., Donovska, T., & Morita, P. P. (2020). Overview of policies, guidelines, and standards for active assisted living data exchange: Thematic analysis. *JMIR mHealth and uHealth, 8*(6), e15923. https://doi.org/10.2196/15923

Fanti, K. A. (2013). Individual, social, and behavioral factors associated with co-occurring conduct problems and callous-unemotional traits. *Journal of Abnormal Child Psychology, 41*(5), 811–824. https://doi.org/10.1007/s10802-013-9726-z

Ganck, A. D. (2019). *The new European interoperability framework.*

Genovese, S., Bengoa, R., Bowis, J., Harney, M., Hauck, B., Pinget, M., Leers, M., Stenvall, T., & Guldemond, N. (2022). The European Health Data Space: A step towards digital and integrated care systems. *Journal of Integrated Care.* https://doi.org/10.1108/JICA-11-2021-0059

Glickman, S. W., Baggett, K. A., Krubert, C. G., Peterson, E. D., & Schulman, K. A. (2007). Promoting quality: The health-care organization from a management perspective. *International Journal for Quality in Health Care, 19*(6), 341–348. https://doi.org/10.1093/intqhc/mzm047

Hofer, T., Schumacher, M., & Bromuri, S. (2015). Compass: An interoperable Personal Health System to monitor and compress signals in chronic obstructive pulmonary disease. In *Proceedings of the 2015 9th international conference on pervasive computing technologies for healthcare, PervasiveHealth 2015* (pp. 304–311). Institute of Electrical and Electronics Engineers Inc. https://doi.org/10.4108/icst.pervasivehealth.2015.259186

Horta, E. T., Lopes, I. C., Rodrigues, J. J. P. C., & Proenca, M. L. (2013). A mobile health application for falls detection and biofeedback monitoring. In *2013 IEEE 15th international conference on e-health networking, applications and services, Healthcom 2013* (pp. 36–40). https://doi.org/10.1109/HealthCom.2013.6720634

Izadi, M., Alemzadeh Ansari, M. J., Kazemisaleh, D., & Moshkani Farahani, M. (2014). Air travel considerations for the patients with heart failure. *Iranian Red Crescent Medical Journal, 16*(6). https://doi.org/10.5812/ircmj.17213

Jara, A. J., Zamora-Izquierdo, M. A., & Skarmeta, A. F. (2013). Interconnection framework for mHealth and remote monitoring based on the internet of things. *IEEE Journal on Selected Areas in Communications, 31*(9), 47–65. https://doi.org/10.1109/JSAC.2013.SUP.0513005

Jimenez, F., & Torres, R. (2016). Building an IoT-aware healthcare monitoring system. In *Proceedings – international conference of the Chilean Computer Science Society, SCCC* (Vol. 2016)IEEE Computer Society. https://doi.org/10.1109/SCCC.2015.7416592

Juen, J., Cheng, Q., & Schatz, B. (2015). A natural walking monitor for pulmonary patients using mobile phones. *IEEE Journal of Biomedical and Health Informatics, 19*(4), 1399–1405. https://doi.org/10.1109/JBHI.2015.2427511

Liu, C. H., Wen, J., Yu, Q., Yang, B., & Wang, W. (2011). HealthKiosk: A family-based connected healthcare system for long-term monitoring. In *2011 IEEE conference on computer communications workshops, INFOCOM WKSHPS 2011* (pp. 241–246). https://doi.org/10.1109/INFCOMW.2011.5928816

Majeed, Q., Hbail, H., & Chalechale, A. (2015). A comprehensive mobile e-healthcare system. In *2015 7th conference on information and knowledge technology, IKT 2015*. Institute of Electrical and Electronics Engineers Inc. https://doi.org/10.1109/IKT.2015.7288802

Moser, L. E., & Melliar-Smith, P. M. (2015). Personal health monitoring using a smartphone. In *Proceedings - 2015 IEEE 3rd international conference on mobile services, MS 2015* (pp. 344–351). Institute of Electrical and Electronics Engineers Inc. https://doi.org/10.1109/MobServ.2015.54

Nawka, N., Maguliri, A. K., Sharma, D., & Saluja, P. (2011). SESGARH: A scalable extensible smart-phone based mobile gateway and application for remote health monitoring. In *2011 IEEE 5th international conference on Internet multimedia systems architecture and application, IMSAA 2011 — conference proceedings*. https://doi.org/10.1109/IMSAA.2011.6156341

Parker, S. J., Jessel, S., Richardson, J. E., & Reid, M. C. (2013). Older adults are mobile too! Identifying the barriers and facilitators to older adults' use of mHealth for pain management. *BMC Geriatrics, 13*(1). https://doi.org/10.1186/1471-2318-13-43

Postolache, O., Girao, P. S., Ribeiro, M., Guerra, M., Pincho, J., Santiago, F., & Pena, A. (2011). Enabling telecare assessment with pervasive sensing and Android OS smartphone. In *MeMeA 2011 — 2011 IEEE international symposium on medical measurements and applications, proceedings* (pp. 288—293). IEEE Computer Society. https://doi.org/10.1109/MeMeA.2011.5966761

Ramesh, M. V., Anand, S., & Rekha, P. (2012). A mobile software for health professionals to monitor remote patients. In *IFIP International conference on wireless and optical communications networks*. WOCN. https://doi.org/10.1109/WOCN.2012.6335565

Sannino, G., De Falco, I., & De Pietro, G. (2015). A supervised approach to automatically extract a set of rules to support fall detection in an mHealth system. *Applied Soft Computing, 34*, 205—216. https://doi.org/10.1016/j.asoc.2015.04.060

Sheikh, M., Qassem, M., & Kyriacou, P. A. (2021). Wearable, environmental, and smartphone-based passive sensing for mental health monitoring. *Frontiers in Digital Health, 3*. https://doi.org/10.3389/fdgth.2021.662811

Shreffler, J., & Huecker, M. R. (2020). *Diagnostic testing accuracy: Sensitivity, specificity, predictive values and likelihood ratios*.

Tamura, Y., Hashida, M., Sannomiya, S., & Iwata, M. (2009). Smart pervasive healthcare-assistance in daily life. In *2009 3rd International conference on pervasive computing technologies for healthcare — pervasive health 2009, PCTHealth 2009*. https://doi.org/10.4108/ICST.PERVASIVEHEALTH2009.6068

Theilig, M. M., Werner, J., Schoffke, F., & Zarnekow, R. (2020). The case for mhealth standardization for electronic health records in the German healthcare system. In *Lecture notes in business information processing* (Vol. 381, pp. 317—330). Springer. https://doi.org/10.1007/978-3-030-44322-1_24

Triantafyllidis, A., Velardo, C., Shah, S. A., Tarassenko, L., Chantler, T., Paton, C., & Rahimi, K. (2015). Supporting heart failure patients through personalized mobile health monitoring. In *Proceedings of the 2014 4th international conference on wireless mobile communication and healthcare — transforming healthcare through innovations in mobile and wireless technologies, MOBIHEALTH 2014* (pp. 287—290). Institute of Electrical and Electronics Engineers Inc. https://doi.org/10.1109/MOBIHEALTH.2014.7015967

Uniyal, D., & Raychoudhury, V. (2014). *Pervasive healthcare — A comprehensive survey of tools and techniques*.

Varshney, U. (2014). Mobile health: Four emerging themes of research. *Decision Support Systems, 66*, 20—35. https://doi.org/10.1016/j.dss.2014.06.001

Wakadha, H., Chandir, S., Were, E. V., Rubin, A., Obor, D., Levine, O. S., Gibson, D. G., Odhiambo, F., Laserson, K. F., & Feikin, D. R. (2013). The feasibility of using mobile-phone based SMS reminders and conditional cash transfers to improve timely immunization in rural Kenya. *Vaccine, 31*(6), 987—993. https://doi.org/10.1016/j.vaccine.2012.11.093

World Health Organization. (2014). *Global status report on noncommunicable diseases (WHO/NMH/NVI/15.1)*.

Zhang, P., Schmidt, D., White, J., & Mulvaney, S. (2018). Towards precision behavioral medicine with IoT: Iterative design and optimization of a self-management tool for type 1 diabetes. In *Proceedings - 2018 IEEE international conference on healthcare informatics, ICHI 2018* (pp. 64–74). Institute of Electrical and Electronics Engineers Inc. https://doi.org/10.1109/ICHI.2018.00015

CHAPTER

15 Hybrid intelligence-based cryptosystem: security and privacy enhancement in telemedicine system

Anirban Bhowmik[1], Sunil Karforma[2]

[1]Department of Computer Science, M.U.C. Women's College, Purba Bardhaman, West Bengal, India; [2]Department of Computer Science, The University of Burdwan, Purba Bardhaman, West Bengal, India

15.1 Introduction

Healthcare systems provide facilities to improve a person's well-being. They may be in the form of surgical, medicinal, or other alterations according to a patient's condition. These services are typically provided by hospitals and physicians through Internet of Things (IoT)-based healthcare systems. The realization of IoT is the most notable advancement in the field of computer science and electronics. At present the healthcare system includes the facility of IoT. As electronic health records, picture archiving and communication system (PACS), and advanced clinical systems are evolving and becoming more prominent, current storage resources are stretched. Many developed countries are establishing healthcare data centers that can help to make data more portable. Due to the sensitive nature of the information contained within electronic health records, it is very significant to impose an advanced security techniques in the system. IoT creates an environment of interconnected devices under single platforms by engaging both virtual and physical world together (Ghazi & Ali, 2018). The medical data transmission becomes very easy with the help of digital healthcare based IoT systems. Healthcare systems widely use the IoT devices for smooth functioning, monitoring, and assessment of patient's conditions and records. But most of these devices and applications are not secure for data communication. The IoT devices are targeted by attackers and this may risk for patients. Therefore, it is necessary to develop an efficient model for ensuring the security and integrity of the patient's diagnostic data in IoT-based healthcare system (Ali, 2018).

Information hiding technique using cryptography has been widely used for wireless communication. Information security guarantees that a secret message is unreadable to a third party, but accessible by the sender and receiver alone while using secret keys. Cryptographic techniques could be symmetric where the same key is used for encryption and decryption or asymmetric where the different keys are used for encryption and decryption. Symmetric cryptographic techniques are

Computational Intelligence for Medical Internet of Things (MIoT) Applications
https://doi.org/10.1016/B978-0-323-99421-7.00010-6

the most appropriate when a large amount of data is to be secured. AES, DES, Triple DES, RC4, IDEA, etc. are different types of symmetric key-based algorithms (Bhalekar & Shaikh, 2019; Kiran & Sharma, 2017). Here we have focused on the design of a hybrid cryptosystem. The following concepts are used in our scheme.

(1) Hopfield Model: A Hopfield net (Kaur et al., 2012; Gentry, 2009) is a fully interconnected net with symmetric weights and without any self-loop. This means that for a Hopfield net, $w_{ij} = w_{ji},$ for all $i \neq j$, and $w_{ii} = 0$, for all i. Because the net is fully connected, the idea of various layers of processing units is no longer meaningful here. Each unit gets input from each of the remaining units, as well as the corresponding element of the input pattern. For the m-unit Hopfield net, the net input to unit Y_j is given below.

$$y\_in_j = x_j + \sum_{\substack{i=1 \\ i \neq j}}^{m} y_i w_{ij}.$$

Here, x_j is the jth component of the input pattern x $= [x_1, x_2, x_3, \ldots, x_m]$ and y_j is the current activation of unit Y_i . The structure of a four-unit Hopfield net is shown below (Fig. 15.1).

The activation of the unit Y_j $Y_j = \begin{cases} 1, \; y_j > 0 \\ Y_j, \; y_j = 0 \\ 0 \quad y_j < 1 \end{cases}$

(2) S-Box: A substitution box or S-box (Ahmad, 2017; Bhalekar & Shaikh, 2019) is one of the basic components of symmetric key cryptography. In general, an S-box takes m input bits and transforms them into n output bits. This is called an (mxn) S-box and is often implemented as a lookup table. Substitution box or S-box in block ciphers is an importance part in public key cryptography. A

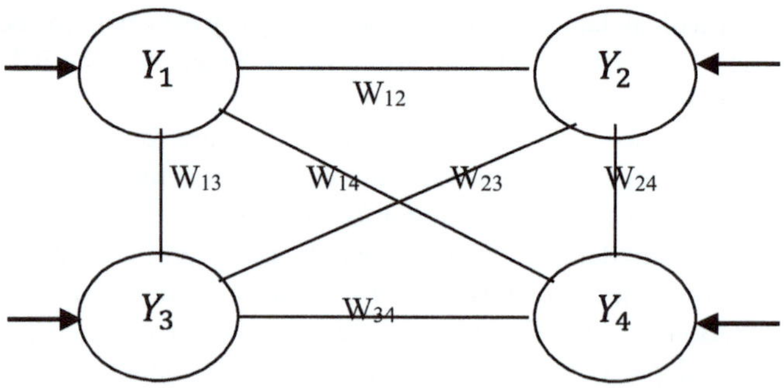

FIGURE 15.1

Structure of a four-unit hopfield net (Kaur et al., 2012).

four-bit S-box has been defined as a box of (2^4 =) 16 elements vary from 0 to F in hex. It is arranged in a random manner. Similarly for eight-bit S-box, number of elements is (2^8=) 256 vary from 0 *to* 255 as used in Advanced Encryption Standard (AES). The S-box performs a byte of the input word. Use of irreducible polynomials to construct S-boxes had already been adopted by crypto community. But the study of IPs has been limited to almost binary Galois field [GF(2^q)] as used in AES S-boxes. So it is important to study four-bit BFs, eight-bit BFs, and polynomials over GF (p^q) where $p > 2$ in public key cryptography.

(3) DNA-Sequence: DNA is deoxyneucleic acid (Barman & Choudhury, 2012; Diallo et al.) which is the starting point of all life. DNA molecules contain strands of nucleotides which are: adenine (A), cytosine (C), guanine (G), and thymine (T). The DNA molecules contain double helix structure combining the complementary strands A to T and G to C. The combination of two bits represents these four bases (Table 15.1)).

(4) Cramer's Rule: Gabriel Cramer obtained a simple method of solution of linear simultaneous equations by using the properties of determinants. Cramer's Rule is a method that uses determinants to solve systems of equations that have the same number of equations as variables (Ao et al., 2017).

Incorporating of the features of DNA in cryptography is a novel concept as for example the DNA encryption technique. In many ways we can use the DNA characteristics. The plain text can be converted into ASCII codes and then into binary code, which can then be replaced by DNA bases A, T, G, and C (Partheeban & Kavitha, 2019; Kazlauskas et al., 2105).

The unique solutions of a 2 × 2 system

(1) $ax + by = e \text{ and } cx + dy = f$ has a unique solution provided $\Delta = ad - bc$ is nonzero, and the solution is given by $x = \frac{de-bf}{ad-bc}$ and $y = \frac{af-ce}{ad-bc}$ this result is called Cramer's rule for $2X2$ systems.

The unique solutions of a n x n system

(2) Cramer's rule can be generalized to an $n \times n$ system of equations $A\overline{x} = \overline{b}$ or

Table 15.1 DNA encoding.

Bits	base
00	A
01	T
10	G
11	C

$$a_{11}x_1 + a_{12}x_2 + \cdots + a_{1n}x_n = b_1,$$

$$a_{21}x_1 + a_{22}x_2 + \cdots a_{2n}x_n = b_2,$$

...

...

...

$a_{n1}x_1 + a_{n2}x_2 + \cdot \cdot \cdot + a_{nn}x_n = b_n$. ... (1) Where $b_i's$ are constants and not all zeros.

Now Δ denotes the determinant of the above system of equations and $\Delta_j = \sum_{i=1}^{n} b_i A_{ij}$ is the determinant obtained from Δ by replacing a_{ij} by b_i. $i = 1, 2, \ldots, n$.

The unique solution is $x_1 = \frac{\Delta_1}{\Delta}$, $x_2 = \frac{\Delta_2}{\Delta}$, $x_3 = \frac{\Delta_3}{\Delta}$,... ,$x_n = \frac{\Delta_n}{\Delta}$, provided $\Delta \neq 0$.

If $\Delta = 0$ and at least one of the determinants Δ_j, $j = 1, 2, 3, \ldots,$ n be nonzero then the aforementioned system of equations do not possess any solutions.

If $\Delta = 0$ and all of the determinants Δ_j, $j = 1, 2, 3, \ldots,$ n be also zero then above system of equations admits of an infinite number of solutions. This is Cramer's rule.

15.2 Background work

The authors of the paper Diallo et al. address the challenges and proposes a new architecture that combines a cloud-based WBANs with statistical modeling techniques in order to provides secure storage

Infrastructure and optimize the real-time user query processing in terms of energy minimization and query latency.

Nabar et al. (2010) proposed a convex optimization framework to design a communication schedule in the body sensor network to achieve an optimal trade-off between energy consumption and the latency. Their main idea is to propose a polling based algorithm that uses time-varying features of individual sensors and gives a decision-tree that helps to resolve scheduling conflicts among devices. It estimates the query results and the sensors only transfer the data if the error is higher than a threshold defined by the query.

Shubhangi (2012) suggests that the system presents a complete unified and mobile platform based connectivity solution for unobtrusive health monitoring. In our proposed work, we focus to use a low power Wi-Fi, (wireless fidelity), to transfer the data between the WBAN and the server that enable a low power consumption.

Kaur et al. (2012) emphasize the fuzzy logic is interdisciplined with data mining that the author had commented as a relatively novel field bringing together various concepts in the network. They had used Fuzzy inference System to derive fuzzy based rules for their measurement. They had also used association rule mining like a priori algorithm which in turn uses breadth first strategy. The synthetic data with various parameters were first processed and fuzzy rules were built related to those data. They had derived Association rules using FIS.

Pandeya et al. (2012) focus on the design aspects of an autonomic cloud environment that collects patient's health data and place them into the cloud repository and also facilitates analysis on the data using Software services hosted in the cloud. They developed a prototype system that could be used as a test bed for the collection of electrocardiogram (ECG) data for ECG beat analysis.

In Gentry (2009), homomorphic encryption is adopted for secure cloud application. The authors have taken the learning with error (LWE) method to record the digital data safely. In this scenario, clients encrypt medical data, while cloud providers process them without decryption. This concept is evaluated by both addition and multiplication in a real-world application. But homomorphic approach is not advantageous for larger volumes of data, especially medical images. Data encryption using this technique is very expensive in calculations and hence cannot be run in practical field.

In Jalali et al. (2019), an access control model is described that secures the medical data of patients against internal cyber security threats. It allows only the legitimate users to communicate via wireless. The proposed model implements authorization in combination with permissions. It removes the discrepancies in the existing access control models.

In Mbonihankuye et al. (2019), Health Insurance Portability and Accountability Act (HIPAA) is discussed. It is necessary to develop a conservational and analytical method so as to keep the medical records of the patients in a well-preserved and adequate environment. The method includes the improvement of working possibilities by delivering all the details necessary for the patient. All the information must be identified clearly. The protection of the privacy of the patient's health data and the security of their information are the most vital issue when considering the adoption of useful health data in the electronic field of healthcare industries.

In Habib et al. (2019), it is found that hacking/IT incidents are the most prevalent forms of attack behind healthcare data breaches, followed by unauthorized internal disclosures. The frequency of healthcare data breaches, magnitude of exposed records, and financial losses due to breached records are increasing rapidly. Data from the healthcare industry is regarded as being highly valuable. To prevent this anomaly, the article employs the simple moving average method and the simple exponential soothing method of time series analysis to examine the trend of healthcare data breaches and their cost. Between two methods, the simple moving average method provided more reliable forecasting results.

15.3 Major problems in telehealth security

There are different types of challenges exists in telehealth system. Different types of attacks or malicious activity may degrade the activity of the medical devices and disrupt the communication system of health care. Active attack and passive attack are mainly disrupting the telehealth security system. An active attack attempts to alter system resources or affect their operation. A passive attack does not affect system resources but attempts to theft vital information from the system. An attack can be occurred by an insider or from outside of the health organization. Based on the target, there are three types' attacks against the telehealth security.

- Attacks against a medical devices which are connected with the Internet.
- Attacks against the communication between devices and users.
- Attacks against the users.

A common method of attack involves tampering or altering of the messages (medical data or image). The medical data and information which are transmitted through wireless environment is very sensitive and vital for treatment. So any changes on these data or information causes risk for patients.

15.4 Objectives and contributions

Our objective is to develop a secure cryptosystem for telehealth security because the security issue is one of the main parameter in health organization. Any cryptosystem has three basic modules: key generation and transmission, encryption-decryption algorithm, and authentication (Barman & Choudhury, 2012). Although the above literatures provide different types of cryptosystem for security issues, all the basic modules are not focused properly. Here we have proposed a symmetric key-based cryptosystem which addresses all the three basic modules and it seems to more secure than above stated systems.

The novelty of the proposed system is pointed out below.

1. Dynamic S-Box generation using Hopfield network model, DNA sequence, and system of equations (solving by Cramer's rule; artificial neural network (ANN)-based dynamic S-Box generation).
2. Key expansion using symmetric key and DNA sequence.
3. Round operation which provides stream cipher using expanded key.
4. Here no key transmission is needed between sender and receiver. The symmetric key is negotiated before the starting of the module-1. The Hopfield network structure with weight vectors is same for both sender and receiver.
5. Authentication check is done by symmetric key-based hash function.

The proposed cryptosystem employs the aforementioned methods in an integrated form, which is more secure and efficient to recognize data as per the priority and sensitivity.

15.5 Proposed methodology

The total concept of our cryptosystem is divided into four parts. The description of each part and a proper flowchart of the system are given below.

MODULE-1

IDEA: In this module we have proposed S-box generation. At first, we used a four-unit Hopfield network model with weight matrix W initial values x $= [x_1, x_2, x_3, x_4]$ to generate four integer values. The initial values are in public mode. The weight vectors of Hopfield network are generated from symmetric key. Using this Hopfield network four integer numbers are generated for solving system of equations by Cramer's rule. Now S-box is generated using the solutions of system of equations and DNA sequence. The algorithms are given below.

Implimentation1.1 (Hopfield Network Model)

Input: Initial values.

Output: Four integer values.

Algorithm:

Step1: Initialize the activations of the units with the input signals. $y\_out_i = x_i$ $i = 1, 2, \ldots, m$

Step2: update the activations of units in random order by executing steps 3 to 4 for each unit $Y_j,\ j = 1, 2, \ldots, m$.

Step3: Find the net input y_in_j to Y_j . $y\_in_j = x_j + \sum y\_out_i * w_{ij}\ (i \neq j)$.

Step4: Find the activation of the unit Y_j . $y\_out_j = \begin{cases} 1, \ if\ y\_in_j > 0 \\ y\_out_j, \ if\ y\_in_j = 0 \\ 0, \ if\ if\ y\_in_j < 0 \end{cases}$

Step5: The values of y_out_j of step 4 are stored in a dynamic array and repeat the step 3 & step 4 16 times to generate four numbers.

Step6: End.

These four numbers are used to generate system of equations and the solutions of these equations are used in S-box generation.

Implementation 1.2 (Solution of system of equations by Cramer's rule)

Input: Four integers, ASCII values of DNA sequence (A, T, C, G).

Output: two integer values.

Algorithm:

a_1, a_2, b_1, b_2 stores the four integers with the condition $a_1b_2 - b_1a_2 \neq 0$

Here we have considered a system of two linear equations in two variables.

$$a_1x + b_1y = c_1$$

$$a_2x + b_2y = c_2 \ldots (1)$$

The solutions using Cramer's rule is given by

$$\mathrm{x} = \frac{D_x}{D} = \frac{\begin{matrix} c_1 & b_1 \\ c_2 & b_2 \end{matrix}}{\begin{matrix} a_1 & b_1 \\ a_2 & b_2 \end{matrix}}, D \neq 0 \qquad \mathrm{y} = \frac{\begin{matrix} a_1 & c_1 \\ a_2 & c_2 \end{matrix}}{\begin{matrix} a_1 & b_1 \\ a_2 & b_2 \end{matrix}}, D \neq 0$$

If we are solving for x, the x column is replaced with the constant column. If we are solving for y, the y column is replaced with the constant column. The c_1, c_2 are replaced by ascii values of DNA nucleotides i.e., *A and A*, *A and T*, *A and C*, *A and G*, *T and A*, *T and T*, *T and C*, *T and G*, ... all combinations.

Now the two s-boxes are generated by using the x values of each solutions and y-values of each solutions system of equations. The following example helps to understand the concept of module-1.

Example:

The integer values 8, 5 10, and 7 are generated from Hopfield network with initial values 4, 6, 5, and 1. Now the system of equations is $8x+5y=1$ and $10x+7y=4$.

Here $D=\begin{vmatrix} 8 & 5 \\ 10 & 7 \end{vmatrix} \neq 0$ so, Cramer's rule can be applied (Table 15.2).

From Table 15.2 we can get two s-boxes. The following s-boxes use hexadecimal number in each cell. The first substitution box is developed from x values of above table (Table 15.2) and second substitution box are developed from y values of Table 15.2.

These substitution boxes are used for key expansion in the next phase (Tables 15.3 and 15.4). These substitution boxes are dynamic and values are depended on output of Hopfield network.

MODULE-2

IDEA: Here two round operations are done. first round takes symmetric key as input and produces an output of 16 bytes hex-data and second round takes the output of first round as input and also produce an output of 16 bytes hex-data. First round uses s-box1 and second round uses s-box2.

Table 15.2 Solution table for the above system of equations.

	A	T	C	G
A	x = 41, y = 123	x = 15, y = 32	x = 37, y = 109	x = 81, y = 29
T	x = 80, y = 253	x = 54, y = 162	x = 76, y = 239	x = 68, y = 211
C	x = 47, y = 143	x = 21, y = 52	x = 43, y = 129	x = 35, y = 101
G	x = 41, y = 123	x = 33, y = 92	x = 55, y = 169	x = 47, y = 141

Table 15.3 Substitution box for x values.

	A	T	C	G
A	29	0F	25	1D
T	50	36	4C	44
C	2F	15	2B	23
G	3B	21	37	2F

Table 15.4 Substitution box for y values.

	A	T	C	G
A	7B	20	6D	51
T	FD	A2	EF	D3
C	8F	34	81	65
G	B7	5C	A9	8D

Implementation 2.1 (Round operations)

Input: symmetric key.

Output: expanded key.

Algorithm for Round-1:

Step1: set symk (Nabar et al., 2010) ← take 8 bytes from symmetric key.

Step2: symk_bin (Habib et al., 2019)← call bin_val (symk(Nabar et al., 2010)). {/* 8 bytes symmetric key is converted into binary form*/}

Step3: Take pair of bits from symk_bin (Habib et al., 2019) and convert it into DNA nucleotide form using Table 15.1.

Step4: Use substitution box-1

Step5: ExpKey1 (Habib et al., 2019) ← generate 16 bytes of hexadecimal data from step4.

Step6: End.

Algorithm for Round-2:

Step1: set tmpkey1 (Nabar et al., 2010) ← take 8 bytes from ExpKey1. // use tmp as temporary key from ExpKey1 in round-2.

Step2: tmpkey1_bin (Habib et al., 2019) ← call bin_val (tmpkey1 (Nabar et al., 2010)). {/* 8 bytes temporary key is converted into binary form*/}

Step3: Take pair of bits from tmpkey1_bin (Habib et al., 2019) and convert it into DNA nucleotide form using Table 15.1.

Step4: Use substitution box-2.

Step5: ExpKey2 (Habib et al., 2019)← generate 16 bytes of hexadecimal data from step4.

Step6: End.

Algorithm for Round-3:

Shift operation is done on ExpKey2 (Habib et al., 2019). The process is as follows.

After shift operation we have got the third key (ExpKey3 (Habib et al., 2019)) from Table 15.5 by arranging the first bytes to 16th byte. The values of a_1, a_2, b_1 *and* b_2 are taken from output of Hopfield model. An example is given below.

Thus three keys i.e., ExpKey1 (Habib et al., 2019), ExpKey2 (Habib et al., 2019) and ExpKey3 (Habib et al., 2019) are generated from symmetric key using above two algorithms. The above three keys are used for encryption -decryption process.

Table 15.5 shift operation.

Left Shift(a_1%4)→	1st byte	2nd byte	3rd byte	4th byte
Left Shift(a_2%4)→	5th byte	6th byte	7th byte	8th byte
Left Shift(b_1%4)→	9th byte	10th byte	11th byte	12th byte
Left Shift(b_2%4)→	13th byte	14th byte	15th byte	16th byte

Example:

First ROUND key generation: Let 6A2BB7AC be the 8 bytes hex value taken from symmetric key.

Now 6A2BB7AC → 01 10 10 10 00 10 10 11 10 11 01 11 10 10 11 00 (Use DNA sequence) → TC CC AC CG CG TG CC GA (S-Box) → 4C2B252323442B3B. Thus ExpKey1 = 4C2B252323442B3B

Now we have taken 8 bytes from above key for second round.

Second ROUND key generation: Let 4C2B2523 be the 8 bytes from first round key. Now 4C2B2523 → 01 00 11 00 00 10 10 11 00 10 01 01 00 10 00 11 (Use DNA sequence) → TA GA AC CG AC TT AC AG (Use S-box) → FDB7516551A26D51. Thus ExpKey2 = FDB7516551A26D51.

Third ROUND key generation:

Left Shift (8%4)	F	D	B	7
Left Shift (5%4)	5	1	6	5
Left Shift (10%4)	5	1	A	2
Left Shift (7%4)	6	D	5	1

⟹

F	D	B	7
1	6	5	5
A	2	5	1
1	6	D	5

So the ExpKey3 = FDB71655A25116D5.

MODULE-3

IDEA: This module describes the process of cipher text generation. The stream ciphering concept is used in our scheme. The XOR operation is done between plain text and three keys for generating cipher text. In recipient end, the plain text is generated using decryption process using same keys. Before encryption-decryption process authentication process must be done. Symmetric key-based MD5 hash function is used for checking authentication.

Implementation 3.1 (Encryption and decryption process)

Input: Encryption keys (ExpKey1, ExpKey2 and ExpKey3), Plain text

Output: Cipher text.

Algorithm (Encryption):

Step1: set pt [ ], ct [ ], tmp1 [ ] as character. // pt [ ] is plain text.

Step2: tmp1 [ ] ← (*pt* [ ] *xor ExpKey*1) *xor* ExpKey2) // round 1 and round 2 encryption

Step3: ct [ ] ← *tmp* [ ] *xor ExpKey*3. // round-3 encryption and ct [ ] is cipher text.

Step4: End.

This ct [ ] is transmitted to recipient end where decryption algorithm (reverse of encryption algorithm) is used for plain text generation.

Algorithm (Decryption):

Input: ExpKey1, ExpKey2 and ExpKey3 and cipher text.

Output: Plain text.

Step1: set pt [ ], ct [ ], tmp2 [ ] as character.

Step2: tmp2 [ ] ← *ct* [ ] *xor ExpKey*2. // round 1 decryption.

Step3: pt [ ] ← *tmp* [ ] *xor ExpKey*1. // round-2 decryption.

Step4: End.

Thus whole cryptosystem is developed by integrating three modules. The flow chat of the proposed scheme is given below for proper understanding (Fig. 15.2).

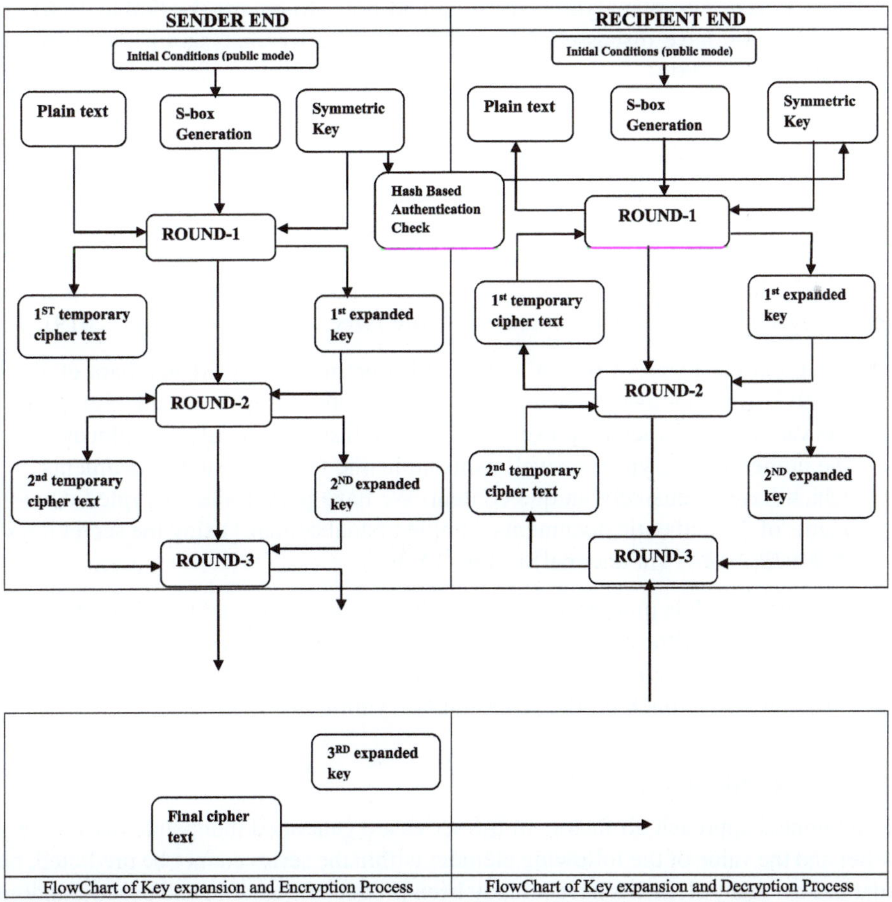

FIGURE 15.2

Flowchart of proposed cryptosystem.

Table 15.6 Specifications of H/w and S/w used in the experiment.

Computer	*Lenovo G80.*
Processor	***Intel*® *Pentium*® *CPU B*950@210*GHz***
RAM	2***GB***
Compiler	***Tubo c, Debc*** ++
Disc drive	SA 9500326***AS*** ATA
Operating system	Windows 7 ultimate (32 bits)

15.6 Experimental results analysis

A good cryptosystem should be designed in such a way that it must robust against different types of cryptanalytic, statistical and brute-force attacks (Table 15.6). In this section, we have discussed different type's security analysis of our proposed scheme (Gentry, 2009).

15.6.1 Statistical analysis

Different sorts of statistical assaults and statistical evaluation are utilized by intruders or hackers to analyze the cipher text for decryption. Therefore, a great cipher text ought to be robust toward any statistical attacks. To prove the robustness of our proposed scheme, we have accomplished the histogram evaluation; avalanche impact evaluation and randomness test (Ayofe Azeez & Van der Vyver, 2019).

(a) Histogram analysis: A textual content-histogram describes (Chenthara et al., 2019) how distinctive characters in a text are disbursed with the aid of graphing the variety of characters at every stage. Here histogram analysis is finished on the numerous encrypted as well as its authentic textual content documents which have extensively unique content. We have proven the encrypted documents of the authentic documents (simple textual content) using the secret keys *ApMn1808AB81* (in decimal) in Fig. 15.3.

Observations: It is plain from Fig. 15.5 that the histograms of the encrypted documents are quite uniform and significantly changed from the respective histograms of the unique files (plain text) and consequently does no longer provide any clue to hire any statistical attack on the proposed encryption process.

15.6.2 Randomness test of key

Randomness approach all factors of the series are generated independently of every other and the value of the following element within the series cannot be predicted, no matter how many elements have already been produced. Random and pseudorandom

Used Keys:- ***ApMn1808AB81***		
FILE TYPE	PLAIN TEXT	CIPHER TEXT
TEXT(.txt)	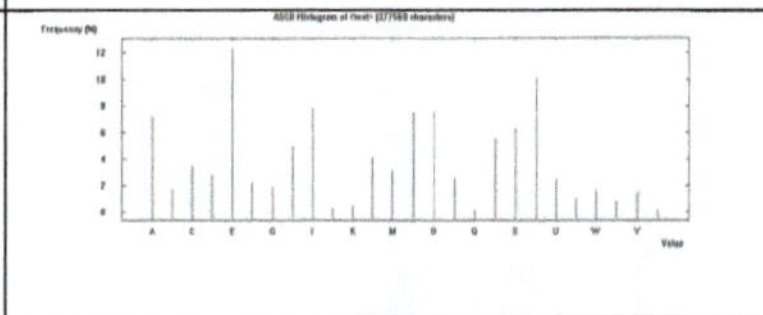	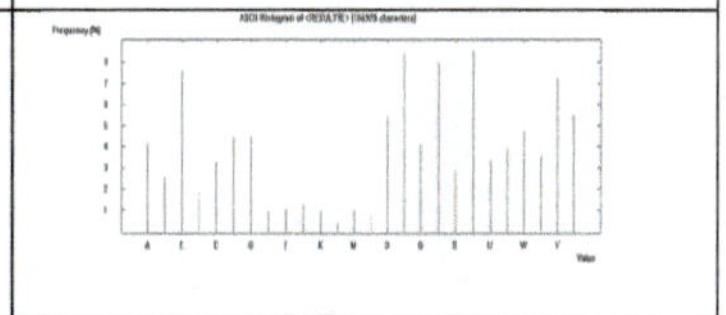
PDF (.pdf)	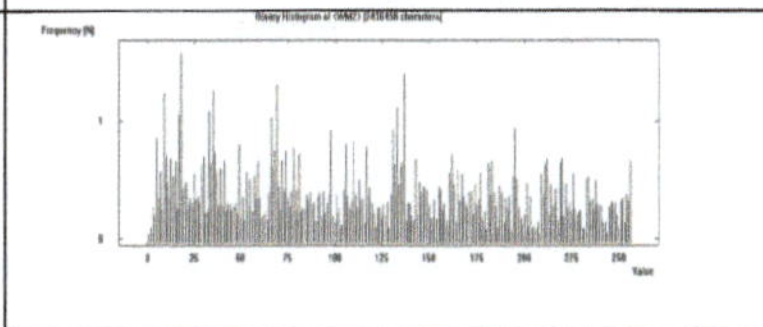	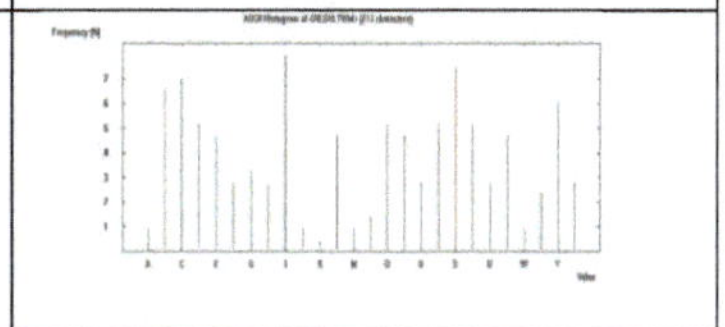
WORD (.docx)	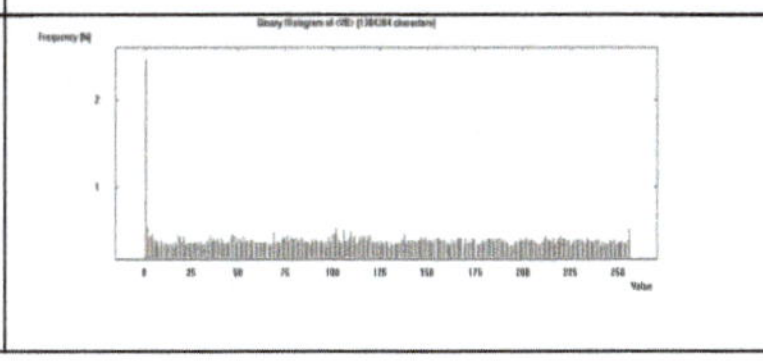	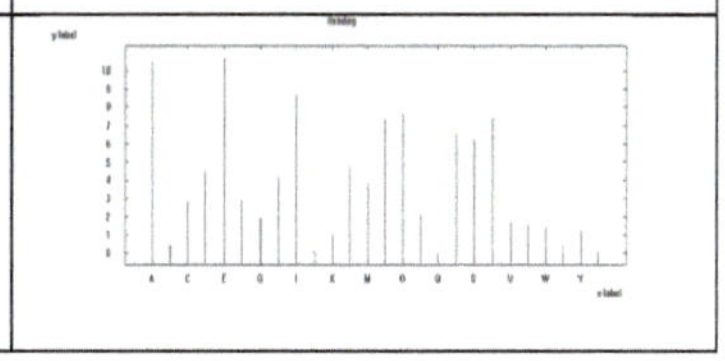

FIGURE 15.3

Histogram analysis.

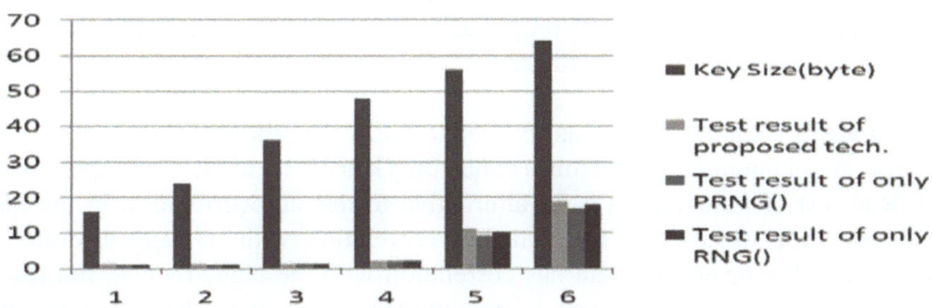

FIGURE 15.4

Graph of above table (taking average value).

numbers that are generated for cryptographic programs have to be unpredictable (ahead and backward). The outputs of a PRNG are deterministic capabilities of the seed; i.e., all authentic randomness is depended on seed generation. An RNG uses a nondeterministic source i.e., the entropy supply. Here we have used RNG for generating weight vectors of ANN and after some learning process the weight values of a particular layer of ANN are used for ROUND key generation. To prove the randomness of our ROUND key we have used a serial test (Seh & et al., 2020; Partheeban & Kavitha, 2019).

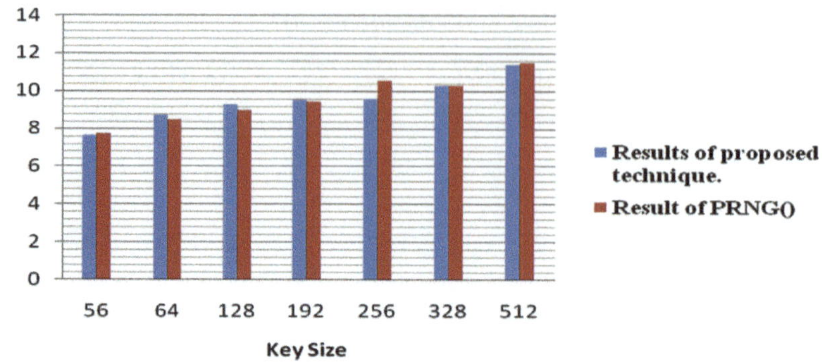

FIGURE 15.5

Graphical diagram of Table 15.8.

Serial Test: The following statics is used for serial test.

$$X = \frac{4}{(n-1)}\left(n_{00}^2 + n_{01}^2 + n_{10}^2 + n_{11}^2\right) - \frac{2}{n}\left(n_0^2 + n_1^2\right) + 1 \ldots (1)$$

Which approximately follows a χ^2 distribution with 2 degrees of freedom if $n \geq 21$ (Barman & Choudhury, 2012). Table 15.7 is given below.

Observation: For a significance level of $\alpha = 0.05$, the threshold values of X for serial test are1.11, 1.2, 1.26, 2.12, 11.01, 19.04 respectively. Thus the sequence generated by the above algorithm passes serial test in each round. Table 15.3 and graphs in Fig. 15.4 prove that our proposed technique is secure against different statistical attacks and differential attacks.

Run Test:

Run test is a statistical test that is used to know the randomness in output data. Run test of randomness is sometimes called the Geary test, and it is a nonparametric test. Run test of randomness is an alternative to test autocorrelation in the data. Autocorrelation means that the data has correlation with its lagged value. To confirm whether or not the data has correlation with the lagged value, run test of randomness is applied. Run test of randomness is basically based on the run. Run is basically a sequence of one symbol such as + or − assumes that the mean and variance are constant and the probability is independent. Procedure for run test for randomness:

Hypothesis: To test the run test of randomness, first set up the null and alternative hypothesis. In run test of randomness, null hypothesis assumes that the distributions of the two continuous populations are the same. The alternative hypothesis will be the opposite of the null hypothesis.

Table 15.7 Serial test on ROUND key.

Key size (Byte)	Proposed tech.	PRNG() (Jegadeeswari et al., 2016)	RNG() (Kaur et al., 2012)	Proposed tech.	PRNG() (Jegadeeswari et al., 2016)	RNG() (Kaur et al., 2012)	Proposed tech.	PRNG() (Jegadeeswari et al., 2016)	RNG() (Kaur et al., 2012)
16	1.11	1.08	1.08	1.12	1.07	1.06	0.99	1.00	1.08
24	1.2	1	1.02	1.21	1.00	1.03	1.23	1.11	1.09
36	1.26	1.25	1.20	1.31	1.19	1.12	1.25	1.18	1.07
48	2.12	2.14	2.13	1.99	1.95	2.01	2.05	1.98	1.99
56	4.01	4.99	4.10	3.01	3.00	3.23	3.12	2.97	2.94
64	6.04	7.02	6.04	5.05	6.08	5.66	5.72	6.03	5.98

Round-1 key test values Round-2 key test values Round-3 key test values.

Table 15.8 Run test data.

Key size (bits)	Results of our technique.	Result of PRNG()
56	7.668	7.771
64	8.747	8.499
128	9.284	9.017
192	9.567	9.456
256	9.622	10.526
328	10.321	10.302
512	11.398	11.501

Calculation of statistics:

The runs test is defined as:

H_0:	the sequence was produced in a random manner
H_a:	The sequence was not produced in a random manner
Test statistic:	The test statistic is $Z = \frac{R-\bar{R}}{s_R}$, where R is the observed number of runs, R, is the expected number of runs, and s_R is the standard deviation of the number of runs. The values of R and s_R are computed as follows: $\bar{R} = \frac{2n_1n_2}{n_1+n_2} + 1$ $s_R^2 = \frac{2n_1n_2(2n_1n_2-n_1-n_2)}{(n_1+n_2)^2(n_1+n_2-1)}$ With n_1 and n_2 denoting the number of positive and negative values in the series.
Significance level:	$\propto$
Critical region:	The runs test rejects the null hypothesis if $\lvert \mathbf{Z} \rvert > \mathbf{Z}_{1-\alpha/2}$ For a large-sample runs test (where $n_1 > 10$ and $n_2 > 10$) at the 5% significance level, a test statistic with an absolute value greater than 1.96 indicates non-randomness. For a small-sample runs test, there are tables to determine critical values that depend on values of n_1 and n_2

If the run test of randomness is sustainable with the null hypothesis, then we can expect the following properties of normal distribution:

Decision run, in run test of randomness: If the calculated value of the run test of randomness lies within the preceding confidence interval, then do not reject the null hypothesis. If the calculated value of the run test of randomness lies outside the preceding confidence interval, then reject the null hypothesis.

Information Entropy:

Entropy measures have gained widespread use in the analysis of complex real-world data. The term "entropy" first originated in the field of thermodynamics and can be interpreted as the amount of information needed to completely specify the physical state of a system. A very orderly and regular system has a low entropy value.

A high entropy score indicates a random or chaotic series, whereas a low score indicates a high degree of regularity.

Entropy measures:

Sample Entropy (m, r) : SampEn is calculated based on the negative natural logarithm of the conditional probability with m length dataset. It is given that it has repeated itself for m points (within a tolerance limit r that is commonly based on the standard deviation of the data) and also for (m+1) points. SampEn can be calculated using the following formula: $SampEn = -\log\frac{A}{B}$, where A is the number of pairs of vector subsets of length m+1 which has a distance function less than r, while B is the number of pairs of vector subsets of length m which similarly has a distance functions less than r (Katiyar & Jeyanthi, 2016).

Permutation Entropy (n): It is used to check the presence of noise in real-world data. For a time series

$\{x_1, x_2, \ldots, x_{N-1}\}$: this entropy algorithm splits the data into overlapping n-tuples, where n is the embedding dimension. Each n-tuple is then sorted in ascending order. Now this sorted tuple generates π (permutation type) according to the ordering of the sorted data. There will be n! Possible permutation types according to embedding dimension n. The relative frequency p (π_i) is determined for each π_i, for $1 \leq i \leq n!$, according to the following equation:

$$\mathrm{p}(\pi_i) = \frac{\text{number of occurrences of type } \pi_\mathrm{i}}{\mathrm{N} - \mathrm{n} + 1}.$$

The permutation $H(n)$ is then calculated as follows:

$H(n) = -\sum_{i}^{n!} p(\pi_i) \log \mathrm{p}\,(\pi_i)$. Where $0 \leq H(n) \leq \log(n!)$. Here 0 indicates a series that ismonotonically increasing or decreasing, and log n! Indicates a completely random series. When experiments occur, $H(n)$ is rescaled by dividing by log n!, thus normalizing $H(n)$ to return values between 0 and 1 with 0 ndicating highly regular data and 1 indicating maximal entropy (Ao et al., 2017).

Permutation Test (t): The permutation test is done for test of randomness. It is performed by first partitioning the original time Series into groups of t elements. When the original time series is not perfectly divisible by t, the remaining data points are discarded. The ordering of the element indices are obtained from the sorted elements of each group. In each group the possible orderings is t! Now the chi-square test can then be performed with t! categories and the probability of each distinct ordering is $1/t$! The chi-square statistic is interpreted as the distance from the expected value given by the null hypothesis and the uniformly distributed input data. Thus a high value indicates a high degree of regularity and a low value indicates a high likelihood of the null hypothesis being true (Chakravorty & Ghosh, 2018). The main difference between permutation test and permutation entropy is that the partitions in the permutation test do not overlap, and the permutation entropy algorithm calculates H (n).

Observations: Tables 15.9a–9c and Figs. 15.6a–6c above show the comparative data analysis and resulting scores of sample entropy, permutation entropy, and the permutation test chi-square statistic. For better comparison, all scores for the various metrics are rescaled in between 0 and 1.4. In addition, the inverse of the natural log is applied to the chi-square statistic from the permutation test. This was done to invert the plots to better correspond with the interpretation of the entropy measures, i.e., a high value corresponds to low regularity and a low value correspond to high regularity.

Table 15.9a Comparative data analysis on uniform (0, 1) series.

	T.val 1	T.val −2	T.val 3	T.val 4	T.val 5	T.val 6	T.val 7	T.val 8	T.val 9	T.val 10
Sample entropy	0.73	0.41	0.50	0.56	0.95	0.61	0.48	0.84	1.14	0.64
Permutation entropy	1.20	0.40	0.72	0.58	1.0	0.88	0.60	0.54	0.69	0.51
p test	0.52	0.98	0.63	0.73	0.82	0.42	0.77	0.59	0.64	0.97

Table 15.9b Comparative data analysis on Gaussian (0, 1) series.

	T.val 1	T.val 2	T.val 3	T.val 4	T.val 5	T.val 6	T.val 7	T.val 8	T.val 9	T.val 10
Sample entropy	0.43	0.41	0.59	0.56	1.3	0.61	0.41	0.74	1.1	0.65
Permutation entropy	1.00	0.92	0.73	0.63	0.41	0.83	0.62	0.52	0.89	0.44
p test	0.61	0.78	0.83	0.45	0.54	0.44	0.93	0.61	0.64	0.71

Table 15.9c Comparative data analysis on exponential (1) series.

	T.val 1	T.val 2	T.val 3	T.val 4	T.val 5	T.val 6	T.val 7	T.val 8	T.val 9	T.val 10
Sample entropy	0.53	0.62	1.4	0.56	0.81	0.62	0.42	0.68	1.0	0.55
Permutation entropy	0.47	0.49	0.74	0.65	0.92	0.85	0.72	0.53	0.49	0.81
p test	0.98	0.78	0.93	0.45	0.57	0.41	0.99	0.61	0.64	0.88

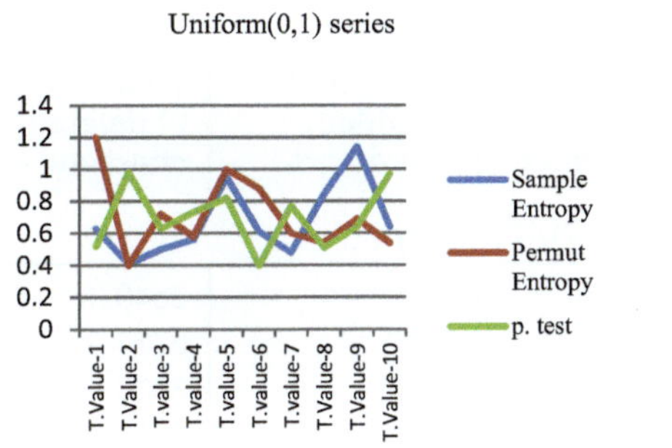

FIGURE 15.6A

Graphical representation of Table 15.9a.

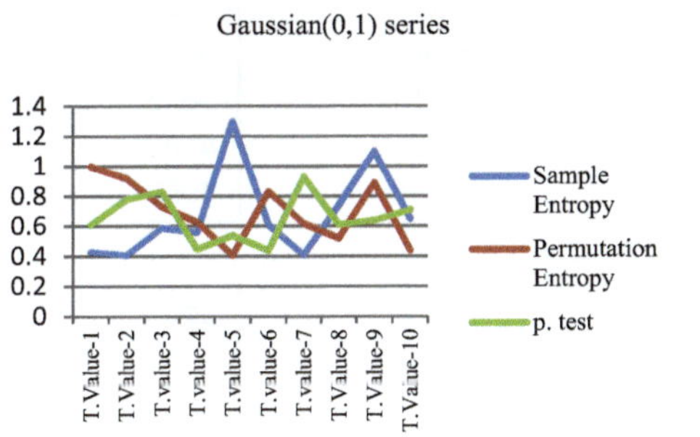

FIGURE 15.6B

Graphical representation of Table 15.9b.

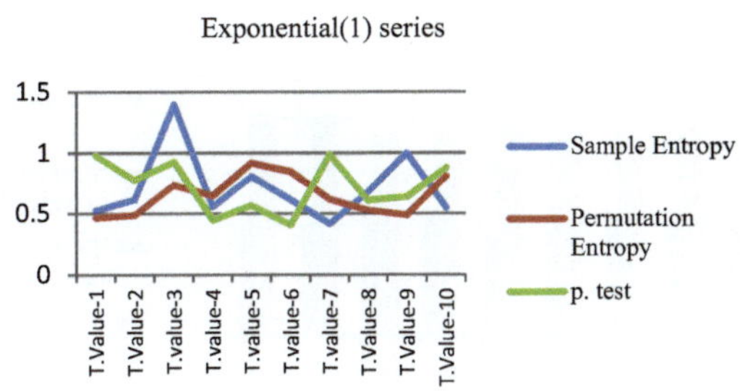

FIGURE 15.6C

Graphical representation of Table 15.9c.

15.6.3 Key sensitivity analysis

An ideal encryption technique should be sensitive with recognize to the name of the secret key, i.e., A single bit trade within the mystery key have to produce a unique cipher text. For checking out the sensitivity of the proposed encryption technique, we've completed the encryption scheme within the documents (.TXT) with moderate adjustments using the secret key. The avalanche effect is shown below only for

Table 15.10 Avalanche effect: change in ROUND key.

Key	Ascii Difference	Total number of added characters	Total number of deleted characters	Total number of changed characters
Avalanche effect on ROUND-1 key				
Abcd@123	0	3526	3540	2541
Abcd@123	8	3717	3714	2363
Abcd@123	9	3862	3836	2272
Abcd@123	108	3929	3878	2219
Abcd@123	30	3614	3612	2456
Avalanche effect on ROUND-2 Key				
AE1CF@725	88	4253	4237	1893
AE1CF@725	8	3694	3676	2325
AE1CE@725	121	3767	3643	2237
AE1CE@725	7	4208	4182	2014
AE1CE@725	70	4034	4059	2031
Avalanche effect on ROUND-3 key				
DEA23$124	78	4261	4243	1793
DEA23$124	18	3793	3779	2115
DEA23$124	110	3864	3853	2147
DEA23$124	40	4106	4072	2244
DEA23$124	90	4095	4099	2131

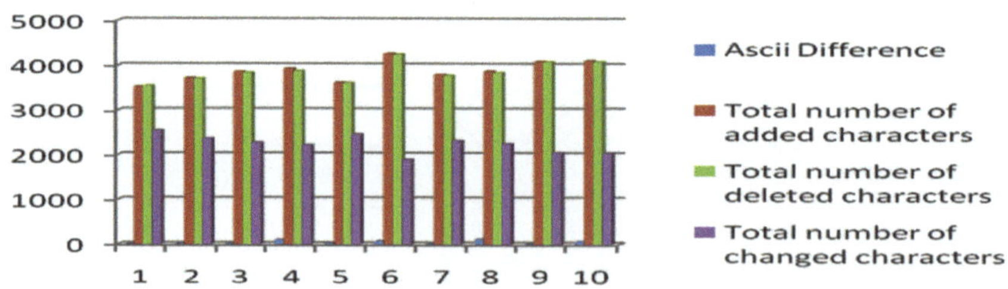

FIGURE 15.7

Graph of above Table 15.10 (taking average value).

changed ROUND key and with fixed ROUND key. The following Table 15.10 and graph (Fig. 15.7) shows the total scenario (Dimitrov, 2020; Abd EL-Latif et al.).

Observation: We've got shown the effects of a few attempts to decrypt an encrypted file with barely three types of round keys than the only used for the encryption of the unique report. The above Table 15.10 shows the added characters, deleted characters and changed characters with slight change (1 byte or 2 bytes) in ROUND key and the above graph (Fig. 15.7) also shows the increasing and decreasing performance among added characters, deleted characters and changed characters for 1 byte change in key. It is obvious that the decryption with a slightly extraordinary key fails absolutely and hence the proposed encryption system is highly key touchy.

15.6.4 Analysis of proposed S-box

Strong s-boxes must satisfy six essential properties which are bijection, nonlinearity, strict avalanche criterion (SAC), bit independence criterion (BIC), input/output XOR distribution, and linear approximation probability (LP).

Nonlinearity: The nonlinearity is defined as the minimum hamming distance between the function $f : \{0,1\}^n \to \{0,1\}$ and a set of its all affine functions (Anonymous, 2020; Katiyar & Jeyanthi, 2016). Nonlinearity specifies the distance to weak cryptographically affine functions.

$nl(f) = \min_{l \in A_n} hd(f, l)$ (9) where A_n is a set of all affine functions over f: {0, 1} A function is said to be perfectly nonlinear if a nonzero vector x = $[x_{n-1};::; x_1 \, , \, x_0] \in \{0,1\}^n$ the values f(y) and f($y \oplus x$) are equal to half arguments y $\in \{0,1\}^n$.

SAC (Balajee Maram & Gnanasekar, 2016) is the concept given by Webster and Tavares in 1985 (Diallo et al.). A function satisfies SAC if 1 bit of the plain text or key is complemented then the output is changed with the probability of $\frac{1}{2}$. SAC is calculated by equation $\alpha := \sum_{x \in z_2^n} f(x) \oplus f(x \oplus e_i)$, where x *and* e are two n bit vectors which differ only in 1 bit i. The Boolean function $f(x)$ accomplishes SAC criterion if and only if $\alpha = 2^{n-1}$ for all $i, \, 0 < i < n-1$.

The concept of BIC was introduced by Webster and Tavares (Diallo et al.). According to BIC, with the change of single bit in plain text or a key for a given set of avalanche vectors, all avalanche variables of respective vectors should be pair wise independent. The correlation coefficient of jth and kth components of avalanche vector. D^{ei} is calculated to measure the bit independence property of overall input pairs P and P_i, which differ only in bit i ($Pi = P \oplus e_i$). $BIC^{ei}(d_j, d_k) = |\, corr\, (d_j^{e_i}\ d_k^{e_i})|$ the overall BIC is defined as: $BIC(f) = max_{1 \le i \le n, 1 \le j,k \le m, j \ne k} BIC^{ei}(d_j, d_k)$, $BIC(f)$ is defined in the range 0 *and* 1. It is ideally equal to zero, and in worst case it is equal to one (Kruse et al., 2017).

Table 15.11 shows the comparative analysis among existing s-boxes and proposed S-box. The above results prove the efficiency and robustness of proposed dynamic s-box.

15.6.5 Security analysis

15.6.5.1 KEY space analysis

The required belongings of a terrific encryption algorithm are the massive key area by way of which algorithm can face up to distinct types of attacks. The total range of various keys in encryption procedure shows the dimensions of key area. The brute-pressure assault is impractical in such crypto structures where key area is huge. Now we don't forget a general case in which the dimensions of secret key's k bits i.e., k

Table 15.11 Comparative study of S-box.

Criteria	Ref. (Partheeban & Kavitha, 2019)	Ref. (Dimitrov, 2020)	Ref. (Abd EL-Latif et al.)	Ref. (Anonymous, 2020)	Ref. (Kazlauskas et al., 2105)	Proposed S-box
SAC	51.3%	49.6%	50.0%	52.1%	48.9%	49.9%
BIC	0.4532	0.3989	0.4010	0.4176	0.4421	0.4215
NL	101	120	112	106	97	100
XOR	$\frac{4}{256}$	$\frac{4}{256}$	$\frac{8}{256}$	$\frac{10}{256}$	$\frac{8}{256}$	$\frac{8}{256}$

the length of key in bits. Now the key space is 2^k and if the important thing space is large then attack is not possible. There is a proportional relation among key space and key size (Ao et al., 2017; Chakravorty & Ghosh, 2018).

15.6.5.2 Brute-force attack:

The massive key space makes the brute-force assault infeasible. In this attack, attacker attempts to translate the cipher textual content into undeniable textual content using every possible key. On common, half of all viable keys are enough for attaining success. Algorithms are recognized to all in maximum networking machine however brute-force assault will not possible if the algorithm uses massive key space.

If an eavesdropper listen this coupled feedforward ANN structure and accessing every public parameter (input values) then it can act as genuine participant. But it is very difficult for eavesdropper to get access of the symmetric key and since the weight vectors of each layer is not publicly accessible then the attacker link weight may not be same at the of time learning process in each iteration (Liu & Ma, 2018).

15.6.6 Performance analysis

15.6.6.1 Comparison on evaluation time w.r.t. standard algorithms

Thc six text files (910 kB, 5, 11, 28, 40 and 80 MB) are used to get experimental results and in each experiment, five cryptography algorithms (AES-256, DES-56, 3DES-168, RC2-128 and RSA- 2048) are used. The Performance of each algorithm is evaluated in terms of speed, memory file size and throughput. The encryption time of any cryptography algorithm means is the time to convert a plain text into a cipher text.

Observations: From Fig. 15.8 and Table 15.12 it is seen that the AES is superior to the other algorithms in terms of processing time. DES consumes less evaluated time than other standard algorithms, so it is the better one after AES. 3DES and RC2 consume approximately same evaluation time for the encryption and decryption processes. But the RSA is the slowest one among the standard algorithms. The throughput of any cryptographic algorithm indicates the speed of algorithm during encryption and decryption processes.

$$\text{Throughput} = \frac{\text{Total Text files size in(MB)}}{\text{Total Evaluation Time of Algorthim in (ms)}}$$

Following Fig. 15.9 and Table 15.13 shows the analysis on throughput among standard algorithms and proposed technique. For any algorithm throughput is a vital parameter as it is inversely proportional to the power consumption of that technique.

15.6.6.2 Comparison on different attributes w.r.t. existing technique

Here we have described a comparative study among different existing techniques and proposed technique through the following Table 15.14.

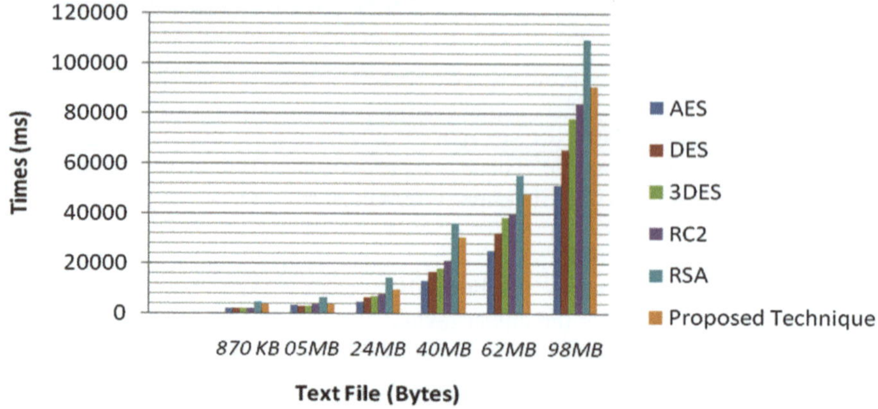

FIGURE 15.8

Graphical representation of Table 15.12.

Table 15.12 The time evaluation of different cryptographic algorithms.

Text file (bytes)	AES (256-Bits)	DES (56-Bits)	3DES (128-Bits)	RC2 (128-Bits)	RSA (2048-Bits)	Proposed technique
910 KB	2,052	2,141	2,225	2,074	4,925	3,912
05 MB	3,605	3,251	3,082	3,862	6,805	4,095
14 MB	4,872	6,484	7,063	7,846	14,540	9,843
33 MB	13,372	16,715	18,327	21,405	36,107	30,762
52 MB	25,038	32,411	38,583	39,858	55,527	47,631
80 MB	51,239	65,731	78,141	83,532	109,237	90,873

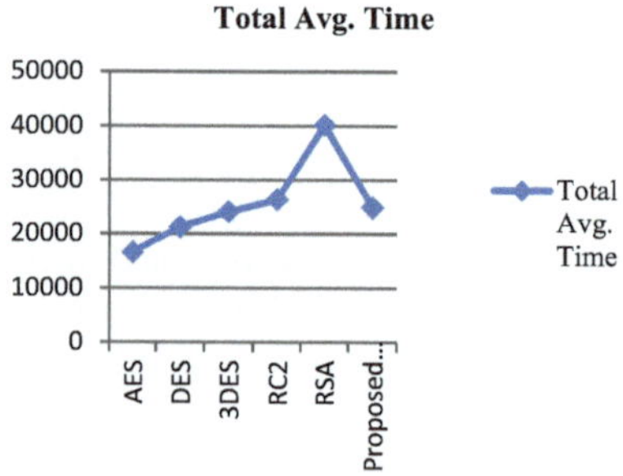

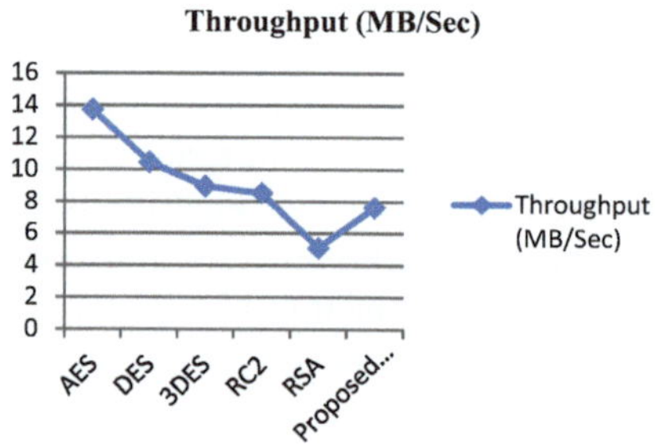

FIGURE 15.9

Graphical representation of Table 15.13.

Table 15.13 Average time and throughput of standard algorithm and proposed technique.

	AES	DES	3DES	RC2	RSA	Proposed technique
Total avg. Time	16,689.33	21,322.67	24,242	26,485.5	40,238.5	25,091.21
Throughput (MB/Sec)	13.75621	10.47412	8.98400	8.54352	5.09712	7.65311

Table 15.14 Comparison w.r.t. different attributes among different techniques.

Attributes ↓	Ref. (Kiran & Sharma, 2017)	Ref. (Diallo et al.)	Ref. (Nabar et al., 2010)	Ref. (Kaur et al., 2012)	Ref. (Gentry, 2009)	Ref. (Hammad et al., 2021)	Ref. (Dey et al., 2021)	Ref. (Sarkar et al., 2021)	Proposed technique
Confidentiality	Yes	No	Yes	No	Yes	Yes	Yes	No	Yes
Integrity	No	No	Yes	No	No	Yes	No	No	Yes
Authenticity	Yes	Yes	No	Yes	No	Yes	Yes	Yes	Yes
Defend against man-in-middle attack	No	No	Yes	Yes	No	No	Yes	No	Yes
Defend against replay attack	Yes	Yes	No	Yes	No	No	No	Yes	Yes
Cryptanalysis	No	No	Yes	No	Yes	Yes	No	Yes	Yes
Session key establishment	Yes	Yes	No	No	Yes	Yes	No	Yes	Yes
Privacy protection	Yes	No	Yes	No	Yes	No	Yes	Yes	Yes
Vulnerability	No	No	Yes	No	Yes	No	Yes	No	Yes

15.7 Discussion and conclusion

The main barrier toward the rapid growth of telehealth applications is the personal information breach. In the COVID-19 era it is seen that telemedicine takes a vital role in the healthcare sector and is very helpful for doctors, nurses and patients. A number of techniques have been proposed for data protection in healthcare informatics and these techniques also attain highest level of data security. However, there are still many gaps in these techniques and need more researches to make these techniques more effective because patient's information is very sensitive and vital for treatment. Our proposed technique shows a novelty in key generation, encryption-decryption and authentication using neural cryptography (Hopfield network model) DNA sequence, and system of linear equations. Different types of analysis prove its robustness in security issues and it also improves various limitations of previous techniques in neural cryptography. It is very effective in medical data security.

References

Abd EL-Latif, Ahmed A., Abd-El-Atty, Bassem, Eman, M., Abou-Nassar, & Venegas-Andraca, Salvador E. (2020). Controlled alternate quantum walks based privacy preserving healthcare images in Internet of Things. *Optics & Laser Technology* Volume 124, 105942. https://doi.org/10.1016/j.optlastec.2019.105942. ISSN 0030-3992.

Ahmad, Ishrat (2017). Cloud computing - threats and challenges. *Journal of computing and management studies*.

Ali, R. A. (2018). Random number generator based on hybrid algorithm between particle swarm optimization (PSO) algorithm and 3D-chaotic system and its application. *Iraqi Journal of Information and Technology, 8*(3), 1–20.

Ao, Tianyong, Rao, Jinli, Dai, Kui, & Zou, Xuecheng (2017). Construction of high quality key-dependent S- box. *IAENG International Journal of Computer Science*.

Ayofe Azeez, Nureni, & Van der Vyver, Charles (2019). Security and privacy issues in e-health cloud-based system: A comprehensive content analysis. *Egyptian Informatics Journal, 20*(2), 97–108. ISSN 1110-8665.

Balajee Maram, K., & Gnanasekar, J. M. (2016). Evaluation of key dependent S-box based data security algorithm using hamming distance and balanced output. *TEM Journal, 5*(1).

Barman, Manisha, & Choudhury, J Pal (November 2012). Fuzzy rule base system for the diagnosis of heart disease. *International Journal of Computer Applications, 57*(7).

Bhalekar, Pallavi D., & Shaikh, Dr M. Z. (March 2019). Machine learning: SURVEY, types and challenges. *International Research Journal of Engineering and Technology, 06*(3).

Chakravorty, J. G., & Ghosh, P. R. (2018). *Advanced higher algebra*. U.N. Dhur and Sons Private Ltd., 978-3- 80673-67-7.

Chenthara, S., Ahmed, K., Wang, H., & Whittaker, F. (2019). Security and privacy-preserving challenges of e-health solutions in cloud computing. In *IEEE access* (Vol. 7, pp. 74361–74382). https://doi.org/10.1109/ACCESS.2019.2919982

Controlled alternate quantum walks based privacy preserving healthcare images in Internet of Things. *Optics & Laser Technology, 124*, (2020), 105942. https://doi.org/10.1016/j.optlastec.2019.105942. ISSN 0030-3992.

Dey, Joydeep, Sarkar, Arindam, & Karforma, Sunil (2021). Newer post-COVID perspective: Teledental encryption by De-multiplexed perceptron. *International Journal of Information Technology, 13*(2), 593–601.

Ousmane Diallo, Joel J.P.C. Rodrigues,MbayeSene,JianweiNiu, Real-time query processing optimization for.

Dimitrov, Miroslav (2020). On the design of chaos-based S-boxes. *IEEE Access*. https://doi.org/10.1109/ACCESS.2020.3004526. PP. 1-1.

Gentry, C. (2009). Fully homomorphic encryption using ideal lattices. In *41st ACM symposium on theory of computing (STOC)*.

Ghazi, A. A., & Ali, F. H. (2018). Robust and efficient dynamic stream cipher cryptosystem. *Iraqi Journal of Science, 59*(2C), 1105–1114.

Habib, M. A., Faisal, C. M. N., Sarwar, S., et al. (September 2019). Privacy-based medical data protection against internal security threats in heterogeneous Internet of Medical Things. *International Journal of Distributed Sensor Networks*. https://doi.org/10.1177/1550147719875653

Hammad, Mohamed, Iliyasu, Abdullah M., Subasi, Abdulhamit, Edmond, S., Ho, L., & Abd El-latif, A. A. (2021). A multitier deep learning model for arrhythmia detection. *IEEE Transactions on Instrumentation and Measurement, 70*, 1–9.

Jalali, M. S., Razak, S., Gordon, W., Perakslis, E., & Madnick, S. (2019). Health care and cybersecurity: Bibliometric analysis of the literature. *Journal of Medical Internet Research, 21*(2), e12644. https://doi.org/10.2196/12644. PMID: 30767908.

Jegadeeswari, S., Dinadayalan, P., & Gnanambigai, N. (2016). *Enhanced data security using neural network in cloud Environment* (Vol. 11, pp. 278–285).

Katiyar, S., & Jeyanthi, N. (2016). Pure dynamic S-box construction. *International Journal of Computers*.

Kaur, Parneet, Singh Khurmi, Dr Sawtantar, & Singh Josan, Dr Gurpreet (December 2012). Fuzzy based analysis of proposed model for physical health standard based on association rule mining techniques. *International Journal of Computer Science and Communication Engineering, 1*(2).

Kazlauskas, Kazys, Vaicekauskas, Gytis, & Robertas, S. M. A. L. I. U. K. A. S. (2005). An algorithm for key-dependent S-box generation in block cipher system. *Informatica, 26*(1), 51–65.

Kiran, & Sharma, Dr S. (November – December 2017). Enhance data security in cloud computing using machine learning and hybrid cryptography techniques. *International Journal of Advance Research in Computer Science (IJARCS), 8*(9), 393–397.

Kruse, C. S., Smith, B., Vanderlinden, H., et al. (2017). Security techniques for the electronic health records. *Journal of Medical System, 41*, 127. https://doi.org/10.1007/s10916-017-0778-4

Liu, X., & Ma, W. (2018). Cdaka: A provably-secure heterogeneous cross-domain authenticated key agreement protocol with symptoms-matching in TMIS. *Journal of Medical System, 42*, 135. https://doi.org/10.1007/s10916-018-0985-7

Mbonihankuye, Scholas, Nkunzimana, Athanase, & Ange, Ndagijimana (2019). Healthcare data security technology: HIPAA compliance. *Wireless Communications and Mobile Computing*, 1–7. https://doi.org/10.1155/2019/1927495, 2019.

Nabar, S., Walling, J., & Poovendran, R. (2010). Minimizing energy consumption in body sensor networks via convex optimization. In *BSN'10: Proceedings of the 2010 international conference on body sensor networks* (pp. 62–67). Washington, DC, USA: IEEE Computer Society.

Pandeya, Suraj, Voorsluys, William, Sheng, Niua, Khandokerb, Ahsan, & Buyyaa, Rajkumar (2012). An autonomic cloud Environment for hosting ECG data analysis services. In *Future generation computer systems* (Vol. 28, pp. 147–154).

Partheeban, Pon, & Kavitha, V. (2019). Dynamic key dependent AES S-box generation with optimized quality analysis. *Cluster Computing, 22*. https://doi.org/10.1007/s10586-018-2386-6

Sarkar, Arindam, Dey, Joydeep, & Karforma, Sunil (2021). Musically modified substitution-box for clinical signals Ciphering in wireless Telecare medical communicating systems. *Wireless Personal Communications, 117*(2), 727–745.

Seh, A. H., Zarour, M., Alenezi, M., Sarkar, A. K., Agrawal, A., Kumar, R., & Khan, R. A. (2020). Healthcare Data Breaches: Insights and Implications. *Healthcare (Basel, Switzerland), 8*(2), 133. https://doi.org/10.3390/healthcare8020133

Shubhangi, M. (June 2012). Verulkar, 2Maruti limkar, "real time health monitoring using GPRS technology. In *International journal of computer science and network (IJCSN)* (Vol. 1), 3 www.ijcsn.orgISSN2277-5420.

Index

Note: Page numbers followed by "*f*" indicate figures and "*t*" indicate tables.

A

B

Kolibri 360 GmbH
Ferdinand-Jühlke-Straße 7
99095 Erfurt, Deutschland
produktsicherheit@kolibri360.de